Importing Care, Faithful Service

Critical Issues in Health and Medicine

Edited by Rima D. Apple, University of Wisconsin–Madison, and
Janet Golden, Rutgers University–Camden

Growing criticism of the U.S. healthcare system is coming from consumers, politicians, the media, activists, and healthcare professionals. Critical Issues in Health and Medicine is a collection of books that explores these contemporary dilemmas from a variety of perspectives, among them political, legal, historical, sociological, and comparative, and with attention to crucial dimensions such as race, gender, ethnicity, sexuality, and culture.

For a list of titles in the series, see the last page of the book.

Importing Care, Faithful Service

Filipino and Indian American Nurses at a Veterans Hospital

Stephen M. Cherry

Rutgers University Press

New Brunswick, New Jersey, and London

Library of Congress Cataloging-in-Publication Data

Names: Cherry, Stephen, author.
Title: Importing care, faithful service: Filipino and Indian American nurses at a veteran's
    hospital / Stephen M. Cherry.
Other titles: Critical issues in health and medicine
Description: New Brunswick: Rutgers University Press, 2022. | Series: Critical issues in
    health and medicine | Includes bibliographical references and index.
Identifiers: LCCN 2021039572 | ISBN 9781978826335 (paperback) | ISBN 9781978826342
    (hardback) | ISBN 9781978826359 (epub) | ISBN 9781978826366 (mobi) |
    ISBN 9781978826373 (pdf)
Subjects: MESH: Nurses, International | Nurse-Patient Relations | Asian Americans |
    Racism | Xenophobia | Catholicism | Hospitals, Veterans | United States
Classification: LCC RT86.3 | NLM WY 88 | DDC 610.7306/9—dc23
LC record available at https://lccn.loc.gov/2021039572

A British Cataloging-in-Publication record for this book is available from the British Library.

For my father and friend, Stephen Paul Cherry.
Thank you for opening the world to me.

Contents

Importing Care, Faithful Service

Chapter 1

Veterans and a Crisis of Care

A year after the Veterans Health Administration scandal in 2014 first broke on national and local news, reporting a wide-spread pattern of negligence in the treatment of American veterans, Rebecca,[1] a foreign-born Indian American nurse in her early forties, agreed to talk to me about her experiences as a nurse at a local Veterans Administration hospital (VA). As we talked about nursing and her career at the hospital, she suggested that working with veterans was immensely rewarding but not without its challenges. "I have worked at the VA for over a decade. I pray and care for my patients as if they were my own family, but every day my faith is tested." When I asked Rebecca to explain what she meant by this, she told me that every foreign-born nurse at the hospital, the majority of whom by her account are Indian and Filipino American, have some story to tell. "Just last week this White veteran got admitted to the hospital, and he didn't want me to touch him." When asked why, she stated that the patient not only refused her care but also blurted out, "I don't want to see you nurses here! You people come and take away the good jobs of our people here. You go back to your country. I don't want you to have anything to do with me and my country!" Shocked by the outburst she described, I asked Rebecca how she responded. She said that she tried to talk to the veteran but eventually got him another nurse, who ironically was Filipino.

Clearly upset after describing this exchange, Rebecca stated that this kind of episode or something like it happens far too often with nurses she knows. "Everyone wants to talk about the scandal, you know it's still all over the news, or [there is] some new scandal, but how many people know our story and what we are willing to tolerate?" Clarifying what she meant, she added, "We are the ones serving this country silently with little recognition. We are the ones taking care of these veterans when no one else will. God as my witness, we really care for these vets." Moved by a mixture of anger and pained frustration, Rebecca stated that her patients have the right to refuse her care, but she also questions the extent to which her patients and even her American-born colleagues really understand her as a person. "I am a proud American citizen. Everyone who works here is an American, but not all of my patients and administrators get that. Maybe we look different from what they think an American should look like, I don't know. Maybe we look like the enemy to them, but I am not their enemy. . . . I am good Christian and I chose to work at the VA. I can get a job anywhere, probably making much better money and with less drama, but I want to serve my country and give back to those who have given so much to me and my family." Apologizing for getting a bit emotional, Rebecca made one last statement before ending our interview: "Sometimes when I sit back and think about it, it hurts deeply, but I guess I just try to keep it to myself. Most of my patients and fellow nurses love me and appreciate what I do for them, but every week or so . . . I tell you, if it were not for my faith in God, I couldn't do this job."

Several months later, I interviewed Lucy, a foreign-born Filipina[2] American in her midforties. Like Rebecca, Lucy suggested that working with veterans is both the most rewarding and most challenging thing that she has ever done in her nursing career. "I love these vets, but wow, sometimes I just have to ask God, What am I doing here?" she stated. Tired from a long day at the hospital, Lucy, like Rebecca, explained that each new shift presents its own unique challenges. "Today I walked into a patient's room, and he just had the most unpleasant look on his face." When I asked what happened next, she explained that the patient, a Black veteran, questioned whether she was a licensed nurse and then refused her care after asking to talk to a supervisor. Lucy said she showed the patient her ID badge and then assured him that she was a licensed registered nurse with advanced degrees, but he kept demanding to see a supervisor. "So, I got my supervising nurse manager, and the next thing I know, because the supervisor is also like Filipina, and she comes in and asks him what the problem is." When I asked her how the patient responded, she said that he said, "Oh no, that's okay, forget it. Never mind. I guess we lost the war."

Understanding how difficult it might be to discuss this situation after such a long shift, I did not want to ask Lucy how the veteran's comments made her feel, but she offered her insights without prompting. "Do you want to know how that makes me feel? Well, we just like laughed it off together later in the lounge. You know, you just have to learn to turn the other cheek—golden rule, you know. . . . Was it racism? Maybe, but if you don't want a Filipino or Indian taking care of you in the hospital, and you want a White nurse, it's like going to be a while for them to find someone else. Sometimes it's really hard . . . makes you want to cry, but after doing it for [many] years, you get used to those situations."

As our conversation continued, Lucy admitted that some cases and patients still trouble her. "Sometimes you never get over the hurt. I know I said we laugh about it, but sometimes it seems so personal. It gets into you and just sticks to your heart." Like Rebecca, Lucy grew noticeably more frustrated as she described her feelings. Explaining one particular case, Lucy stated that she was doing bed-side intensive-care nursing with a recovering open-heart surgery patient, who served in World War II, when things took an unexpected turn. The veteran was White and had several of his family members with him at the hospital for support. Lucy describes the circumstances as a challenging case, but it was not the patient that posed a challenge or the technical aspects of the surgery:

> So, he was on a vent, but when he started waking up he was kind of rest-less, and I sedated him, and he calmed down and went back to sleep. So, the family came and they kind of saw me, and so they went to the charge nurse, but the charge nurse was also like Filipina and was kind of nicely requesting that I need to be relieved with someone else because that patient's family has seen me as Asian and their father has PTSD [post-traumatic stress disorder]. They were afraid that when he wakes up, he will see me as Japanese or something and will be rambunctious [anx-ious] and scared.

When I asked Lucy how she responded to the request, she stated that she un-derstood and immediately switched assignments with another nurse. She then added, "I wanted to honor this man for serving in WWII and helping to save my Philippines from the Japanese, but all his family saw was my Asian face. I wanted to be in that surgery. I wanted to hold his hand and pray for him, let him know that God was with him, and that everything was going to be alright." Visibly upset, Lucy tried to summarize how she sees herself versus how these situations make her feel. "I am a proud American citizen and a good Christian. I do work in the community for homeless veterans. Despite doing everything God and this country asks of me, I am still like the enemy. I am like a foreigner to them. I wish they could just see me for my service and just appreciate me for who I am. I'm not asking for much, just what I've earned!"

Introduction

Every year thousands of nurses like Rebecca and Lucy immigrate to the United States. Their visible presence in hospitals across the country reminds us that American healthcare increasingly depends on them to help mitigate its seemingly endless nursing shortages. As alarming as this might sound, it is nothing new. For over a century, the United States has struggled to meet the demands of its nursing care shortages domestically and has turned to foreign-born nurses. Today, the major sources of this so-called imported care remain the same as they have been historically—India and the Philippines.[3] However, it is not just any Filipino or Indian[4] becoming a nurse and immigrating, as we will see in subsequent chapters, but largely devout Catholic women.[5] They enter the country well trained, often with advanced degrees from prestigious universities using American standards and with considerably more years of experience than the average recently graduated American-born nurse. Despite these qualifications and the fact that these nurses are so desperately needed,[6] they enter the country at a time, not unlike previous eras, when the American social and political climate is once again increasingly hostile or at the very least unwelcoming to many of them as immigrants.

The brief but raw and impassioned narratives that open this chapter reveal the challenges foreign-born nurses can encounter while working in American hospitals. Although every nurse, regardless of nativity and background, is likely to experience some of these challenges, the Filipino and Indian American nurses in this study, and likely elsewhere, face the added pressure of being foreign-born women and ethnic/racial minorities in an increasingly xenophobic and racist America. This book analyzes the complex relationships between foreign-born nurses and their patients amid these circumstances. It does so by looking at nurses working at a VA hospital—an intense work environment that has historically magnified broader American sentiments about new immigrants. The Veterans Health Administration and its facilities are not your typical hospitals. They represent the largest integrated healthcare system in the country, a complicated network of government hospitals that have been the subject of ongoing scandal and investigation. Its patients are also not your typical patients. American veterans often have compounding mental and physical problems, and in many cases are also dealing with the harsh realities of PTSD. This, as we have already seen, can complicate foreign-born nurses' relationships and interactions with their patients.

Race matters in American healthcare. The caregiver-patient relationship is the cornerstone of any treatment regimen or long-term health goal. Prejudiced and discriminatory interactions can threaten this therapeutic alliance and can impact the mental and physical health of both the patient and their care provider. Every American hospital has policies protecting its employees against workplace discrimination at the hands of colleagues and administrative supervisors, but when a patient is racist or biased in some way toward a healthcare provider, there is often little to no recourse. This is the dilemma that Rebecca and Lucy painfully describe. What do you do when your patient is a racist or xenophobe? Patients have the legal right to refuse any care provider that they believe does not meet their needs. They also have the right to choose their care providers as they see fit. Research suggests that most patients want care providers who look like them, if available, but that is the problem. What happens when there are no nurses on a given shift that look like the patient? Likewise, and perhaps even more troubling, what happens when a patient or their family views their nurse to be a foreign enemy or a threat, despite the fact that the countries they emigrated from have never been at war with the United States?

Although Rebecca states that she attempts to keep how she feels about these difficult interactions to herself, often turning to prayer, and Lucy suggests that she tries to laugh it off, the agony of these experiences, even though they are not the daily norm, have clearly made a deep impact on them. Momentarily sad or angry, they continue to work at the VA seemingly with great joy and resolve—stating that they find more reward than challenge in their daily rounds. Compared to other private or public hospitals, the VA requires all of its full-time employees to be American citizens, excluding students and those in medical residency. Due to this policy, the overwhelming majority of its foreign-born nurses have previously worked at other American hospitals. They know what the so-called other side looks like because they left it to work at the VA. Many foreign-born nurses left their previous hospitals for better pay and opportunity, but many also stated that they quickly found that the VA was not what they were expecting. It was and is worse. So why do they stay? Why do they state that they want to finish their careers serving American veterans when the work is seemingly so challenging and possibly not as financially rewarding or opportune as at other hospitals? More importantly, and the central focus of this study, what motivates their daily care and deep commitment to American veterans both inside and outside of the hospital?

This book answers these questions through an intimate and critical analysis of the words and lives of foreign-born Filipino and Indian American nurses, licensed professionals from two of the largest immigrant populations in the country today. Their stories provide distinctive insights into the often-unseen roles race, religion, and gender play in the daily lives of new immigrants employed in American healthcare. Previous studies have documented the role race and gender play in American hospitals, including their impact on foreign-born nurses, but few have looked at the role of religion, specifically Catholicism, within these intersecting contexts. None have done so looking comparatively at foreign-born Filipino and Indian American nurses caring for American veterans. It is a unique case study with far-reaching implications.

Admittedly, the answers to the questions posed by this study can be messy, often unsettling, and further complicated by trying to make visible what is often invisible and very private or difficult to discuss. The deeply emotive conversations that open this chapter are a testament to this. Despite how anguishing they may be to read at times, the subjective experiences of foreign-born nurses such as Rebecca and Lucy reveal a side of American healthcare that many are blind to or simply choose to ignore. At the heart of this book are stories of perseverance and strength amid the most difficult of circumstances and work conditions. Yet, the nurses in this study do not see their work at the VA as a secular job, something they tolerate simply for a paycheck. Instead, they see it as a career that has deep religious meaning and sacred purpose.

When Rebecca and Lucy state that they are good Christians, they do not say this merely as a casual identification but as a declaration of faith that they say motivates and shapes every aspect of their personal and professional lives. For these women, like the overwhelming majority of the other foreign-born Filipino and Indian American nurses I interviewed, nursing is described as a religious calling. Serving American veterans specifically is seen as a patriotic duty, a moral obligation to give back to their adopted country. Despite emigrating from countries with distinct languages and histories, the majority of these nurses share a common cultural understanding and belief in the universality of the Catholic family. This is how they were raised. It is also how they were trained in their nursing programs. As a result, they say that they turn to their Catholic faith in the face of hardship—whether it is the normal daily challenges of being a nurse, the added pressures of coping with veterans who suffer from PTSD, or the racism and xenophobia from both their American-born peers and patients. Beyond revealing the role of religion as an important coping mechanism, their stories also demonstrate how Catholicism and their faith more generally powerfully influences and shapes their approaches to care both inside and outside of the hospital.

Research increasingly points to the benefits of religion and spiritual care on health. Yet, American healthcare continues to debate not only how to best teach spiritual care to healthcare professionals but the extent to which religion and spirituality should be engaged, if at all, in institutional settings with patients.[7] There is little debate for the foreign-born nurses in this study. Foreign-born Filipino and Indian American nurses are trained with a cultural understanding that complete patient care must include a holistic approach to the mind, body, and soul (spirit). Putting this training into practice, these nurses say that they readily engage their faith as an integral part of their care for American veterans. Although they do not deny science or the more biological causes of illness, as we will see in subsequent chapters, they see them through the lenses of their Catholic faith—a complex set of cultural and spiritual frameworks that can and do come into conflict with the secular norms of the government hospital in which they work. As a result, these nurses often find themselves caught between what they were taught about religion and spiritual care in their churches and nursing schools in another country, under vastly different cultural circumstances and norms, and what American nursing standards and hospital policies mandate. This is not completely unique to these nurses, but something American Catholics and other nurses of faith have historically had to confront both personally and professionally.

Studying the ways foreign-born nurses engage spiritual practice at a secular hospital such as the VA allows us to understand the tensions that can exist between the legal separation or disestablishment of religion in public institutions and the lives of people who are religious, both those working at a hospital and the patients they serve.[8] It also provides greater insight into the ongoing debates over the role of religion and spirituality in American healthcare. Throughout this book, the private and at times deeply intimate conversations with foreign-born Filipino and Indian American nurses demonstrate how Catholicism animates their approaches to patient care while at the same time compelling them to take civic action on behalf of American veterans both inside and outside of the hospital. As they extend their care into the community on issues such as poverty, community health, and homelessness, their stories reveal a rather serious predicament. More than forty-four million people living in the United States today are foreign born. They represent nearly 14 percent of the American population but 16 percent of all registered nurses and 22 percent of all nursing assistants—disproportionate shares, and this does not include doctors and other healthcare professionals.[9] The country appears to increasingly depend on foreign-born nurses' faithful service and is seemingly made better by their care and community engagement, as subsequent chapters will demonstrate, but despite this fact, highly vocal segments of the country today grow increasingly fearful of how they and other immigrants might forever change America.

The American Nursing Shortage Crisis

With the passage of the Affordable Care Act in 2009, health insurance coverage was expanded by an estimated thirty-two million Americans. This dramatically increased the need for doctors, nurses,[10] and other healthcare providers.[11] Many people responded to this demand by flocking to the nursing profession.[12] In fact, nursing is one of the few industries in the United States that is still experiencing employment growth and projected to continue to grow.[13] Today the United States has the largest professional nursing workforce in the world, over three million workers or nearly one-fifth of the world's supply of nurses.[14] Nursing is also one of the fastest-growing occupations in the nation.[15] However, despite nursing's relative size and growth as an occupation, the demand for more nurses is currently outpacing supply.[16] Hospitals across the country, including VA hospitals like the one Rebecca and Lucy work at, are in desperate need of nurses.[17]

According to the Bureau of Labor Statistics, over one million vacancies for nursing positions will emerge over the next four years.[18] By 2025, this shortage is expected to be more than twice as large as any nursing shortage since the introduction of Medicare and Medicaid in the mid-1960s.[19] Even more alarming, some estimates suggest that by 2030 upwards of two million nurses will be needed to fill projected nursing needs—a 28.4 percent increase in demand with few immediate solutions in sight.[20] Although some states are expected to be able to meet their needs or exceed them by 2030, many are projected to be hit much harder. Texas, for example, the location of this study, looks to be one of the states with the greatest projected need—a nearly sixteen-thousand-person difference between the projected supply and demand for nurses.[21] It is a potentially catastrophic problem, but historically speaking, it is nothing new as chapter 3 will further demonstrate.

Every policy briefing, study, and speech about the current nursing shortage claims that the circumstances are far different than any shortages in the past, but there are some contributing factors that remain the same.[22] The economy still plays a major role in the supply and demand of nurses, as does the general perception of the nursing profession. Nursing continues to be seen as a demanding profession with poor or challenging working conditions.[23] Any temporary gains in the numbers of American-born nurses during shortages are typically made by nurses returning to work during high unemployment periods or new students entering the field when no other jobs or better jobs can be found.[24] Once the economy rebounds, many of these gains are lost as nurses who originally reentered the labor force during these times reduce their hours or return to non-nursing jobs. This creates a new void, and the shortage cycle inevitably starts again.

What makes the current nursing shortage unique and, in some ways, unprecedented in the history of American healthcare is a matter of age. Today there are more Americans over the age of sixty-five than at any other time in the country's history. By 2030, the number of senior citizens in the United States is expected to increase by 75 percent—over sixty-nine million people.[25] One in five Americans will be a senior citizen, and by 2050, an estimated eighty-nine million Americans will be aged sixty-five or older.[26] As people age, they often need more care. Two-thirds of current Medicare beneficiaries aged sixty-five years or older, for example, have multiple chronic conditions.[27] More than four million have at least six long-term ailments, and this is expected to only get worse with time as the population continues to age. As previous studies have demonstrated, higher patient-to-nurse workloads, such as those predicted in the coming years, are associated with an increase in medical errors, longer hospitalizations, lower patient satisfaction, and an increase in mortality rates.[28] If more nurses do not enter the workforce, nursing leaders fear that people may die at higher rates or possibly receive poor and substandard care because there are simply not enough nurses to keep up with the increasing number of patients.

Further complicating this trend, nurses who stayed in the profession after the so-called Great Recession of 2008 are beginning to reach the end of their careers. In 2010, nearly 30 percent of American-born registered nurses were fifty-five years of age or older.[29] As they reach retirement age in the next five to ten years, it is expected that nearly one-third of the current nursing population will leave the workforce.[30] By 2030, roughly one million nurses are projected to retire.[31] Who will replace them? Although nursing is still dominated by women, with each passing decade women continue to have more career choices than they did in the past. This, in and of itself, is not a problem, but it makes finding a solution increasingly difficult when fewer women are becoming nurses or remaining nurses and men are not entering the field in high enough numbers to replace them.[32] Today, men represent fewer than 10 percent of registered nurses and fewer than 12 percent of students enrolled in nursing programs.[33]

One obvious way to relieve nursing shortages is to educate more nurses domestically and make the field more attractive to new recruits, but there are several significant barriers to this solution, despite its necessity and utility.[34] Nearly one hundred and fifty-five thousand new nursing graduates entered the workforce in 2015.[35] Although the number of nursing students and graduates has continued to grow over the last several years, the American nursing education system has not been able to keep pace with the demand for more nurses. According to the American Association of Colleges of Nursing, some eighty thousand qualified nursing-school applicants were turned away from programs due to insufficient numbers of faculty, clinical sites, classroom space, and other budgetary constraints.[36] People want to become nurses, but nursing programs simply do not have the resources to keep up with number of people who apply to their programs or the federal and local support they need to expand their programs as needed. As a result, the demand for American-born nurses remains significantly higher than the current supply of graduates. It remains to be seen how interest in nursing as a profession will be fully impacted by the coronavirus pandemic (COVID-19) or force changes in federal support for nursing programs but about one in five healthcare workers has left their job since the pandemic started.[37] If staffing shortages continue as projected, or even worsen in the future, and American nursing schools are unable to meet these needs, foreign-born Filipino and Indian American nurses are likely to play an important role in helping to mitigate these shortages—just as they have done in the past.[38]

Importing Care?

Although there is considerable debate about the historical and current causes of American nursing shortages and the degree to which international recruitment of nurses is the solution or even part of the solution, it is clear that foreign-born nurses' presence is growing in response to these circumstances. Over the last several decades, American hospitals have successfully lobbied Congress for migration policies that facilitate the importation of foreign-born nurses to provide critical and temporary relief during acute shortages.[39] During the late 1980s, for example, Congress passed the Immigration Nursing Relief Act of 1989 in response to severe nursing shortages and an urgent call for temporary relief. The act created the H-1A nonimmigrant visa category for nurses and placed no limits on the number of visas that could be issued. Subsequently, the Immigration Act in 1990 created the H-1B category for skilled temporary workers who hold bachelor's degrees, which also aided nurse migration.[40] Nurses such as Rebecca and Lucy from the opening narratives of this chapter, for example, entered the country under this legislation. Almost ten years later, the Nursing Relief for Disadvantaged Areas Act of 1999 also created the H-1C nonimmigrant visa category to relieve hospitals with acute nursing shortages serving disadvantaged areas with a minimum share of Medicaid and Medicare patients.[41] When these emergency acts expired in 1995 and 2009 respectively,

H-1B and H-1C visa types were not renewed. However, in 2005, President George W. Bush signed into law the Emergency Supplemental Appropriations Package that reallocated over fifty thousand unused employment-based immigrant visas to registered nurses and other critical healthcare professionals in short supply.[42]

Since 2005, several emergency nursing relief bills have been introduced in the United States Congress and sent to committees for study, but none have advanced to a vote. In 2009, for example, H.R. 4321 or the Comprehensive Immigration Reform for America's Security and Prosperity Act of 2009 was introduced to the House of Representatives with the hope of lifting visa quotas for foreign nationals seeking to work in shortage occupations such as nursing.[43] Like many recently proposed bills, it died on the floor with little discussion. Although recruiting foreign-born nurses is less expensive and takes less time than educating American-born nurses, the effectiveness of this strategy continues to be widely discussed.[44] Nursing leaders also continue to suggest that importing foreign-born nurses does not address larger and more serious workplace problems that are driving American-born nurses away from the profession.[45] Hence, injecting foreign-born nurses into a dysfunctional system that is not capable of sufficiently recruiting and retaining domestic nurses will not solve the crisis.[46]

Echoing these concerns, President Obama stated in 2009 that, "the notion that we would have to import nurses makes absolutely no sense."[47] Although the point of Obama's message, and perhaps that of nursing leaders more generally, was to explore the creation of new jobs for American-born nurses in the wake of a recession, many immigrants working in healthcare, including the nurses I interviewed, suggested that they took the message as an indication that Obama, and the nation as a whole, did not appreciate them or that the doors of opportunity for others to immigrate and seek employment in healthcare were starting to close.[48] Adding to this perception several years later, in 2012 former District of Columbia mayor Marion Barry in a speech after his victory party for the Democratic nomination for the DC Council Ward Eight seat complained about "dirty" Asian business and then singled out Filipino nurses as a problem in local hospitals. "It's so bad, that if you go to the hospital now, you find a number of immigrants who are nurses, particularly from the Philippines. And no offense, but let's grow our own . . . so we don't have to be scrounging around in our community clinics and other kinds of places—having to hire people from somewhere else."[49] The election of President Trump in 2016 and the subsequent enactment of emergency anti-immigrant legislation, including the temporary suspension of expedited H-1B visas and the threat to bar all immigration

during the COVID-19 pandemic, heightened these fears as new waves of xenophobic concerns continued to rise. Although some bipartisan legislation has
actually made it through the House into the Senate in recent years, nothing has
been passed. Many in Congress continue to argue for importing more foreign-
born nurses[50] but have yet to convince a majority.

It is a complicated problem. Many nursing leaders, including those in the
American Nursing Association (ANA), question the ethics of international
nurse recruitment—fearing that continually drawing nurses away from India
and the Philippines will only replace one crisis with another by creating
staffing shortages in these countries. Likewise, many argue that foreign-born
nurses are only a short-term solution at best that serves the interest of the
hospital industry but does not necessarily serve the interest of patients or
create better incentives and work conditions for both foreign and domestic
nurses.[51] Beyond these issues and debates, and in some cases within them,
much of the more public rhetoric that surrounds discussions about importing
care today, as in the past, often takes on a nativist and xenophobic tone that
reflects increasing public concerns about immigrants. Will continual waves of
immigration lower wages and worsen conditions for American-born workers?
If so, will this reduce incentives for industries such as healthcare to recruit
American-born workers? Are immigrants a national security risk or a threat to
their patients? Can they be trusted? And with time, will these immigrants
assimilate and become average American citizens, or will their loyalties forever remain foreign—never becoming real Americans?[52] These questions are
not new but seemingly timeless in the fears they express. American history is
replete with examples, highlighted by a long cycle of xenophobic responses to
increased Catholic and Asian immigration.[53]

Historicizing Immigration Concerns

The United States has always been a nation of immigrants. It has also always
been a nation of xenophobic fears.[54] Since the beginning of the twentieth
century, over eighty million immigrants have settled in the country. With each
successive wave, public and political sentiment has often turned against immigrants. In 1820, for example, hundreds of thousands of Irish Catholics began
to enter the United States alongside waves of Germans, Poles, and Italians.
Over the next thirty years, the number of Irish would grow to represent roughly
40 percent of all immigrants in the country.[55] As Catholic immigrants established new communities and built institutions within them, including hospitals to care for the rapid influx of new Catholic immigrants, they experienced
significant Protestant hostility.[56] Many Americans saw the Irish and other

Catholics as dirty, diseased, and unfit to be citizens. They also saw them as a threat to jobs and to the continuance of an American Protestant majority. Throughout the mid-1800s, mobs killed Irish Catholics and burned their homes to the ground. Catholic churches were vandalized, and a host of social sanctions across the country led to the privatization of schools, social clubs, and civic associations that further prevented Catholics from joining and participating fully in American society.[57]

In 1849, amid this turmoil, a fraternal society of American-born Protestant men formed the Order of the Star Spangled Banner in New York to rally against the so-called threat of Irish Catholic immigration. As chapters of this secret society increased in popularity across the country, the society eventually coalesced into the American Party, also known as the Know Nothings—a political movement built on a rabidly anti-Catholic immigrant platform. In 1854, the American Party, running on the slogan "America must rule Americans," won fifty-three seats in Congress.[58] Two years later, Millard Fillmore, the former 12th vice-president and the 13th president of the United States (1850–1853), who took over the presidency after the death of President Zachary Taylor, garnered nearly 22 percent of the national popular vote when he ran for president with the endorsement of the Know Nothing Party.[59]

During this rise in national popularity, what would eventually be the peak of the movement just before the American Civil War, a new chapter of the Know Nothings was founded in San Francisco, California, to oppose Chinese immigration.[60] This intensified the harassment of Chinese immigrants, who were not Catholic but over time replaced the Irish as the object of nativist fears. This would change with the mass migration of Filipinos, who were both Asian and majority Catholic. After the Spanish-American War and subsequent American rule of the Philippines, Filipinos entered the United States as colonial nationals, but their increasing presence in agricultural labor led to fears that they were taking jobs from American-born workers. Like the Irish and Chinese prior, Filipinos were widely demonized, and violent anti-Filipino outbursts erupted throughout states such as California and Washington.[61]

Whether it was the arrival of large waves of Chinese immigrants in the late nineteenth century or subsequent waves of Filipino immigrants in the early twentieth century, to name a few, Asian Americans have long been considered a threat to the United States. Labeled as savages or the so-called Yellow Peril, they were largely characterized as uncivilized, potentially disease ridden, and thus unfit for American citizenship.[62] These views, like those levied against the Irish, led to widespread persecution, mass killings, anti-miscegenation laws preventing Asians from interacting with White Americans, and the eventual barring of all Asian immigration to the United States through the Chinese Exclusion Act and other subsequent legislation throughout the late nineteenth century.[63]

Not much changed at the turn of the century. The Immigration Act of 1917, also known as the Literacy Act because it imposed literacy tests on new immigrants, for example, effectively barred all Asians from entering the country. Where earlier acts largely focused on the Chinese, subsequent legislation sought to curb the growing presence of other Asians, including Filipinos and Indians, as the country saw a revival of nativist and anti-Catholic sentiments.[64] The Supreme Court verdict in *United States v. Bhagat Singh Thind* in 1923 made Indians ineligible for citizenship and further restricted their migration. Likewise, the Tydings-McDuffie Act in 1934, some ten years later, answered the specific call for Filipino exclusion by granting the Philippines gradual independence while stripping all Filipinos of their American citizenship and ending their migration. In the 1950s, as the country formally removed race/ethnicity as grounds for exclusion, subsequent legislation allowed a limited number of visas for Chinese and other Asians to enter the United States. The country was changing, and so were its needs, particularly in healthcare.

Concerns over Imported Care

After the passage of the 1965 Immigration Act and the increased migration of degreed Asian professionals to the United States, including doctors and nurses called on to help mitigate emerging healthcare staffing shortages, Asian Americans were labeled a model minority, the ideal immigrants because of their relative economic success.[65] However, this model status did not necessarily make them any more accepted as so-called real Americans.[66] This includes foreign-born health professionals such as the nurses in this study. Despite the passage of the Civil Rights Act in 1964, nursing, especially its national lobby and administration through the ANA largely remained dominated by White women.[67] When foreign-born nurses began to migrate to the United States in larger numbers in the 1960s, they entered a highly racialized field that was stratified along Black and White lines.[68] Given that the majority of these nurses were neither Black nor White, their growing presence in American hospitals was foreign in every sense of the word.[69]

The Exchange Visitor Program (EVP), instituted some two decades earlier as part of the 1948 Information and Educational Exchange Act, allowed thousands of agencies, hospitals, and ANA itself to sponsor foreign-born nurses to increase cultural exchange through/with the International Council of Nurses. But the program did not ease American concerns over subsequent waves of foreign-born nurses, including the first sizeable migration of Indian nurses, or warm American hospitals to their eventual increased presence.[70] In fact, the majority of exchange nurses during these early years were from northern Europe and Scandinavia.[71] They were foreign but White, which meant that their presence was seen more as a novel curiosity than a major challenge to American nursing racial stratification. When European nursing shortages forced the American EVP system to shift its geographic focus to Asia in the late 1950s through the early 1960s, ANA issued a position statement in the *American Journal of Nursing* that expressed its apprehensions over the use of foreign-born nurses for American labor needs.[72] Although ANA's opposition included ethical concerns that foreign-born nurses might be exploited in the American labor market or that their continued migration would lead to a so-called brain drain in their own countries, it was clear that considerable debate existed over the importation of foreign-born nurses for one reason or another.[73]

Newspaper coverage of foreign-born nurses was sparse throughout the 1970s. The few articles that were published often portrayed them as a temporary solution to the growing problem.[74] While these stories also highlighted the frustration and vulnerability foreign-born nurses faced in their new work environments, any sympathetic tone was quickly erased by reminding readers that foreign-born nurses were in imminent danger of deportation, were not as competent as American-born nurses, and posed a potentially hazardous threat to their patients.[75] Reports about their professional care from nursing supervisors also suggested that foreign-born nurses were timid, noncaring, unable to converse in English, indifferent to death, and impersonal toward the financial and emotional problems of their patients.[76]

Nursing journals at the time often tried to dispel these generalizations by chalking them up to misconceptions and cultural difference. Yet, they also highlighted the fact that nurses from countries such as Ireland and England, White nurses, were easier to assimilate into American hospitals.[77] Any attempts to counter public perceptions or assuage nursing leaders' concerns seemed hollow, especially when you consider that foreign-born nurses continued to receive lower pay than American-born nurses and were given the worst shifts, often with the most difficult patients.[78] Foreign-born nurses entering the United States in the 1970s faced several difficulties in adjusting to their new careers. They often felt lost and alone with only their faith to comfort them. This was particularly true of foreign-born Indian American nurses who, unlike foreign-born Filipino American nurses, had fewer numbers in their respective hospitals and hence less peer support in their own native languages.[79]

Speaking in a language other than English in front of patients was/is universally against American hospital policies, and foreign-born nurses followed these regulations. In private or during breaks, they were free to speak with their peers in their native languages, but they also faced intense scrutiny for doing so—and still do today, as we will see. Beyond further alienating them from their American-born peers, speaking in their native languages also raised concerns about their English comprehension as it related to other technical proficiencies or the ability to interact with doctors and patients. Questions about foreign nurses' ability to effectively communicate were often reportedly justified by pointing to the high rate at which many foreign nurses failed the State Board Test Pool Examination (SBTPE) nursing exam.[80] However, nurses from English-speaking nations such as Ireland and England fared only slightly better on the SBTPE exam than nurses from non-English-speaking nations such as India and the Philippines but were treated far better by their American-born counterparts.[81] Race mattered, as did the degree to which their other cultural differences were seen as foreign. Filipino and Indian American nurses, at least in the 1970s, epitomized what Americans perceived to be a foreign threat. They were Asian at a time in which many native-born Americans were increasingly anti-Asian after the Vietnam War.[82] As a result, they were often seen as disposable labor—never fully trusted and largely considered unequal in every conceivable way to American-born nurses.[83]

During the early 1970s, much of the debate over the employment of foreign nurses remained out of the public eye. This dramatically changed in 1977 when Filipina Narciso and Leonora Perez, both foreign-born nurses from the Philippines, were convicted for supposedly murdering patients at a Veterans Administration hospital in Ann Arbor, Michigan.[84] With no murder weapon, fingerprints or direct eyewitnesses to the crimes, the Federal Bureau of Investigations (FBI) relied on highly circumstantial evidence to question the nurses who worked in the same intensive care unit where the failures and deaths occurred. Knowing that both women were devoutly religious, the FBI called on them to act on their faith and admit before God that they had conspired to kill American veterans, but they both maintained that they were innocent.[85] During the trial, the nurses explained that they were angry about staffing shortages at the hospital. Although the prosecution never attempted to establish a clear motive, some task force investigators suggested that the only plausible reason that two seemingly dedicated and hardworking nurses would kill their patients was to dramatically demonstrate the need for more nurses at the hospital.[86] After deliberating for thirteen days, the jury found the nurses guilty on three counts of poisoning.[87] In February of the following year, the case was overturned on an appeal, citing several instances of misconduct by the prosecution during the trial. The prosecution was given permission for a retrial, but the case was eventually dropped.

A decade after the Narciso and Perez case, Filipino and other ethnic nurses were better organized and had created institutions and associations to protect themselves from further discrimination and unfair treatment.[88] However, nursing leaders and journals throughout the 1980s and early 1990s continued to depict them as ill-prepared for careers in American hospitals, passive, and unable to converse clearly in English.[89] For all that foreign-born nurses had gone through to prove their worth and loyalty to their profession and the United States, they were still seen by many as too foreign or not fully American.[90] Today, foreign-born Filipino and Indian American nurses continue to report being treated as inferior, often stating that they are talked down to by peers and superiors or treated like children for asking questions.[91] From California to Baltimore and Michigan to Florida, foreign-born nurses report being made fun of for their accents or harassed in front of other employees for being or acting "culturally different."[92] When they attempt to rally together to support one another, they are at times accused of being cliquish, or coded jokes are made about how they all might be related because they look alike.[93] Beyond these caustic experiences with their peers and superiors, the frequency of which is difficult to ascertain, they also report being treated like "servants" by their patients or rejected by them or their families based on the color of their skin or the sound of their names.[94] These same nurses also routinely report getting blamed for taking jobs away from so-called real Americans or being told to go back to India and the Philippines.[95]

The United States is one of the, if not the, largest receiving country of foreign-born nurses in the world today.[96] Their presence has helped the country mitigate its perennial staffing needs, even if temporarily, but this has not necessarily improved the way they are treated.[97] Forty percent of foreign-born nurses in one study, for example, report that they are discriminated against in shift assignments, wages, and benefits.[98] Although the limited research in this area often gives the false impression that racism and discrimination do not exist in healthcare and are not the cause for these trends, this is debatable, especially for foreign-born nurses given the history discussed in this chapter[99] and the fact that ANA itself has actually drawn attention to and condemned the exploitation of immigrant nurses in recent years.[100]

Like other Asian immigrants historically, foreign-born nurses today face a host of rather complex challenges living and working in the United States. When things become difficult, many foreign-born Filipino and Indian American nurses say that they turn to the support of a higher power and their faith.[101] Just as Narciso and Perez were known by their peers at the time for being devout Christians, the same is true today for the majority of foreign-born nurses like Rebecca and Lucy interviewed for this book. They see their faith as an active and vital part of their professional care. Like Catholic immigrants in the past, the foreign-born nurses in this study struggle with the tensions between how to be both good Catholics and patriotic Americans in an environment that is at times very unwelcoming to them as immigrants. They also struggle, as we will see, with the disconnects between how they were raised and trained to understand Catholic approaches to nursing as spiritual care, and the separation of church and state in American secular hospitals such as the VA.[102]

Faith, Hidden in Plain Sight

Since 2002, the Veterans Administration has struggled with implementing policies regarding the public display of religious symbols in its hospitals, especially during Christian holidays. The antireligious display policy, based on the Supreme Court ruling in the case of *County of Allegheny v. ACLU* in 1989 (492 U.S. 573) that stipulated that any public display cannot advance or inhibit religion or favor one religion over another and must have a secular purpose, has continually drawn criticism and incited the anger of veterans and their families.[103] In 2014, these complaints came to a head when administrators at a VA hospital in Michigan ordered Christian symbols and statues in a chapel to be covered up. Although this was only done temporarily to meet federal religious-freedom requirements during chapel off-hours, and the covering was eventually taken down after numerous complaints, the story went viral, causing even greater concern on veteran blogs and message boards.[104] One year later, administrators at a VA hospital in San Antonio, Texas, tore down Christmas holiday decorations put up by a veteran of the Vietnam War because they were deemed offensive and overly religious, and Christmas trees were banned in all public spaces at a VA hospital in Virginia.[105]

In 2019, the VA changed its policy after the Supreme Court verdict in the case of *The American Legion vs. American Humanist Association*. Arguing first that the verdict reaffirmed the role religion plays in the lives of many Americans, the VA then suggested that it had been inconsistent on the place of religion at its facilities in recent years and was working to simplify and clarify its policies governing religious symbols and spiritual and pastoral care. The new policy allowed (1) the inclusion in appropriate circumstances of religious content in publicly accessible displays at VA facilities; (2) patients and their guests to request and be provided religious literature, symbols, and sacred texts during visits to VA chapels and during their treatment; and (3) acceptance of donations of religious literature, cards, and symbols at its facilities and distribution to VA patrons under appropriate circumstances or to a patron who requests them.[106] This effectively reversed prior policy but still raised serious questions over the separation of church and state—and the best ways, if any, to implement the new policy, particularly at the point of care.[107]

Despite often being hidden in plain sight, religion and spirituality have historically been a vital part of healthcare, especially nursing.[108] Starting with Florence Nightingale, considered by most to be the founder of modern nursing and the person who singlehandedly elevated the profession to what it resembles today, nursing grew from charitable and religious roots into a profession that carried considerable social respect and admiration. From 1837 to 1850, Nightingale had a series of experiences she believed were messages from God to serve the sick and the poor.[109] Since nursing had not yet emerged as a proper profession and was largely seen as a dirty and menial job, Nightingale struggled to answer these calls given the expectation for women of her social status. However, against the wishes of her parents, Nightingale rebelled against Victorian cultural and class expectations, and revolutionized the nursing profession in the process.[110]

When Nightingale began formally nursing in the 1850s, she worked with both Protestant and Catholic sister-nurses.[111] This significantly influenced her conception of nursing not only as a religious duty but as a disciplined and organized practice.[112] After volunteering as a field nurse during the Crimean War and reporting back to Great Britain about the deplorable conditions of English soldiers, Nightingale wrote *Notes on Nursing* (1859). The book not only created the foundations for contemporary nursing theory but also became the basis for Nightingale's nursing curriculum at the Nightingale Home and Training School for Nurses established in 1860—the world's first formal nursing program connected to a hospital. This curriculum emphasized knowledge and practice, not faith and spirituality, but Nightingale also believed that nurses needed ongoing spiritual nourishment to deal with the challenges of nursing, especially in dealing with issues surrounding dying patients.[113]

Despite Nightingale's often rocky relationship with the Anglican church, she believed that moral science was the ultimate goal of nursing care and that nursing education was synonymous with the study of God's character or the nature of God's laws.[114] Many who later followed Nightingale or graduated from her nursing program were torn between nursing as a profession and a religious calling. They drew on their faith as an integral part of their professional practice.[115] This was especially true and continues to be the case, as we will see, in countries such as India and the Philippines, where the Nightingale model of nursing historically spread through the support and instruction of Protestant missionaries.

Today, religion and spirituality remain important to nurses both personally and as an inseparable part of their professional care. Roughly 91 percent of nurses in a recent study, for example, stated that they consider themselves to be spiritual, and 42 percent consider themselves to be religious.[116] Beyond self-identifying as spiritual or claiming a religious affiliation, these nurses also stated that there is something spiritual (84 percent) or religious (24 percent) about the type of care they provide their patients. Moreover, 85 percent subsequently stated that they believe that their spirituality and religiosity can improve the quality of patient care.[117] This is true not only for American nurses nationally but for foreign-born Filipino and Indian American nurses who grew up in religious homes, largely attended religious schools—including religious nursing training programs—and entered the nursing profession with a belief that they were called by God to do so. However, as we will see in subsequent chapters, they often struggle to find the best ways and opportunities to engage their faith in the secular settings in which they work—despite the fact that research suggests that patients want more spiritual discussions with their healthcare providers and believe that spiritual health is as important as physical health.

The United States remains one of the most religious countries—if not the most religious country—in the world.[118] Understanding this, we should not be surprised that patients want or at the least are open to discussing their faith with healthcare providers.[119] Yet, patients report that these discussions rarely take place.[120] There are several possible reasons why healthcare professionals are reluctant or do not want to engage in any form of spiritual care with their patients. First, many healthcare professionals question whether or not they have a relevant role in providing spiritual care or prefer to defer to chaplains.[121] Second, part of the reason for this deferment may be due to the secular settings in which many healthcare professionals work and interact with patients. Understanding patients' rights and the legal separation of church and state, healthcare providers are often afraid to talk about these issues or are not sure when and if it is appropriate. Third, the reason that healthcare providers do not talk about these issues or engage in spiritual care more is because they say they have not been adequately trained to do so.[122] Although the overwhelming majority of the nurses interviewed for this book stated that they prefer to keep their faith private unless a patient asks, they do engage their faith, and frequently with great reward and at potential professional risk. Their perspectives on spiritual care can and do lead to conflict with the secular environment in which they work.

How they navigate these tensions and disconnects plays an important role in shaping not only how they see themselves as Catholic nurses but their perceived place in American healthcare and the United States more generally.

Studying amid Scandal and Scrutiny

Research for this study was conducted in the Houston metropolitan area over a four-year period (2014–2018) through the participation of a snowball sample of foreign-born Filipino and Indian American nurses who are currently or formerly employed at the Houston VA hospital. Houston, Texas, was selected for several reasons. First, Houston is the most racially and ethnically diverse, rapidly growing metropolitan area in the United States. Much of this diversity and growth has occurred as a result of immigration.[123] From 2000 to 2013, for example, Houston's immigrant population grew at a rate nearly twice that of the national average (59 percent versus 33 percent).[124] As a major emerging immigrant gateway city and a model of what the country is expected to look like demographically in the next thirty years, Houston poses a unique and important case for study.

Second, the Texas Medical Center (TMC), of which the Michael E. DeBakey VA Medical Center (Houston VA) is a part, is the largest medical complex in the world and the largest single employer in the city. The TMC serves over eight million patients a year through the care of over one hundred and six thousand healthcare workers.[125] Although the nativity of these employees is not fully known,[126] like other medical centers and hospitals across the country, the TMC depends heavily on foreign-born workers to maintain its steady institutional growth and meet the needs of an increasingly diverse and aging population.[127] Third, Texas has the second-largest veteran population in the country, roughly 1.5 million veterans, and the Houston VA is in the top twenty largest veterans hospitals in the country by number of staffed beds.[128] The Houston VA is also a teaching hospital, providing clinical training for healthcare professionals through one of the largest VA residency programs in the country.[129] Each academic year, almost two thousand students are trained through one hundred and forty affiliation agreements with colleges and programs in nineteen states.[130] How the Houston VA operates at all levels, from its complicated point-of-care negotiations between church and state to managing the racial/ethnic and nativity tensions among and between staff and their patients has far reaching impacts on those whom they train and who go on to work at other hospitals across the country.

Although the original study was conceived as an ethnography, the timing of the project quickly changed both its scope and direction after the 2014 national VA scandal. The Veterans Health Administration scandal of 2014 broke when a widespread pattern of negligence in the treatment of U.S. military veterans was reported at VA hospitals across the country. Not only were VA hospitals not meeting their target of getting patients appointments within fourteen days, in some hospitals, staff reportedly falsified appointment records to make it appear that they had met this target.[131] Even more troubling, some patients died while they were on the waiting list to be seen at a VA hospital.[132] The scandal was not the only problem to draw attention to the VA system in recent years, but the investigation was the largest in over a decade. Since my research protocol was still working its way through the VA review process prior to the investigation, my status as a nonpaid researcher was eventually revoked, and I was asked to leave the hospital. Even as the investigation ended, I was never able to get back into the Houston VA system to directly observe foreign-born nurses as they care for American veterans.[133]

Despite these emergent limitations, the scandal did not deter foreign-born nurses from participating in the study. On the contrary, as the opening narratives of this chapter highlight, it seemed to embolden their desire to talk about their experiences. Although the original project had nothing to do with larger systemic VA problems, it was an unavoidable subject moving forward as the study shifted from the hospital to a snowball sample largely drawn from associations that represented the two largest groups of foreign-born nurses working in the hospital—the Filipino Nurses Association (FNA, pseudonym) and the Indian Nurses Association (INA, pseudonym). Over the next several years, I interviewed over one hundred and sixteen healthcare providers, of which eighty-seven were foreign-born nurses originally from India and the Philippines. I also conducted several focus groups and panel discussions at the general meetings of both associations.

All of the nurses in this study are U.S. citizens, which is not the case nationally.[134] This is a function of site selection and VA employment requirements. However, in relation to other demographic characteristics, the interview sample is representative of the wider demographic profile of foreign-born Filipino and Indian American nurses across the United States with the exception of age. The sample is older by an average of five years. This is also a product of site selection.[135] Drawing on the same sample frame, I also surveyed foreign-born Filipino and Indian American nurses on issues ranging from work life and experience to religious and community engagement.[136] Like the interview sample, the survey sample is representative of the wider demographic profile of foreign-born Filipino and Indian American nurses across the United States with exception of citizenship and age.[137]

In addition to interviewing and surveying foreign-born Filipino and Indian American nurses, I interviewed thirty-five American veterans about their experiences at the Houston VA hospital. I also monitored and engaged foreign-born Filipino and Indian American nursing blogs and veterans blogs, as well as other relevant online groups. Triangulating this unique and original data collection, I historically situated and contextualized the central arguments of this book within an exhaustive exploration of the current literature on race, gender and nursing, immigrant religious life, and the ongoing debates over the role of spirituality and religion in American healthcare.[138]

Book Overview

Chapter 2 historicizes Filipino and Indian nursing migration to the United States. It analyzes the impact of Western colonial states, the Rockefeller Foundation, and Protestant medical missionaries on the development of nursing as a paid profession in India and the Philippines. The chapter concludes by theorizing how Catholic cultural frameworks motivate and shape foreign-born nurses' professional and community lives as they care for American veterans and work for the betterment of their health both inside and outside of the hospital. Chapter 3 further contextualizes the current American nursing shortage and explores the unique and challenging character of the VA hospital and its patients. The chapter demonstrates that foreign-born Filipino and Indian Americans' stated desire to stay at the hospital and serve veterans is not about opportunity or economics but their faith and an ardent belief that it is their patriotic duty as American Catholics to serve God and their country.

Chapter 4 defines and explores the dimensions along which foreign-born nurses say they experience various forms of discrimination with their patients, coworkers, and administrators. It then unpacks the important ways in which foreign-born nurses say they use their Catholic faith to cope with the challenges of working at the VA—reframing the realities of their daily rounds into a deeply held belief that their labor is God's work. Chapter 5 begins by exploring the ways in which matters of faith are addressed in some of India and the Philippines's top nursing programs today. It then engages the current debates over the role of religion in American healthcare and analyzes the ways in which foreign-born nurses see Catholicism as a vital part of their care for American veterans.

Chapter 6 widens the theoretical lens of previous chapters. It demonstrates how faith and Catholicism compels foreign-born Filipino and Indian American nurses to extend their care for American veterans from the hospital into the community by acting on issues such as poverty, community health, and homelessness. Chapter 7 explores the implications of this study in the wider context of ongoing political and popular concerns over the state of American healthcare. It evaluates the utility of importing care amid perennial nursing shortages and then demonstrates the possible roles that immigrants might play in not only serving an increasingly diversifying country but helping to shape the new American story from a Catholic perspective.

Chapter 2

Colonialism, Christian Culture, and Nursing Care

Every month, the Filipino Nurses Association (FNA, pseudonym) holds their general meeting in an auditorium of a local hospital. Each meeting, or at least those I observed over a four-year period, started with a prayer. However, at one particular meeting a moment of silence for the victims of the massive earthquake that struck Bohol in Central Visayas in the Philippines preceded the prayer. Leading the meeting was Emmy, a foreign-born Filipina American nurse in her early fifties. "Let us take a moment of silence to remember those who have died or been injured in the Philippines and pray for their speedy recovery."

After a moment of silence, Emmy thanked the members and asked them to bow their heads in prayer: "Dear Lord, we are daily reminded of why we are here and how much is asked of us. We understand our responsibility as Christians and the charity we must show to our brothers and sisters here in the United States and those in the Philippines." Pausing, Emmy then stated, "Heavenly Father, we come to you today asking for your guidance, wisdom, and support as we begin this meeting. . . . Allow us to grow closer as a group and nurture the bonds of community. Fill us with your grace, Lord God, as we make decisions that might affect others. Continue to remind us that all that we do here today, all that we accomplish, is for the pursuit of joy for the greater glory of you, and for the service of humanity. We ask these things in your name, Amen."

In response, the majority of the members in attendance made the sign of the cross or nodded their head and replied, "Amen." Immediately following the prayer, Emmy asked for an update from various members about their own families and friends in Bohol and then inquired about their various efforts to raise money for the region's disaster relief. Moving on to the broader agenda, the members updated Emmy on the successes of their health fair held the previous week at a local Chinese church, and then strategized about their upcoming flu shot roundup at a local Catholic church. The meeting lasted another hour and became rather technical in its discussion of nursing issues, but throughout the meeting, religion or faith more generally appeared to be important to the nurses.

Not long after the meeting, I interviewed Emmy and asked her why she thought there were so many Filipino nurses in the United States and why they appear to be predominately Catholic. "The U.S. needs nurses and the Philippines is a Catholic nation. It's that simple," she stated. She then explained, "We have to leave the Philippines because they [family] depend on us nurses to help. That's why there are so many of us here in the U.S. It's not just because we see nursing as a calling to be good Samaritans but for the remittances we can send home. My mother made me a nurse, really. I had no choice. She said go for nursing and then you can go to the U.S." When I asked Emmy why her mother wanted her to go to the United States specifically, she stated that her family already had relatives working in the United States as nurses. She then added, "Nursing is your passport out of poverty, and the U.S. is the dream of every Filipino. . . . So, I enrolled in a private school, it was a Catholic School. It was good for me because it combined my Catholic faith and upbringing with my future profession. I wasn't happy with my mother at the time, but she was right. She made me pray on it, and well, here I am. It's kinda of hard to explain. It just felt right, and I still think it's what God wants me to do." Asking her why she thought her mother's advice was good or why she thought things worked out for the best, Emmy explained, "Nursing allowed me to stay a good Catholic and put my faith into practice by giving back to those in need. What more could you ask for? I am living my faith and earning a good living that allows me to help so many people."

Two weeks later, I attended an annual dinner meeting for the Indian Nurses Association (INA, pseudonym)[1] at a local Indian restaurant. Like the monthly FNA meeting, the INA meeting started with a moment of silence led by Joy, an Indian American nurse in her late fifties. As Joy later explained during an interview, "We usually start with a moment of silence so that we can properly dedicate our efforts to God in our own ways and our own prayers." As the meeting progressed, the association's annual accomplishments were outlined in vivid detail. In response to a PowerPoint presentation that highlighted their local community health clinics for Bhutanese and Nepali refugees and their raising money for victims of the earthquake in Nepal, salutations and applause for each project echoed throughout the banquet hall for the next hour. Toward the end of the meeting, Joy announced the names of students who were the recipients of INA's nursing scholarships that year and then reminded members that they could receive a 15 percent discount to attend the College of Nursing and Health Care Professions at Grand Canyon University—a private Christian institution in Phoenix, Arizona, if they were looking to continue their nursing education. Drawing the formal meeting to a close, Joy concluded, "I hope and pray that we can all continue working for the betterment of this country through our profession as nurses. . . . God bless America!"

After everyone had eaten, I asked Joy privately, in a room adjoining the banquet hall, why she thought Indian nurse migration to the United States was on the rise and why so many of them were Christians, specifically Catholics of various rites from the Kerala region. "Well, part of it is historical. Do you know the history of nursing in India?" she questioned. Explaining that I was familiar with some of the history, Joy then stated, "Nursing is our passport out of India, and it's a profession that allows women to earn money and stay true to their faith." This sentiment was shared or expressed similarly by many foreign-born Indian American nurses I interviewed. Kareena, for example, an Indian American nurse in her mid-fifties, like Joy, tried to explain nursing migration patterns from her home country by telling her own story in a subsequent interview:

> As a child I went to a Catholic school run by the nuns, and some way or another I was inspired by them. And then when my father had surgery, I was about fifteen years old, and I remember how the nuns came to us to console us. . . . This left a big impact on me. I wanted to be like them, not just saving people but doing God's work. I told my dad how much I wanted to be like them, but he told me that he did not want to me to become a nun. So, I prayed on it and decided that I could at least become a nurse like Florence Nightingale and join my aunt in America. It was my calling to do this, but it was still women's work—lower class women. You have to remember that women of upper classes looked down on us nurses back then. But it still felt like the right path for me.

When I asked Kareena if Indians' perceptions of nursing had changed since her migration, she stated, "Much has changed since my time. Everyone wants to be a nurse now, even the Hindus and Muslims but it's still kinda looked down on as lower class compared to doctors. One thing that hasn't changed is the fact that Christians still dominate the profession in migration."

Pushed and Pulled

Nurses such as Emmy, Joy, and Kareena have been immigrating to Western countries like the United States for over a century. Searching for opportunity and a better life for themselves and their family,[2] they are pushed and pulled to leave their home countries by a host of complex forces and factors.[3] For some, especially for women, nursing is seen as a passport out of poverty, one that provides financial stability and security for themselves and their family. For others, immigrating to Western countries provides greater opportunities for professional development and better working conditions that they cannot find otherwise by remaining in their own countries.[4] This is particularly true for women in India and the Philippines.

Recent nursing strikes in several Indian states, for example, have drawn greater attention to the poor working conditions and low pay of nurses in the country.[5] Combined with a lack of mobility and opportunity for further training due to restrictive multiyear contracts, these conditions can serve as a powerful motivation for many nurses to leave India. Yet, in other cases, nurses may be pulled to another country by the appeal of better wages and a higher standard of living, despite being happy with their current living or working conditions.[6] The average pay for a registered nurse in Texas, for example, is roughly twenty times greater than that of a nurse in metropolitan Manila in the Philippines, and Texan nurses' salaries are on average below the national average for the United States.[7] Ostensibly, this vast difference in pay makes individual decisions to immigrate rather easy. However, these decisions are often far more complex, based on more than how much money a nurse can make.[8] New economic models remind us that it is not just isolated individuals who are making these decisions but families who collectively weigh in on how taking a job in another country will impact everyone, not just the individual in question.[9]

As we have already seen with the cases of Emmy and Kareena, family plays a major role in these decisions.[10] Whereas Emmy states that her mother forced her into nursing and wanted her to join her family already in the United States, Kareena explains how her father shaped her desire to care for others by steering her away from becoming a nun and how she instead became a nurse like her aunt living in America. In both cases, faith appears to have shaped these decisions within the larger context of family. The majority of the nurses I interviewed, whether they are from India or the Philippines, all described the importance of family in their decisions to go into nursing and eventually immigrate to another country. Many explained how they felt pressured, if not forced, to go into nursing because of the opportunities it provides.[11] Others described how family networks not only financed their nursing education but played an important role in managing which sibling in the family got to go to nursing school, where they eventually immigrated, and how the monetary remittances they send back are spent or allocated among family members.[12] This places an enormous burden on nurses individually to succeed and support their family, but they say they are willing to continually make these sacrifices out of a sense of duty and a lifelong obligation to their family.[13]

Poverty, family, and better opportunities abroad in Western countries all can shape the context in which people choose nursing and then make the difficult decisions to immigrate to another country, but understanding this context does not necessarily explain who they are or where they are from. The overwhelming majority of the foreign-born nurses in the United States are women from Asia.[14] The Philippines is by far the leading country of origin for foreign-born nurses in the United States (29 percent) followed by India at a distant second (7 percent).[15] This is nothing new; in fact, women from these two countries have been the top sources of American nursing migration for decades, but the question remains why.[16] Why women, and why women from these particular countries?

Nursing as Women's Work

For all of the changes nursing has experienced over the last two centuries, it has largely remained feminized labor—women's work. In the United States, as in much of the world, nursing remains dominated by women, with only a small but historically increasing number of men entering the profession. The current ratio of American women nurses to men is roughly ten to one, and this disparity is largely driven by patients' gender preferences and stereotypical views of gender roles that directly lead to discrimination against men or obstacles to men entering nursing schools in the first place.[17] Although this helps to explain why women become nurses—and perhaps why the profession is still seen as feminine—it does not necessarily answer where foreign-born nurses come from or who they are beyond women.

The concept of global care chains, for all its merits in linking structural circumstance to personal dimensions of work migration, has often been criticized for its narrow focus on the feminized migration of domestic workers.[18] By expanding the scope of analysis for global care chains to nurses, scholars such as Nicola Yeates[19] help us understand how nursing chains have lengthened and multilateralized care work over time, while remaining very rooted in migration flows from poorer to richer nations (developing to developed nations). Regardless of push and pull factors, individual and collective decisions to immigrate must also be understood within a broader global context that recognizes the complex interplay of political, economic, and sociocultural forces.[20] By focusing exclusively on push and pull factors, many studies have lost sight of the larger historical and global contexts that situate these decisions.[21] There is a historical reason why India and the Philippines are the largest sources of nursing migration to the Western hemisphere. It is tied to their colonial past and their ongoing postcolonial relations to nations such as the United States[22] that continue to play significant roles in shaping global care chains and the various forms and flows they presently take.[23]

Over the last decade, scholarship has increasingly acknowledged this. However, with a few exceptions,[24] it has largely ignored the fact that religion has also played and continues to play an important role in nursing migration.[25] It is not just all or any women from India and the Philippines who are becoming nurses, as we saw in chapter 1, but devout Christian women, largely Catholics from lower socioeconomic circumstances, whose decisions to become nurses and immigrate to countries such as the United States are reified and then justified and interpreted through religiously oriented cultural frameworks. Understanding this necessitates comparative historical analyses and a deeper understanding of the psychological and sociological forces that motivate people and their daily decisions both at work and in their homes and communities.

Drawing heavily from the scholarship of Barbara Brush, Catherine Ceniza Choy, Sheba George and Sujani Reddy [26] among others, in the coming pages I demonstrate how the impact of Western colonial states and the presence of Protestant medical missionaries in India and the Philippines were not just cultural but also geographic. These forces gave rise to nursing as a women's profession and reoriented women's aspirations outward, internationally, instead of inward toward their own communities.[27] Rather than providing an exhaustive comparative history of nursing in India and the Philippines, something that is well beyond the scope of this study, I outline shared contexts and themes in their histories that help answer why these nations remain the top sources of nursing migration to the United States. Doing so also allows me to contextualize why the majority of these nurses were and continue to be Catholic. I conclude the chapter by defining my theoretical use of cultural frameworks. I specify how consciously held religious beliefs and commitments not only reframe the nursing profession as a calling for these women but motivate and shape their professional and community lives.

Religious Roots of the Empire of Care

The globalization of nursing as a women's profession finds its historical origins in Western imperial expansion and colonialism.[28] Although the sociocultural circumstances and structural paths of how this unfolded over time obviously vary greatly from country to country, especially in India and the Philippines, many of the general contours are the same, at least as they relate to the emergence and ongoing flow of nursing migrants to the United States.[29] Medical missionaries, largely Protestants from the United States, entered colonized territories, either those under American control or the British Crown, and immediately set out to evangelize its people through concerns over public health. Within a few decades, they not only introduced and spread the idea of nursing as a paid profession for women, often in the face of staunch cultural opposition, but paved the way for international organizations such as the Rockefeller Foundation to develop university-based nursing programs and exchange fellowships that initiated a flow of nursing students to the United States. Over time, this ensured that the United States would have a readymade international workforce trained using American standards and willing to immigrate if or when the country faced nursing shortages.[30]

Prior to British colonial rule of India (1757–1947)[31] and American colonial rule of the Philippines (1898–1946), nursing was not seen as a culturally acceptable profession for women in either country.[32] Several factors contributed to this perception. In India, the complex relationships of religion to caste and class presented one of the greatest obstacles to the development of nursing as a women's profession. Specific cultural beliefs about purity and pollution in Hinduism, the dominant religion of the country, led many Indians to stigmatize nursing as a so-called dirty job because it often required working with bodily fluids and excretions.[33] Since nursing also required working outside of the home with men who were not relatives, both as peers and patients, and often hands-on in the latter case, it was seen not only as an unclean profession but as one particularly unfitting for women.[34] Among the Christian and Muslim minority populations of India, this was also the case to some extent, but going to school and working outside of the home were actually of far greater concern than issues of shame and modesty.[35] Whereas midwifery was seen as an honorable duty of Indian women in their own households, a natural extension of their womanhood regardless of their religion, as a paid profession it was almost universally seen as a lower-caste/class job across the country prior to and throughout much of British colonial rule.[36]

In the Philippines, women of all classes actually enjoyed greater mobility and relative equality to men prior to Spanish conquest and influence in the islands. Before the Spanish arrived, which preceded American colonial rule by several hundred years, women could own land, engage in commerce, and hold political power.[37] After almost four hundred years of Spanish colonial rule

(1523–1898), women's statuses were largely pushed back in all public and private spheres.[38] Although lower-class women still played a significant role in retail trade and commerce during this time, particularly in Manila, Spanish influence increasingly limited women to domestic arenas and framed their aspiration as subordinate to that of men.[39] As in India prior to British colonial rule, midwifery in the Philippines prior to American occupation and colonial rule was seen as something women undertook only in order to care for their own families in their own homes.[40] However, Catholicism did not instill the same widespread cultural norms about purity and pollution in Philippine society as Hinduism did in India. In fact, early Spanish attempts to proselytize in the Philippines (in the 1580s) were largely unsuccessful until local chieftains encouraged families, specifically its matriarchs, to seek out priests because they believed baptism could cure illnesses.[41] Becoming Catholic was seen as literally healthy for the family. As a result, the spread of Catholicism in the Philippines was uniquely tied to women and health, but this did not necessarily facilitate the entrance of women into nursing as a degreed profession.

Opportunities to enter higher education were limited for Filipinas in the Spanish university system.[42] Midwifery outside the home was still largely seen as something undertaken by the lower class.[43] Women were lauded as the so-called natural helpers of men, but nursing as a profession, like the circumstances in India, was undesirable and thought to hurt or limit a woman's chances to marry.[44] This changed, to a greater extent, with the arrival of American Protestant medical missionaries and then shifted even further with the eventual acceptance of the Nightingale model of nursing and the spread of its values both in the Philippines and India.

Nursing and Christian Womanhood

Florence Nightingale had a tremendous impact on global nursing, as we saw in chapter 1, but in some ways this impact was even more pronounced in India and the Philippines. As single, Protestant medical-missionary women entered these countries, inspired by Nightingale's example, they sought to reshape and liberate foreign women by training them as nurses and making them so-called proper ladies through the ethos of a noble profession.[45] From the early 1900s through the late 1970s, for example, magazines in Kerala, South India, published short biographies of Florence Nightingale to inspire Malayalee women to take on her life and profession as a model for their own.[46] Seeking to transform the view of nursing as a dirty profession, these missionaries reframed it as an extension of Victorian femininity—pulling it from the private sphere of the family into the public one, much as Nightingale had done in England. However, in doing so, they also further cemented nursing as women's work.[47]

Although this helped to remove some of the stigma surrounding nursing by reframing it as noble and virtuous, it was only successful because it amplified existing cultural understandings of women as natural caregivers.[48] This is not to say that Filipinos and Indians did not resist some or all foreign images of womanhood. In fact, many people accused medical missionaries of putting too much emphasis on the money women could earn as nurses rather than how they might be perceived doing the work.[49] As such, Filipinos and Indians did not passively accept colonial values but had agency and played major roles in the development of nursing in their own countries through their own cultural and religious understandings.

Despite all the press medical missionaries received back in their home countries, they were relatively unsuccessful at proselytizing. This was particularly true of efforts to convert Hindu Indians in the upper and elite castes.[50] Missionaries had greater success among those in the lower castes, but it is important to note that the majority of young Indian women who became nurses during this time were largely already Christian, specifically Syro-Malabar and Syro-Malankara East Syriac rite Catholics from Kerala.[51] According to many historians, Indian Christians were far less bound to Hindu caste-based cultural norms and mores that would have prevented them from working with men outside of the home.[52] However, it is more likely that a complex mix of cultural norms, class statuses, and socioeconomic circumstances explain this better, given that lower-caste women had been working outside the home well before missionaries tried to convince them to do so.[53] Christian women were also available in large numbers in areas where nurses were needed—poor states with higher rates of disease and bad sanitation that often already had a long historical relationship with Christianity.

The Catholic church in India, tracing its origins back to the evangelism of Thomas the Apostle in the first century CE, was well established before Protestant medical missionaries arrived under British colonial rule and played an important role in building hospitals in places such as Goa.[54] Hence, when Protestant missionaries were less successful in proselytizing among Hindus or Muslims, they often turned to existing Christian communities to staff their hospitals and build nursing programs that were rapidly spreading across the country. It was a matter of supply and demand, and subsequently, states like Kerala,[55] which had historically been more successful educating and encouraging women to pursue work for pay outside the home than anywhere else in

India, ended up being major centers for nursing.[56] By the mid-1940s, 90 percent of Indian nurses came from Christian communities, largely in Kerala, and well over 80 percent were trained in mission hospitals and programs established by both Catholic and Protestant missionaries.[57] Since the start of its independence from British colonial rule, Kerala has produced more nurses than any other state in India, and roughly 85 percent of those immigrating to the United States are Christian.[58] Today, despite the fact that only 3 percent of the total Indian population is Christian, an estimated 30 percent of all nurses are from traditional Christian households, largely Catholic ones of Roman/Latin or East Syriac rites.[59]

As in India, the Catholic church was firmly established in the Philippines well before American Protestant missionaries landed during the Spanish-American War. The key difference was that Catholicism was the majority religion of the Philippines and had become an integral, if not inseparable, part of all facets of its culture.[60] Unlike Protestant missionaries evangelizing in India among a Hindu-majority population, in the Philippines Catholic missionaries directed their proselytizing efforts toward converting Christians. Since the Philippines had been Catholic longer than the United States had been a country, it was a daunting task, but, in some ways, they were much more successful than in India. The one advantage that Protestants medical missionaries had was not in matters of faith but essentially in institutional openness and the opportunities for education that they could provide women specifically. However, the Catholic church, seeing these successes unfold as Protestant missionaries flooded the Philippines during American colonial rule, countered Protestant efforts by revamping their existing institutions, opening them to women and sending in the Redemptorists, the Benedictine Sisters, the Congregations of San Jose, and the Missionary Sisters of the Immaculate Heart to create a new image for the church.[61]

Frank Laubach, a well-known Protestant American missionary at the time, noted that the influx of these new, highly trained priests and nuns reinvigorated Catholic universities with young enthusiastic scholars and sparked a Catholic counterreformation that had far-reaching effects, especially for women seeking nursing education.[62] In 1907, for example, St. Paul University Philippines was founded on the island of Luzon by the Sisters of St. Paul of Chartres, who came to Cagayan Valley upon the invitation of Bishop Dennis Dougherty with the explicit mission of recruiting Filipinas.[63] One year later, the same group of Sisters, under the direction of the archbishop of Manila, Jeremiah Harty, established Saint Paul's Hospital School of Nursing in Iloilo City, a little over a mile from the Protestant-run Union Mission Hospital Training School for

Nurses.[64] Wherever Protestants made inroads, the Catholics countered, often with more competitive incentives and with the added benefit of being Catholic institutions seeking to serve Catholics, not convert them. Today, slightly more than 10 percent of Filipinos in the Philippines are Protestant.[65] Although data on the religiosity of nurses leaving the Philippines in migration to the United States is sketchy at best, the overwhelming majority appear to be Catholic, with the second-largest group being Protestant.[66]

Whether in India or the Philippines, Protestant medical missionaries historically were most successful at spreading nursing as a women's profession among those who were already Christian. As such, the greatest impact Protestant medical missionaries ultimately made was not necessarily religious but cultural and geographic. American medical missionaries reoriented women's understandings of womanhood in India and the Philippines and directed them out of their homes into a profession largely shaped by foreign Victorian cultural values.[67] Nursing emerged in both countries as a foreign or Western profession but was still largely seen as lower-class women's work.[68] Hence, most Filipinas and Indian women seeking to advance in their new careers found more opportunities abroad in colonial or former colonial empires than within their own countries. This did not happen by mere coincidence, but in fact, it grew by colonial design—the training and indoctrination of an empire of care, as Catherine Ceniza Choy so astutely defines it.[69]

From the moment the United States began its colonial rule of the Philippines, Protestant medical missionary efforts were already heavily aligned with wider American special interests and institutional aspirations. Over the next several decades, the Rockefeller Foundation, under the direct support of John D. Rockefeller, became the single largest source of capital for the development and spread of medical sciences in the world.[70] Rockefeller not only funded American medical missionary efforts around the world but also played a central role in advising American public health projects both directly in the Philippines and indirectly in India.[71] In 1922, the foundation sponsored a nursing graduate from St. Luke's Hospital School of Nursing in the Philippines to study at Columbia University's Teachers College in New York City.[72] This further laid the foundation for the Exchange Visitor Program (EVP) for nurses after World War II that not only expanded the foundation's efforts in the Philippines but cemented Filipina nursing migration to the United States for decades to come.[73] Several decades later, the same connections were established in India.

In 1952, for example, the Rockefeller Foundation assigned Lillian Johnson to upgrade the Trivandrum School of Nursing in the capital city of the state of Kerala.[74] Seven years later, the foundation funded a four-month American travel

grant for Kumari Lakshmi Devi, the first Indian general secretary of the Trained
Nurses Association of India. When Devi returned to India, the positive reports
of her experience helped the foundation extend the EVP established in the
Philippines to include India.[75] It is under the auspices of the EVP that the first
wave of Indian nurses migrated to the United States.[76]

Today, of the two hundred and seventy-three active nursing recruitment
firms in the United States, 45 percent have recruiters operating in India, and
62 percent have recruiters in the Philippines. This is by far the two largest targets
for nation-based recruitment operations, and these numbers do not include individual hospitals and other private healthcare companies who are also actively
recruiting in these two countries.[77] This is not just a matter of historical interpretation but something nurses still actively recognize and acknowledge today. For
example, Lucinda, a foreign-born Filipina American nurse who immigrated to
the United States in the late 1980s, explained during an interview, "After graduation I worked in the Philippines for about three years, and then I was fortunate,
and I think it was a blessing that I was recruited after less than three years to
come to [the] U.S. and work. God was really looking out for me, not everyone is
this fortunate, but you know it is the dream of all Filipinos to come here." Likewise, Alma, a foreign-born Indian American nurse who in another interview
shared her own path to the United States during the late-1980s, stated, "When
I grew up my neighbors who were coming to the U.S. worked in the medical field.
So as a young kid I wanted to come to the U.S., so I chose the medical profession.
I saw so many wonderful things about the United States. It seemed like the land
of opportunity—especially when going through an American nursing magazine
that we were getting in the [school] library. . . . Everything American seemed
perfect. . . . I truly believe that I was called to care in this country." These sentiments or something similar to them echoed throughout my interviews with
foreign-born nurses.

Calling, Caring, and Cultural Frameworks

> It is true that the usefulness of a calling, and thus its favor in the sight of
> God, is measured primarily in moral terms, and thus in terms of the
> importance of the goods produced in it for the community
> —Max Weber, The Protestant Ethic and the Spirit of Capitalism

Max Weber's provocative historical argument in *The Protestant Ethic and the
Spirit of Capitalism* suggests that early sixteenth- and seventeenth-century Calvinist Puritans not only viewed their secular careers as a religious calling, a
fulfillment of God's purpose for them on earth, but engaged the world through

an ethic that instilled sacred meanings and moral motivations into their understandings of work and community life.[78] At its core, Weber's work asks us to consider how culture provides the normative ends toward which people act.[79] Building on or at least influenced by Immanuel Kant and other early German idealist philosophers, Weber suggests that religiously devout people engage the world with a sacred purpose and a sense of moral duty—a set of deontological ethics that compel them to seek out action that is right or just.[80] However, it is not the consequences of these actions that necessarily make them morally right or wrong but the deeply felt religious motives of the person who carries them out.

Motives matter. They represent an important means by which culture is operationalized in our lives and can often reveal how people think and feel about the relationship between their faith and the daily decisions they make. To fully understand the powerful influence cultural frameworks can have in motivating social action through consciously held beliefs, such as those expressed by the nurses in this chapter, we must make shared cultural values a fundamental part of our scholastic inquiry.[81] At the same time, we must also empathize with individual psychologies and emotions through an analysis of life histories because these very subjective and internal feelings often shape our interactions with the social world.[82] Although these aspirations continue to be the central aims of contemporary cultural theorizing, previous studies have paid little to no attention to how cultural frameworks shape immigrants' understandings of their secular careers or the ways in which faith and moral commitments animate their daily lives both at work and in their communities.[83] None have done so looking comparatively at foreign-born Filipino and Indian American nurses.

Cultural frameworks are schemas of interpretation, knowledge structures that mediate and give form to our daily experiences and decision-making.[84] Their compulsive power lies in the fact that they equally constitute who we are and how we see ourselves and others. They are not only external to us but internal, finding emotional resonance within us. They do not just act on us but through us. They permeate all aspects of society from our socialization into cultural norms to our understandings of self.[85] As such, cultural frameworks are intrinsic to the way we conduct our lives because they give meaning to social life. They shape and bias our memory, pattern our behavior, and provide the deeply felt motives that compel or empower us to act—whether this action is consciously and rationally planned or a more unconscious reaction to social circumstance.[86] Doing what is right, for example, can be motivated as much by a rhetoric of good versus evil or a set of deeply held religious beliefs, as an unexplainable feeling or gut instinct.[87] Thus, whether or not the motives for our social actions are fully conscious or unconscious to us in any given situation or context, they are deeply constrained and enabled by cultural frameworks.[88]

Acknowledging this presents a challenge to theorizing about culture and the motives for social action and behavior. Whereas some theorists might understand the decisions to become a nurse and emigrate to another country for employment as rather rational deliberations—grounded in a cost-and-benefit analysis of what is best economically both for the nurse in question and their larger family[89]—the overwhelming majority of the foreign-born nurses in this study, as we have seen thus far, state that they either could not explain why they became a nurse beyond it just feeling right morally or had little to no say in the decision. Other nurses acknowledged that parental expectation and economics played a major role in their decisions but also suggested that going into nursing and subsequently immigrating was one of the only ways for them to put their faith into practice given the opportunities that were available to women seeking paid labor in their country.

Similar to the Calvinist Puritans Weber describes, the foreign-born nurses in this study, although Catholic and not Protestant (an important distinction), describe nursing as a calling. For them, nursing is not simply a secular job but a career that they say has deep religious meaning and purpose regardless of its economic utility. They did not necessarily choose nursing but rather, as Emmy, Joy, and Kareena state in the opening narratives of this chapter, say that God chose it for them. As we will see, these nurses are moved by the powerful influence of this calling and the cultural frameworks that motivate their care ethic to serve others despite the high cost or professional debates associated with acting on them.[90] We must not forget that a secular work environment like a VA hospital is often wary of the legal ramifications of its employees expressing their religious beliefs. This can impact not only how they see or understand their faith in the context of best nursing practices but the extent to which they engage in spiritual care.[91] Despite institutional constraints or ever-changing policies, many of the nurses I interviewed stated that they pray for or with their patients. They do so because it feels right—a practical sense of how things should be done.[92] These nurses see some level of spiritual care as an equally important part of physical care. From their perspective, the two are inseparable. It is a holistic view of medicine that they suggest makes as much sense to them professionally as it does religiously.

The majority of the nurses I interviewed initially went to the VA after working at other hospitals because the VA, as a government institution, ostensibly offered greater benefits, flexible hours, and numerous opportunities to train or advance in their career. Yet, as future chapters will demonstrate, these are not the reasons why they say they continue to work at the hospital. Many nurses stated that they found that the opportunities they were promised did not exist and that work conditions were in some cases worse than at their previous hospitals. In response to these circumstances, they state that they turn to their faith to guide them through their days and inspire them to fulfill their duties with Christian purpose and joy. When things get truly rough, they also report turning to prayer and then describe how they remind themselves daily that nursing is their God-given calling.

It is important to remember that hospitals in general tend to be high-stress environments with high turnover rates among their nursing staff. However, it is equally important to point out that VA hospitals have the added challenge of serving U.S. military veterans who often have unique physical and psychological needs because of their experiences in war. Complicating matters, being a foreign-born nurse caring for veterans with PTSD or racial and xenophobic biases against people who may or may not look like their enemy in war adds further stressors to their work environment, and might lead most so-called rational people to find another job. Despite the potentially high cost of working at the VA, the nurses in this study do so because they say they feel morally called to serve veterans. It is not just a patriotic duty as they describe it but a moral obligation—a call to act on what is right and live life accordingly.[93] This reminds us that people are not just rational calculators or purveyors of social capital but also moral beings whose deeply held religious beliefs can not only constitute who they are but shape their daily lives and the decisions they make. We might still infer that economics and capital gains are some of the underlying reasons why nurses in this study went into nursing and eventually sought employment at the hospital or that the desire for salvation in due course by seeking out good works ultimately patterns their care for their patients, but this is not exactly how they describe it. It is far more complicated from a more phenomenological perspective.

Had Weber been able to interview the Calvinist Puritans that are the subjects of his historical study of rational capitalism's emergence rather than analyzing the writings of their churches' founding fathers, he most likely would not have found that their calling to a secular career and the subsequent manner in which they attempted to integrate their faith into daily work was done solely to achieve a heavenly reward or obtain signs of the likelihood of that reward. This is simply not how most pious people would consciously respond. In fact, answering in such a way may actually signal to others quite the opposite of achieving that future reward. The same may be said of the nurses in this study.

While some level of rational deliberation plays a part in their decisions, morality and faith ultimately shape their narrative understanding of these decisions.[94] Serving others is thus seen as a moral obligation. Although this is how the nurses in this study often describe their care, we must also recognize that it is not just consciously held beliefs and moral commitments that animate their service to veterans or the ways they see and understand their own career but a host of cultural frameworks, embedded in competing and blended social orders.[95]

Tensions between Church and State?

The Catholic church has long held that healthcare is a human right.[96] Calling on the example of Jesus and his ministry, the church continues to assert that health from a biblical perspective is predicated on wholeness, not just of the physical body but also of the social and spiritual body.[97] This understanding of wholeness has always been a major part of the guiding mission of the Catholic Health Association in the United States from its inception in 1915 to the present—the largest group of nonprofit healthcare providers in the nation today, comprising over six hundred hospitals and one thousand and six hundred long-term care and other health facilities in all fifty states.[98] It has also played a major role in shaping the views and approaches to care of Catholic nurses and either directly or indirectly influenced students of all religious backgrounds (or none) in Catholic nursing programs around the world.[99] The majority of these nurses, as we will see in subsequent chapters, do not deny science or the more biological causes of illness but also see it through the lenses of their spiritual frameworks, which may or may not come into conflict with the norms of the environments in which they work.[100]

The church is well aware that despite a belief that it has historically made significant contributions to society's care of the sick on both a personal and institutional level, its perspectives on religion, spirituality, and healthcare are increasingly at odds with or at the very least being challenged by larger secularizing trends and other forces, particularly in the United States.[101] American Catholic hospital leaders have reacted to these challenges by extending their religious values into national debates over universal healthcare, abortion, and reproductive services, but this, in many cases, has only led to further tensions between the values of the church, the government, and American society.[102] The merger of Catholic and non-Catholic hospitals in recent decades has only heightened these tensions.[103] Whereas fields such as medicine were once closely tied to religion in the public sphere, modern authorities have increasingly debated and then legislated a separation of church and state, while also attempting to respect patients' religious and spiritual beliefs. As we might expect, this separation can and does break down. The values of secular medicine and religion, which are not necessarily mutually exclusive, can come into conflict in certain circumstances, possibly leaving patients and healthcare providers alike in contention or struggling to collectively and individually find the proper place, if any, of religion and spirituality at the point of care.[104]

Every social system and institution is defined and made meaningful by overlapping and competing cultural frameworks.[105] A hospital is no exception. Foreign-born nurses working at a VA hospital, for example, inhabit specific social locations. Despite the fact that the nurses in this study are actively religious with deeply held beliefs and moral commitments, the VA is a secular government institution with strict albeit ever-changing policies regarding religion—as we saw in chapter 1. As licensed professionals, nurses understand these policies or at least try to keep up with the changes but are also aware that medical studies increasingly demonstrate the benefits of incorporating religion and spirituality into their care beyond what they say feels right from their own faith perspectives. As a result, they find themselves caught between what they were taught about religion and spiritual care in another country—both in their churches and nursing schools, under vastly different cultural circumstances and norms, and what American nursing standards and hospital policies mandate. Likewise, they struggle to reconcile their own cultural understandings of what it means to be women and nurses in the United States, both in the VA system and within the broader context of community norms—the potentially competing worldviews of their American-born peers.

In many ways, these nurses find themselves foreign in more ways than just their nativity. As they learn to craft their own place within these countless competing and overlapping social orders, they often strategically appropriate different cultural frameworks depending on the circumstances and contexts, while also consciously and unconsciously following their hearts—doing what they state feels right. Obviously, this can and does lead to conflict, as we will see, especially when these nurses' deeply internalized cultural frameworks lead to understandings or meanings that do not match the institutional or social orders in which they are embedded. How they cope with these tensions and disconnects, as we will see in subsequent chapters, plays an important role in shaping not only how they see themselves as Catholic nurses but their place in the new American story.

Conclusion

The United States is facing an unprecedented healthcare crisis.[106] As healthcare expands to cover more Americans and the country continues to age at an unprecedented rate, the demand for new nurses has dramatically outpaced supply. Thus far, American nursing schools have not been able to meet emerging staffing shortages by producing enough new graduates, often because of forces that are well beyond their control. As a result, the country will likely continue to turn for help in mitigating these perennial shortages where it always has historically—internationally. However, understanding these circumstances, we can see that it is not just any and every country that the United States will likely call on to supplement its nursing needs but specifically India and the Philippines. This is not a random phenomenon or a mere coincidence. There is a clear historical reason why the United States is the top destination for Filipino and Indian nurse migration. It is tied to their nations' colonial pasts and their ongoing postcolonial relations to American geopolitical interests. Acknowledging this, we must point out that it is not just any person that is becoming a nurse and migrating from these countries but largely still women, specifically Catholic women.

Despite the fact that women such as Emmy and Kareena come from different countries with vastly different cultures, even within their own Catholic communities their paths to the United States and the way in which their faith shaped and continues to inform their careers is strikingly similar—at least as they describe it. This should not be all that surprising. The general contours of Emmy and Kareena's paths to nursing and their eventual migration to the United States fits into a larger framework that is typical of the majority nurses from their countries, especially women. Looking at figure 2.1, women from India and the Philippines often come from fairly impoverished circumstances with large families in communities that limit the opportunities for women to gender-specific labor. Inspired by their Catholic upbringing and motivated by a dire need to find a job that can help provide better lives for themselves and their family, they typically say that they went into nursing out of necessity and a belief that they were religiously called to the profession. They often then go on to select nursing programs at top Christian universities where the curriculums, largely based on American standards and texts, also reinforce these beliefs and further reify their understanding of nursing as not only women's work but God's work. In some cases, their programs do not explicitly teach religion as part of the nursing curriculum, but religion is often widely available through other campus resources and groups, and these women typically say they actively sought it out during their training.

When they graduate, often at the top of their classes, they usually have already been recruited by American agencies or specific American hospitals. They generally state that they really did not know what to expect when they

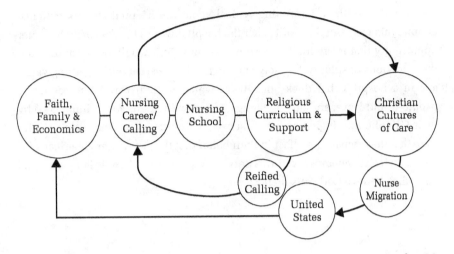

Figure 2.1 Development of Foreign-Born Nursing Care Frameworks. Source: Stephen M. Cherry.

arrived in the United States, but report that they had faith that this was where they should be and that God had a plan for them. After spending time in various public hospitals, becoming American citizens in the process, while also continuing to send money home to their families in India and the Philippines, some of them, like Emmy and Kareena, eventually take jobs at VA hospitals. Those that do, often remain there through the duration of their careers, despite the challenges of being foreign born and serving American veterans.

Through it all, these women suggest that their faith and every aspect of their career from coping with death to their approach to patient care has been and continue to be informed by deeply held religious beliefs. This faith not only reframes the ways they describe their nursing profession as a calling but motivates and shapes the way they see their professional and community lives. This in turn reinforces their cultural understandings and further inspires the next generation of nurses in their home countries. Much like the stories about Florence Nightingale that missionaries used to inspire Filipino and Indian women to go into nursing, stories of challenge, faith, and success from the United States not only are spread among their family back home but are highly editorialized. It is a self-reinforcing cycle, and it is not unique to Emmy and Kareena but a pattern shared by the majority of the foreign-born nurses in this study.

In the next chapter, I further establish the foundation for subsequent analyses in the remainder of the book by demonstrating the unique character of the VA hospital as well as the daunting challenges veterans can present as patients.

As we will see, there is nothing typical about the hospital and its patients. Despite this fact, and the reality that the hospital was not necessarily the better opportunity that many foreign-born nurses thought it would be when they left their previous hospitals, they stay and are making a career out of serving veterans in a hospital that does not always welcome their care. Whereas many people would leave, and do, the foreign-born nurses in this study, influenced by their Catholic upbringing and their subsequent nursing training, emphatically state that they remain steadfast in their belief that they are better Americans for their service to veterans. And this service, regardless of how it is received, is what they believe God calls them to do.

Chapter 3

New American Battlefields

"So, is this your first time at the VA?" Betty, a White nursing administrator and researcher in her late fifties asked me. I respond that it was indeed my first visit to the hospital, and she then suggested, "Well, the VA is not like any other hospital you will ever visit. You're going to find that out very quickly. . . . Thank you for reaching out to us. I really enjoyed speaking with you about your study on the phone. I so want this research to happen because I worry much about my foreign-born nurses." When I asked why Betty was concerned about the foreign-born nurses working at the VA, she stated, "So many of them come from countries where women are second-class citizens. They have no power, no voice. It is a different view of who or what a woman is. . . . It's cultural, religious, and it's something they bring with them that must be unlearned. They are just too passive and in order to be a good nurse you must be assertive. It's like being on a battlefield. Soldiers have to be strong and disciplined and speak up if they are going to win the day."

Although Betty went on to tell the success stories of many of the foreign-born nurses she has mentored over the years, adding that she could not be prouder of them, it was clear throughout our conversation that she was concerned about not only cultural differences but the increasing number of foreign-born nurses at the hospital. "I don't understand why we can't get more nurses born in this country to work at the VA. . . . We shouldn't have to depend on foreign[-born] nurses to take care of those who fought for our freedom. It's really sad. I don't think they [foreign-born nurses] get what it means to serve vets." Betty was clearly frustrated, but she was not alone. Many of the American-born nurses and administrators I spoke with during the early formation of this study

expressed similar sentiments. Susan, a White nurse in her late forties, for example, stated that she thought that most of the foreign-born nurses working at the
VA were there just for the benefits. "They could [not] care less if a patient is a
veteran. It's about money. I don't think it's so much a matter of disrespect as it is
with just not valuing the service they [veterans] have done." She then stated,
"They're just another patient to them, and that's not right. These men are heroes.
They have unique needs. The hospital should not be a place that reminds them
of war but [one] staffed with people who care for them with the peace and understanding they deserve."

When I asked Susan what she meant by this statement, she paused for an
uncomfortably long period of time and then said, "Look, I don't really want to
get into it but some of these doctors and nurses remind our veterans of their
enemies in war. I hate to say it but it's true." Seeing that I was a bit confused,
Susan explained:

> It's post traumatic stress disorder—PTSD. Their accents and behaviors
> remind veterans of those they fought. Not always but too often. Is that
> right, no, but I don't think it's so much about racism as unfamiliarity. The
> country looks a lot different today than when many of them fought. More
> recent vets, well . . . they question the names of doctors and nurses that
> remind them of the Middle East. They are not so quick to trust people
> with names that seem foreign. That's what I mean. Depending on who
> their doctor is or who their nurse is, coming to the VA can trigger the
> trauma they experienced in war. It doesn't mean that they [foreign-born
> nurses] are bad at their job. I actually think they are very competent.

At first, I did not fully understand Susan and Betty's battlefield references or
the difficult challenges they say foreign-born nurse might face in their interactions with veterans. I had certainly not yet observed these challenges firsthand,
but a few weeks after speaking with the two of them, after yet another meeting
to process my WOC (Without Compensation) researcher application at the hospital, I got onto the fifth-floor elevator heading down, and these unique circumstances became much clearer.

Walking onto the elevator, I was greeted by a White Vietnam veteran wearing
a shirt and hat that had the words "Vietnam Veteran" written on them. I casually
said hello, and he replied hello back. As the elevator stopped on the next floor,
another White Vietnam veteran got on. Although I could not be certain that
the veteran served in Vietnam, I assumed by the Vietnam War patches on his
leather vest and the acknowledgment between the two men that this was the
case. As the men began to talk to each other, asking where they served and for

how long, the elevator stopped again, and a Vietnamese doctor, or possibly a nurse, got on. I assumed she was Vietnamese from the traditional Vietnamese surname on her white coat. Regardless of her name, she was Asian in appearance, and as she entered the elevator the veterans who were standing loosely across from each other at the front of the elevator took a dramatic step back and moved to one side of the elevator. Nothing was said, but the men looked at each other, looked at the doctor (or nurse), and then looked at me. Their glares and body language were not friendly, as they crossed their arms and frowned. The doctor (or nurse) did not respond, or perhaps she did not even notice, but simply got off on the next floor.

Alone with each other in the elevator, they looked at me, a White man, and appeared to want to talk or have me acknowledge the situation in some way. Curious about what had just occurred, I asked, "Did ya'll know that doctor?" To which one veteran replied, "No, and I don't want to." "Here, here, brother," the other veteran responded while tipping his Vietnam Veteran hat, drawing more sympathetic attention to his veteran status. When I asked if the doctor (or nurse) had a bad reputation, the other veteran responded, "I don't even know who she is. I'm sure she is very good at what she does, but you just don't get it. You're just a young pup with no clue about the shit we went through. Didn't your dad ever tell you stories about 'Nam?" I was not sure what to say.

As the elevator opened at the bottom floor and we started to get out, one of the veterans grabbed me by the arm and said, "Look, I don't know you from Adam, but someone needs to realize that this hospital has way too many foreigners working in it." Releasing my arm as I pulled away, he continued, "It's hard on us, but I guess you wouldn't understand that . . . sometimes it feels like we lost the fucking war! It's like walking into a battlefield every time I come to the VA. Why are there so many damn foreigners? For God's sake can't we get some Americans working in here? I can't even say the name of half the doctors who supposedly want to help me. . . . I don't trust them. . . . Do you work here? You know people die around here just waiting to see a doctor they can't even understand? Can you fix this or are you just another suit?" I was at a complete loss for words. I explained that I was not a VA employee but had just attended a meeting at the hospital that day, to which he said, "Well, good day to you." And with nothing more to say, we simply parted ways.

VA Nursing Shortages

The Government Accountability Office (GAO) estimates that roughly 9 percent of the VA's registered nurses left in 2014, the year this study began.[1] The GAO estimates that upwards of 20 percent of the VA's current nurses will become eligible for retirement over the next five to ten years, adding to the problem.[2] From 2011 to 2015, 42 percent of all nurses who left the VA retired. Beyond this, and perhaps even more troubling, another 51 percent of those who left the VA during this same time quit or voluntarily transferred to another government agency.[3] Like other hospitals across the United States, the VA is having difficulty recruiting and retaining nurses. Nursing shortages are seemingly universal. However, the VA faces some unique challenges, as Betty alludes to in the opening pages of this chapter. Given the distinctive character of the hospital as a government facility and the often-unique needs of its patients, the VA is also at a distinct disadvantage to address these challenges. This is nothing new but part of a larger historical problem the VA has faced for many decades.

As early as 1936, if not earlier, hospitals across the United States who once found nurses in plentiful supply began to report severe shortages.[4] It was the first of several shortages that persisted through both world wars and lasted until the mid-1960s. When the United States entered World War II, the crisis hit a critical point. Without enough nurses to serve both civilian and military needs, the federal government began to subsidize nursing education, but it was not enough to increase the number of nurses needed to meet the growing demand.[5] In 1943, Congress passed the Bolton Act that created the Cadet Nursing Corps. The act provided over $160 million for nursing education and financial support for over one thousand and six hundred nursing students who joined the corps.[6] Although participants in the program were not required to join the military, federal efforts during this time, in addition to the general call of the war effort itself, drew over seventy-seven thousand nurses to enlist in the military. This severely reduced civilian nursing numbers. Healthcare and hospital officials hoped that when these nurses returned from the war they would enter or return to civilian positions, but they did not.[7] This not only hurt the ability of public hospitals to care for their patients but crippled the revamped VA's ability to open and run the newly commissioned hospitals for returning WWII veterans.[8]

In 1946, President Truman signed the Hospital Survey and Reconstruction Act, also known as the Hill-Burton Act, which provided money to expand state and local hospitals and health facilities.[9] At the same time, employers across the nation increasingly began to offer health insurance as a nontaxable wage benefit—dramatically expanding the number of Americans with health insurance.[10] The combination of these two circumstances created a heavy demand for more nurses. Compounding the problem, enrollment in nursing schools dramatically fell from roughly one hundred and twenty thousand students in 1946 to less than ninety-nine thousand by 1949, as incentives and support for nursing education were no longer federally funded.[11] Nurses worked long hours with low pay, no retirement pensions, and limited opportunities for promotions and advancement.[12] Nursing schools were also expensive. As a result of these cumulative factors, many potential students no longer saw nursing as a good profession, and the shortage continued to worsen through the early 1960s.[13]

In 1964, President Johnson signed the Nurse Training Act to once again provide incentives for nursing education and increase the supply of nurses,[14] but the subsequent boom in nurses seeking employment was less a result of federal incentives than of the rise in nursing wages public hospitals were able to offer after the expansion of the American healthcare system with the passage of Medicare and Medicaid legislation in 1964.[15] This ultimately hurt government hospitals, who found it difficult to compete with the wages and opportunities for advancement that other hospitals were able to offer. One year later, Congress passed the Hart-Celler Act, also known as the 1965 Immigration Act, which dramatically expanded the nation's ability to import nurses under provisions for immigrants with specialized skills in high demand.[16] However, throughout the 1970s, an era of conservatism in federal spending on healthcare began to emerge, starting with Nixon's presidency, that hurt domestic nursing and recruitment.[17] This was especially problematic for the VA. After the passing of the Civil Service Reform Act in 1978,[18] just one year after the Narciso and Perez murder trial involving two foreign-born Filipina nurses working at the VA discussed in chapter 1, all nurses applying for positions at the VA were required to be citizens prior to being employed. This once again crippled the VA's ability to compete with nongovernment hospitals.

By the mid-1980s the supply and demand for nurses was fairly balanced across the United States, surprisingly even at the VA, and for a brief time in the mid- to late 1990s there was actually a surplus of nurses.[19] It did not last long, as yet another series of shortages emerged in the early 2000s.[20] Today, nursing shortages at the VA are not just about a national lack of nurses but continued competition with the private sector. 28 percent of registered nurses who resigned from the VA between 2011 and 2015, for example, stated on exit surveys that they felt like there was no opportunity for advancement at their hospital.[21] Another 21 percent said that they were dissatisfied with the job for various reasons including certain obstacles that prevented them from doing their job using best practices, a lack of administrative support, and troubling leadership in the wake of the 2014 VA scandal.[22] And medical center directors within the VA seem to agree that these factors are indeed impacting their recruitment efforts. An Office of the Inspector General (OIG) report, for example, states that widespread severe nursing shortages are not just a result of a lack of qualified applicants (35 percent) but also noncompetitive salaries (33 percent) and private sector competition (25 percent).[23] Considering the weight of these compounding factors, we can discern that many nurses believe that they can find more satisfying jobs elsewhere and get paid better or, at the least, find better opportunities to advance in their careers in an environment that is more supportive than the VA.

The 2014 scandal only further hampered VA recruitment efforts.[24] In response to the scandal, Congress passed the Veterans Access, Choice, and Accountability Act (VACAA), which appropriated five billion dollars to address mounting concerns in the VA. Among other things, an urgent call to hire more nurses by the end of 2016 was provisioned within the Act.[25] In 2017, Congress passed a modified and amended version of VACAA, titled the VA Choice and Quality Employment Act of 2017. The law requires the Office of the Inspector General to report a minimum of five clinical and five nonclinical VA occupations that have the largest staffing shortages at each medical facility. In 2018, nursing was the second-highest occupation in need.[26] This was a slight improvement from 2014 but still a critical concern. Two years later, the coronavirus (COVID-19) pandemic has only further complicated VA nursing needs.[27]

Broken System?

Despite some evaluations that suggest the VA system provides healthcare that is second to none in the United States,[28] scandal, controversy, and veterans care have gone hand in hand since the founding of the country. From the neglect of disabled Revolutionary War veterans who were promised payment by Congress but largely did not receive anything to hundreds of thousands of American combat veterans from WWII who found themselves with limited access to services after returning home or experienced widespread instances of poor care when they finally did get services, the VA has had a long history of systemic problems.[29] Even after President Carter signed the 1980 Veterans Rehabilitation and Education Amendment, attempting to correct problems with veterans care, and President Reagan subsequently signed legislation elevating the Veterans Administration to cabinet status, creating the Department of Veterans Affairs in 1989, the VA continued to face problems with denied benefits, accounting errors, increased wait times, and numerous cases of ethical violations or substandard care.[30] The 2014 scandal only further highlighted these problems and the abundance of negligence the system has historically wrought when it comes to ensuring the well-being of American veterans. In many ways, the system has repeatedly failed American veterans—shuffling them from place to place, burdening them with bureaucratic red tape and unnecessary hassle, and they are more than angry about it.[31]

Veterans want change. They want a hospital that better serves their needs with honor and respects their service to the United States, while also allowing them to remain together as a community. Part of the solution to the numerous problems the VA system faces, as we have seen, is hiring more nurses. Yet, as the VA largely continues to struggle staffing its hospitals—more so in some regions of the country and states such as Texas, the question remains: Who will continue to care for America's veterans? According to Betty and Susan, foreign-born nurses' presence in the hospital is growing, and the veterans I spoke with in the elevator seem to share this view. However, as we will see, this may be more perception than reality. Although foreign-born nurses may in fact be increasingly employed at the hospital, serving an important role in caring for veterans, it is not clear that they are now a majority. The more important question is not whether foreign-born nurses' presence has grown or the extent to which the Houston VA depends on them, but, given the perceptions and sentiments of veterans or nurses such as Betty and Susan, why would foreign-born nurses seek employment at the hospital when other hospitals seemingly offer better pay and opportunities and in a more welcoming environment? Even more important, why do they stay?

The remainder of this chapter sets out to answer these questions, further setting the foundation for analyses in subsequent chapters. Although the VA does not keep records on the nativity of its employees, including nurses, due to the fact that everyone who works at the hospital must be an American citizen, the chapter will demonstrate that foreign-born nurses from India and the Philippines do serve an important role in caring for American veterans. This, in and of itself, should not be a surprise given what we have learned in previous chapters. What is more remarkable is the reason they say they stay at the VA. White nurses and administrators such as Betty and Susan are at least partially correct in their perceptions and subjective assessments of foreign-born nurses' motivations for working at the hospital, but, as we will see, the foreign-born nurses in this study who left the public and private sectors to find better opportunities and benefits at the VA stated that those opportunities were often hollow or that promises of better benefits were not always what they expected. As the data cited in previous pages reflect, foreign-born nurses are a part of the high nursing turnover rate and crisis the hospital faces.

Those I interviewed who stay and are making a career at the VA, however, are not just foreign born but also largely devout Catholics. This has a tremendous impact on their perceptions of their care and patients. They see their careers as a religious calling and a patriotic duty. By engaging their medical training through the lenses of these cultural frameworks, they state that they are compelled to care for American veterans with a sense of moral obligation and sacred purpose. They navigate the so-called new American battlefields at the hospital, as Susan and Betty describe it, with faith and deeply felt motives—despite the unique challenges that being foreign-born and working with veterans at a secular government hospital can and do present.

Unique Hospital with Distinct Challenges

Ask any nurse at the VA, foreign born or not, and they will tell you that there is nothing typical about the VA hospital and its patients compared to other hospitals where they have worked. "Veterans come in all shapes and kinds. Much depends on their wartime experiences. I see a big, big, big, big, big difference in their needs depending on where they served and when," explains Aami, a foreign-born Indian American nurse who has been working at the VA for over five years. When I ask her if the patients are about the same as those she cared for in other hospitals, she quickly responded, "Absolutely not, they're unique in every way imaginable, and I might add much more difficult or perhaps challenging is the better word."

Echoing this sentiment in another interview, Gabby, a foreign-born Filipina American nurse in her late forties stated, "The patients are really very challenging. They are very, very difficult patients in terms of their disease and all the issues of war they bring with them and not just PTSD [post traumatic stress disorder]. You can't even imagine what we see. God only knows the challenges we [nurses] face daily." Giving his own thoughts, James, another foreign-born Filipino American nurse and U.S. veteran added in another interview, "The veterans can be difficult. I think it's just how the vets are like, trained to begin with, like, in the military way." James then explained that he sees a great deal of turnover among nurses at the VA because they are not prepared to work with veterans. "If they [nurses] are coming from a private hospital and coming here [VA], for them it's a change because at the private hospital it is you that dictates the patients. . . . With the vets, no, you cannot do that. You gotta explain to them. It's kind of like finding the common ground. . . . Now whether or not you are prepared for all the physical and emotional issues they bring is another matter."

The average American veteran is a White (77 percent) man (91 percent), married, ages fifty-five or older (68 percent), and considerably less healthy than your average civilian American—as the nurses in previous pages point out.[32] Veterans have higher rates of coronary heart disease than those who have not served in the military (5.5 percent versus 3.4 percent).[33] They also have higher rates of heart attack (6 percent versus 3.6 percent), higher rates of cancer (11.1 percent versus 9.8 percent), and higher rates of functional impairment (24.9 percent versus 20.9 percent).[34] Additional factors further complicate their overall physical health. Those who served in the military are more likely to get insufficient sleep than nonveterans (43.1 percent versus 35.1 percent), drink alcohol excessively (20.4 percent versus 18.1 percent), and smoke (21.8 percent versus 17.8 percent); all of which can lead to other health problems or a worsening of existing diagnosed conditions, including mental health ones.[35]

Data on the mental health of veterans is complicated by a host of factors or often inaccurate given poor tracking of veterans' health after they retire.[36] However, what we do know suggests that those who served in the military face significant challenges.[37] Roughly 19 percent of veterans have a traumatic brain injury (TBI) compared to less than 1 percent of the civilian population.[38] 7 percent of veterans have both TBI and PTSD.[39] Although PTSD can and does occur in the general civilian population after the experience of any traumatic event, it is one of the greatest challenges facing American veterans. Further complicating the treatment of PTSD is the common co-occurrence of alcohol use disorders, which are more likely to occur among veterans given their tendencies to drink alcohol excessively.[40] Depression is often not considered a combat-related injury, but it is also highly associated with combat exposure and is part of the wide spectrum of post-deployment mental health issues that impact veteran suicide rates,[41] which are significantly higher than the general civilian population, especially among those who served and who are now ages fifty or older.[42] Every day roughly twenty veterans commit suicide, and this rate, while better than it has been at some points in the past, continues to rise.[43]

Collectively, what does this all mean? It suggests that what nurses working at the VA say about their patients is true. American veterans are unique patients who face inimitable physical and mental health challenges. VA hospitals are their primary sources of care. From 2001 to 2014, the number of veterans enrolled in and using VA Healthcare more than doubled (from 20 percent to 42 percent).[44] Some 9.7 million veterans used at least one VA benefit or service in 2016, an increase of roughly 10 percent since 2007.[45] As the number of veterans needing or seeking care increases, this increase obviously places an added burden on the VA to recruit and retain nurses. However, who they are able to recruit, who stays, and how they are perceived can be a point of contention.

Foreign-Born Crutch?

In an odd, widely circulated article titled "Foreign Medical Graduates Are Major Crutch for VA System," posted and reposted on several veteran and healthcare blogs and veteran advocacy group forums, Joan Mazzolini, journalist and chief of communications for the Cleveland city council in Ohio, claims that Veterans hospitals are using the excuse of ongoing staffing shortages to pass over qualified American doctors and hire thousands of part-time foreign doctors through residency programs.[46] Although this practice happens elsewhere, according to Mazzolini, it is more common at the VA because many hospitals are teaching hospitals. As such, the practice of hiring part-time, foreign-born doctors, who may or may not be citizens is not necessarily a matter of preference but need, money, and convenience. Citing sources within the VA, Mazzolini states that hiring foreign doctors "allows (the) VA to hire exceptionally well-qualified physicians who otherwise would not be available to care for veterans."[47] Since these foreign-born doctors are already working at the hospital through residency programs, and American-born doctors with more experience can get more lucrative positions elsewhere, the VA not only uses foreign-born doctors to mitigate its perennial staffing needs but has become increasingly dependent on them.

As the article continues, claiming that upwards of 50 percent of doctors at some VA hospitals are foreign born, the tone becomes increasingly critical of these doctors. Highlighting supposed problems with English proficiency or the need for VA hospitals to use accent-reduction programs because patients cannot understand foreign-born doctors, the article turns from critical analysis to laying blame for VA problems on foreign-born care providers.[48] In response to the article, one blogger, a self-identified veteran in closed comments actually defended his foreign-born doctors, highlighting the fact that we "need them" because of the shortages.[49] Others quickly posted links to other pages so he could "better educate" himself. These other forums were not as positive.

One forum in particular stood out in the ongoing linked dialogue. "Why can't they [VA] hire American doctors," a self-identified veteran commented. He then posted, "Don't get me wrong I am not a racist but they have extreme difficulties with communication and are used to living a different life than we are. Did they put Vietnamese doctors there right after the Vietnam veterans came back from war? Please give me your opinions but no bashing I am just looking to see what other veterans think!"[50] Responding, another self-identified veteran stated, "I think the VA should be giving preference to doctors that are American. If not for the communication, for the stress and other symptoms that can be caused by going to a doctor that you were at war with, lost buddies/family over or at least the same type of people. And if someone takes that the wrong way I don't care unless you were shot at by them too!!!"[51]

Most responses echoed this sentiment, but another veteran posted a partial defense for his foreign-born doctors while also calling on the VA to hire more supposed Americans. "My doctor at the VA is a Filipino with Asian features and a Spanish name. Very knowledgeable and respectful, actually has good doctor manners. My heart doctor is from India, fantastic man, very respectable and knowledgeable and is a winner of some medical citations for inventing techniques. . . . At the VA I go to, Americans park my car and my Filipino doctor does the doctoring. Shouldn't be this way but Americans caused it to be so. . . . I just wish that they'd hire more Americans who served like us."[52]

Agreeing, yet another self-identified veteran stated, "Most American doctors certainly don't want to work at the VA. Too many ridiculous rules, and the past history of the VA abusing doctors and providers has caught up with them. The VA pay is not up to par with the money to be had in private practice. The VA is a good hospital, despite the lack of quality doctors. They have excellent mid-levels and a great nursing staff. Vets can complain all they want, but where else can you get a LIFETIME [his emphasis] free or low-cost health coverage for only 2 years of service."[53] Responses to this comment took a violent turn with many in the forum questioning whether the person was in fact a veteran or a so-called real American. One supposed veteran, for example, stated, "Go jump on a camel and get your ass back over to [the] desert where you belong. Hell I have probable [sic] shot a couple of your cousins."[54] Others quickly commented, "Just hire more fucking veterans, those that served in medical units. . . . They're one of us, they get us, not like some back-ass foreigner here to take jobs away from good Americans."[55]

Clearly, the employment of foreign-born health providers at the VA is a contentious issue for many veterans—just as we saw in the case of the Vietnam veterans I spoke with on the elevator. Although PTSD may further complicate these circumstances and their perceptions, it is important to note that the only nationalities specifically mentioned in the linked blog dialogue above, positively or negatively, were Filipinos and Indians, neither of which have ever been at war with the United States. As such, racism and xenophobia, as we will continue to see, appear to play a role in shaping veterans' perceptions of their caregivers at the VA. Foreign-born doctors and nurses do not simply remind veterans of their former combatants, which may actually be the case in some circumstances, but are seen as foreigners who are supposedly less qualified, backwards, and a national threat—taking jobs away from so-called good Americans.

Despite the fact that the VA system strategically attempts to be an inclusive institution by hiring and promoting diversity,[56] White women remain the most employed demographic in in the VA workforce, as figure 3.1 demonstrates.[57] However, from 2014 to 2015, the first years of this study, the demographic representation of Asian women in the VA workforce did grow slightly. Although this numeric growth is small, the proportion of Asian women working in the

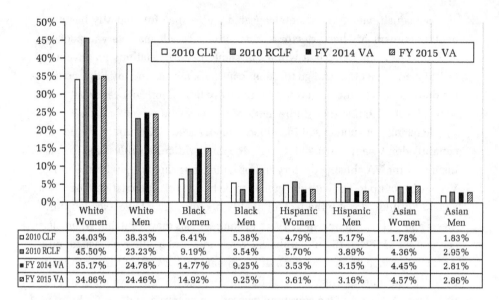

	White Women	White Men	Black Women	Black Men	Hispanic Women	Hispanic Men	Asian Women	Asian Men
2010 CLF	34.03%	38.33%	6.41%	5.38%	4.79%	5.17%	1.78%	1.83%
2010 RCLF	45.50%	23.23%	9.19%	3.54%	5.70%	3.89%	4.36%	2.95%
FY 2014 VA	35.17%	24.78%	14.77%	9.25%	3.53%	3.15%	4.45%	2.81%
FY 2015 VA	34.86%	24.46%	14.92%	9.25%	3.61%	3.16%	4.57%	2.86%

Figure 3.1 VA Workforce Diversity versus Civilian Labor Force Diversity for Select Groups. Source: Veterans Health Administration (VHA) Support Service Center (VSSC) Human Resources (FY 2014 and FY 2015) and U.S. Census Bureau (2010). See Office of Diversity & Inclusion, Human Resources & Administration, U.S. Department of Veterans Affairs, "Diversity & Inclusion Annual Report FY 2015, accessed December 2020: https://www.va.gov/ORMDI/DiversityInclusion/Workforce_Analysis.asp

VA workforce in 2015 is significantly higher than the relative proportion of Asian women in the Civil Labor Force (CLF)[58] in 2010 and is slightly higher than that of the Relevant Civil Labor Force (RCLF) in the same year.[59] The Office of Diversity and Inclusion for the U.S. Department of Veterans Affairs in their 2015 annual report suggested that this higher proportion of Asians, along with a higher proportion of Hispanics, was a positive indication of their work-force diversity efforts.[60] How much veterans could actually perceive this change at their local VA is not clear, but perhaps in comparison to their daily interactions with people and populations outside of the hospital, it was more noticeable—and dramatically so, as the online blog narratives in this chapter might suggest.

Since the VA does not officially track the nativity of its staff, it is difficult to know just how widespread the practice of hiring part-time foreign-born doctors really is at any given hospital. The same is true for other medical staff such as nurses. This is made even more complicated, as noted in chapter 1, by the fact that the Houston VA is a teaching hospital with one of the largest VA residency

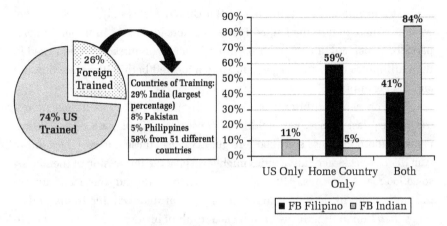

Figure 3.2 Country of Education for Non-Nurse VA Healthcare Professionals (Left) and Country of Education for Foreign-Born VA Nurses (Right). Sources: Analysis of Houston VA Healthcare Provider Portal (2015), left, and Stephen M. Cherry, Foreign-Born Nurse Survey (2015), right.

programs in the country.[61] However, by going onto the health provider portal at any local VA hospital webpage, you can find information on the degrees earned by each full-time physician working at that hospital and from which colleges and universities.[62] Out of nearly eight hundred and fifty full-time physicians posted on the portal at the beginning of this study, roughly 26 percent of those working at the local VA were trained at foreign universities and colleges.[63] Among those trained abroad, 29 percent were trained in India, 8 percent in Pakistan, 5 percent in the Philippines, and 58 percent were trained in some fifty-one other countries. This does not necessarily mean that these doctors are foreign born nor does it give us any indication about the backgrounds of other medical staff, including doctors in residence or nurses. That said, perception is everything, as we will see in coming chapters. When a veteran logs on to their health provider portal to find a doctor, they are presented with a list of so-called foreign names that, regardless of where these doctors' degrees are from or where they were trained, give the added impression, perhaps falsely, that the VA hires more foreign-born doctors than so-called Americans.

Although the VA health provider portal does not post the same information for most nurses or other medical staff, many veterans often look up the credentials and educational backgrounds of their nurses after meeting them during appointments or longer stays at the hospital using the Texas Board of Nursing webpage.[64] Perception, again, is important but not always accurate. As figure 3.2 shows, 11 percent of the foreign-born Indian American nurses in this study, for example, were educated in the United States only, and 84 percent were educated both in the United States and abroad, largely in India. By comparison, 59 percent of foreign-born Filipino American nurses were educated in the Philippines only, and 41 percent were educated both in the United States and the Philippines.[65]

Seen on paper or through the health provider portal, some Indian American nurses' last names, particularly of those from Kerala, are often Biblical names—and hence less so-called foreign. Likewise, these nurses' education in American colleges and universities might also give the impression of their being so-called real Americans. Although the reason that Filipino Americans are significantly more likely to have done all or most of their training in the Philippines than Indian Americans in India is a result of history—as we have seen in the previous chapter—and the fact that there are two hundred and eighteen U.S. credentialed programs in the Philippines that the VA has on its approved list for employment education compared to zero in India. Both populations of nurses are equally as likely to heighten veterans' perceptions that the VA hires more foreign-born medical staff than those born in the United States once they see them or interact with them at the hospital.[66]

Many of the veterans I interviewed, for example, stated that they do in fact look up their care providers online before coming to the VA for an appointment, but they also suggested that it is often hard to know just by names or where they went to college whether they are foreign born or not. John, for example, a White, twenty-eight-year-old veteran who served in Afghanistan, explained, "Seeing is believing and American is American. You don't always know by names who you're going to get [caring for you]. It helps you avoid the obvious foreigner whose names you can't pronounce but not always. But you can also tell immediately when you see them or talk to them." Expressing a similar sentiment, Mike, a Black veteran in his late thirties, who also served in Afghanistan among other places, stated, "You just don't know who is true red, white, and blue, if you know what I mean."

Asking for clarification, Mike then explained, "Look I'm not trying to be racist, I just don't trust people with names I can't pronounce, or sometimes when I see them and I can't tell where they're from or I talk to them and I don't understand them, or they have a real thick accent, it makes me wonder if they're really American, you know. I need to know they love this country not just want to get a job. I want to know they care about me and respect my service. It's a trust issue." When I asked Mike what "one of us" means to him, he stated, "Well I guess it's folks I'm used to being around, but if I had my way I would make the VA hire vets to work at the hospital. They're true to this country, and I trust my fellow soldiers." Mike was not alone in this belief, as we saw in the blog post in previous pages, but the VA does hire veterans and even has special incentives to recruit them to the hospital.[67] However, this does not mean that these veterans were born in the United States. In fact, it is just as likely that they were born in the Philippines or somewhere else, and no one knows that they served, including their fellow veterans.

Many American-born nurses who served in the U.S. military complain about VA hiring practices on local blogs. It is a recurring theme for discussion. One veteran nurse who served in the military, for example, stated, after ranting about how she and her friends were not able to get a job at the Houston VA, "Forgot to mention, the entire RN staff and manager were Filipino. My colleague, who was an air force officer, stated that he began speaking Tagalog during her interview, which she told them was highly inappropriate."[68] The nurse did not mention whether the Filipinos were military veterans or not, but the tone of the blog and its responses seem to indicate that she did not ask.

In 2016, there were approximately five hundred and eleven thousand foreign-born veterans of the U.S. armed forces living in the United States, accounting for roughly 3 percent of the 18.8 million veterans nationwide.[69] Of these foreign-born veterans, the second-largest population was born in the Philippines, roughly 13 percent of all foreign-born serving veterans.[70] By comparison, Indians are the fifth-largest foreign-born veteran population.[71] Currently, one of the fastest ways, if not the fastest way, to become an American citizen is to join the U.S. armed forces through the Military Accessions Vital to the National Interests program (MAVNI), which recruits heavily from certain countries based on linguistic needs and skills to fill critical shortages in areas such as healthcare. Despite this fact, it is not clear that foreign-born veterans once out of the military, who specialize in medicine, like James in this chapter, will continue to work at the VA or find better opportunities elsewhere. The VA is reportedly not an easy place to work, especially if you are foreign born or perceived to be so.

Lure of a Better Job

When you ask nurses at the VA about their own impressions about who works at the hospital, most suggest that there is indeed a large foreign-born presence. Miriam, for example, a foreign-born Indian American nurse who has worked at the hospital for over ten years, stated, "I really don't know the statistics, but there are a lot of foreign nurses and doctors—especially the nurses I work with on the floor. I don't know who has more, you know, who's prevalent—Indian or Filipinos, but there is a lot of them, I mean us." Adding to this perception in a separate interview, Lettie, a foreign-born Filipina American nurse who has worked at the hospital for over twenty years, explained that when she was first hired by the VA in the late 1990s there were not many so-called American nurses working at the hospital. She went on to suggest, however, that "now, there [are] a lot of White nurses, but they are all in administrative. The median nurses and the nurses that really do patient care are mostly foreigners—Filipinos and Indians. There's a lot of foreign-born doctors at the VA right now too. . . . A lot of them [are] Middle Eastern and then from Pakistan and India."

When I asked foreign-born nurses why they originally took jobs at the VA, the reasons were in fact the same as what Betty and Susan suggested in the opening narrative of this chapter—money, benefits, and opportunity. Sarah, for example, a foreign-born Indian American nurse, stated, "Actually at that time I started I was not really thinking about what the VA really was. You know, just a government facility, that's what I thought. It was a good opportunity, good pay, and I was not really aware of a lot of things." Agreeing, Esther, a foreign-born Indian American nurse, who was at Sarah's house when I interviewed her, added, "When I came to the VA, when I wanted [a] 10 percent raise [compared to where I was], they gave half, but it was much better than just pay [because] they have so many other good things like disability, they have a good vacation plan, a lot sick leave, a lot of holiday . . . not to mention all the opportunities for training and advancement."

The lure of a better job with better pay and benefits echoed across my conversations with many Filipino American nurses as well. Maricar, for example, a Filipina American nurse who has worked at the VA for over five years, suggested, "There was a lot of opportunity at the VA, you know, pension and holidays, and I had friends who worked there, other Filipinos. Because when they work at the VA and she recommended me to work over there, [she] said it was better benefits so that's why I ended up at the VA." The average VA nurse nationally makes roughly $79,300 a year compared to $71,730 for all nurses in the United States (VA and non-VA).[72] However, much depends on what grade you enter the VA system at and to what step you have advanced in your career. In Texas, for example, the average VA nurse at grade one across all steps makes $70,642 a year (ranging from the step 1 base salary of $60,637 to the step 12 salary of $80,646) compared to grade five across all steps, which makes $165,347 a year (ranging from the step 1 base salary of $159,894 to the step 12 salary of $170,800)—a significant difference.[73] This likely determines the extent to which your salary is better or worse than the private sector where in Houston, the average nurse makes roughly $70,642 annually—lower than the national average.[74] As Lisa, a foreign-born Filipina American nurse, pointed out in an interview, "I went to the VA for the retirement and benefits. It's a government job, so, you know, it offers more." However, after a brief pause, she emphatically added, "At least that is what I thought."

Lisa's comments highlight an ongoing theme in my conversations with other nurses working at the VA. Many nurses stated that they initially went to the hospital for opportunity and advancement but found that it was not what they expected and, in some cases, not what they were promised. Explaining this, Yvonne, a foreign-born Filipina American nurse, stated with visible signs of irritation, "I thought the VA had better health insurance, better benefits, and all that. But it appeared that it wasn't true. They do have a good list of things that are available but when it comes to quality, it's not as good as what we had at another hospital], you know, the choices of doctors." She then added, "You gotta have a deep faith and thick skin to keep the job or you would go mad and quit. . . . I'm not sure it's worth it. I was just looking for a better job, not saint-hood. I was promised more and it hasn't been produced." Expressing a similar sentiment, Bev, a foreign-born Indian American nurse, commented in another interview, "I think the structure of the VA makes it so difficult to get things done quickly, I don't know. I cannot explain much about it, but I feel doing things are much easier in the private hospital. But otherwise up to two years or three, it was really difficult for me to transition from private to government. It's just kinda backwards in getting things done. I'm pretty sure, thinking back, this is not what I was expecting. I thought it would be better."

Some of those who went to the VA solely for better opportunities or training and advancement often expressed disappointment in the realities of their jobs. Others, particularly those with a military background, stated that they knew better in what to expect from a government facility. Roughly 10 percent of the foreign-born nurses in this study either served in some branch of the U.S. military or are still active reservists in comparison to little over 7 percent of the general public. They came to the VA because of their military service. Stan, for example, a foreign-born Filipino American nurse in his late fifties, stated with a bit of pride in his voice, "I came to the VA because [of] the patient population that kind of like impressed me and mostly the veterans because I served in the [U.S. armed forces]. I enjoyed working with the vets." In other cases, some nurses might not have served in the military themselves but sought employment at the VA to honor a relative in their family that did. Explaining this, Cheri, a foreign-born Filipina American nurse who was about to retire, stated, "My father was in the U.S. Army. He served in WWII. . . . In fact, he was going to be commissioned to go to Washington after the war, but my mother did not want to go so we stayed in the Philippines and that's where I was born. So, well, um, working at the VA is kind of a way to recognize my father and his service."

Being the child of someone who served in the military or growing up around someone in the family who did had a tremendous impact on many of the foreign-born nurses I spoke with, whether their relatives served in the U.S. military or in the military in the countries from which they immigrated. Aliana, for example, a foreign-born Indian American nurse whose father was in the Indian military, explained that she was looking for better opportunities than those available in the private hospital she was working at prior to the VA and was also looking to honor her father, at least subconsciously. "I didn't have much opportunity in the private office, so I kept looking and for me the VA turned out to be a very good spot. . . . I don't know how, but when I came [here] the VA was always in the back of my mind. Unfortunately, my father passed away actually when I was in school. He did not live to see me working at the VA. So, he never saw any of this. . . . He would have been so proud of me and my dedication to veterans." Although nurses' active military service or their family's history might have drawn some of them to the VA more than solely looking for a better job, it does not necessarily mean that they stayed or plan to make a career at the hospital. Like other foreign-born nurses who are not veterans and making a career at the hospital, the reasons they stay make them rather unique.

Why Stay?

The overwhelming majority of the foreign-born nurses I interviewed (87 percent) who have worked at the VA five or more years and stated that they intend to finish their career at the hospital are largely not staying because of money, scheduling, or advancement, contrary to what many veterans or White administrators have suggested. These reasons represent only a small percentage of the overall reasons they give for staying at the hospital. When asked to give only one key reason why they have stayed or plan to stay, 9 percent of foreign-born Filipino American nurses and 11 percent of foreign-born Indian American nurses suggested that "money and advancement" was it (see figure 3.3). Jane, for example, a foreign-born Filipina American nurse who has worked at the VA for five years, stated, "I'm not happy here [at the VA] but I plan to stay because I have children and can work at times that allow me be home when they need me. I care about the veterans but it's hard." Likewise, Eliza, a foreign-born Indian American nurse in her late fifties, simply suggested, "I'm here to collect a government retirement. This place is backwards and racist, but I'm sticking it out to end my career. God knows I don't have long to go."

An additional 2 percent of both foreign-born Filipino and Indian Americans stated that they planned to stay at the VA for so-called other reasons (see

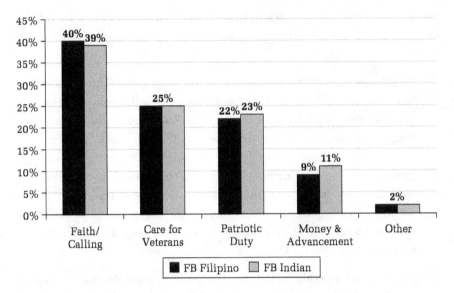

Figure 3.3 Why Stay at the VA Hospital? Foreign-Born Nurses' Top Reasons. Source: Foreign-Born Nurse Interviews (Coded Themes).

figure 3.3). In most cases they did not specify what these other reasons were. Some told me that it involved a desire to stay working with close friends or relatives. Loli, for example, a foreign-born Filipina American nurse, stated, "My girlfriend who works at the VA, she kept bugging me for years. She said go to the VA, it is better benefits, but I guess I wasn't ready then so maybe it took two or three years before I said okay. . . . I just didn't go for the benefits but want[ed] to work with my girlfriend. We are like sisters." In all the cases above, nurses were brutally honest in describing why they intend to stay at the hospital. They were also more than willing to point out problems at the hospital such as issues of organizational inefficiency, xenophobia, and racism or lament the degree to which their expectations in going to the hospital were not always met. However, this is not to say that the VA has not been a good career move for foreign-born nurses. It also does not mean that the hospital fails to recognize them for their achievements.

Maria Mendoza (actual name), for example, a foreign-born staff nurse in the eye clinic from the Philippines, was honored with the Outstanding Service Award for her disaster-relief efforts in helping victims of typhoon Ondoy (Philippines) and the Haiti earthquake victims.[75] Likewise, Lissy Joseph (actual name), a thirty-three-year-old foreign-born nurse from India, was nominated by her fellow nurses for the honor of being a "Top Ten Houston Area Nurse." [76] In both cases, it is not clear that either nurse has stayed at the VA purely for advancement or recognition, but at least in the case of Lissy, the way she describes her upbringing and path into nursing to a local reporter provides a better context for understanding why she has decided to make a career at the hospital:

> Back home in the little village where I grew up, my mother cared for the sick and delivered babies. At the end of someone's life, she would sit and hold their hand. I don't know how she knew how to do all these things, but she was a wonderful lady. . . . When I started learning, I would think of my mom, wondering how she knew how to do all those things, and when I was caring for patients, I incorporated my mother's ways of caring, along with what I learned. Like many new nurses, it was a job at first, but now it is my calling. . . . We care for men and women who have taken care of us without looking for repayment. . . . Now it's my turn to pay them back.[77]

Lissy sees nursing as a calling. She also sees working at the VA as a way to give back or pay back veterans, as she puts it, for their service to this country—and she is not alone in her reasoning. The top three reasons foreign-born nurses in this study gave for staying at the hospital were a care or love for veterans, a sense of patriotic duty, and their faith—specifically a stated belief that they have been called by God to serve veterans.

Looking at figure 3.3, we can see that 25 percent of both foreign-born Filipino American and Indian American nurses stated that they plan to stay at the hospital because they care for the veterans and are concerned that if they leave there will be no one else to care for them. Explaining this concern in greater detail, Carol, a foreign-born Indian American nurse who has worked at the VA for over five years, stated rather emphatically, "I can't leave the VA! Who would care for them [veterans] if I do? Don't get me wrong, they are difficult sometimes but I really love them, like my own family." Expressing a similar concern in another interview, Missy, a foreign-born Filipina American nurse also in her mid-forties, stated, "We [Filipino] nurses have a special place in our hearts for these vets. They can be ornery as hell but we treat them like family. You don't always like your kin but you always love them. I think that is why there [are] so many of us from other countries working here long time. It's cultural, how we were raised, and that's why I worry about who comes in after me. Americans [native-born] don't share this same love and concern. They learn nursing is about machines and numbers and then they forget about the heart aspect." From these nurses' perspectives, American-born nurses are technically proficient but supposedly lack the heart to care for vets the same as they do—a constructed image of their peers as somehow different or lesser. Understanding this perception, regardless of whether measurable differences do indeed exist,[78] foreign-born nurses say they are making a career at the VA not only because of their love for their patients but also from a stated fear that the same care they provide will be lost if they leave. At the same time, many nurses see their care as a way of giving back to their adopted country.

Twenty-two percent of foreign-born Filipino American nurses and twenty-three of foreign-born Indian American nurses stated that they plan to stay at the hospital because it was their patriotic duty (see figure 3.3). When I asked nurses to explain to me what patriotism means to them, the answers largely revolved around serving the country in some way or giving back to those who have served. Gina, for example, a foreign-born Indian American nurse in her midforties, explained, "Serving veterans is a patriotic duty, period. I feel like if you serve in the Veterans Medical Center you are caring for those who gave us freedom. They've done so much for us, so giving back to them I feel like I am serving my country." Echoing this sentiment in another interview, Sarah, a foreign-born Indian American nurse stated, "You know, I don't feel stuck between two countries like some people say about us foreigners. I took my citizenship immediately. I wanted to be an American. So yeah, I am still Indian, but this is my country, and I feel obligated to give back to the country that has done so much for me."

Among the nurses I interviewed who are former or currently active reservist in some branch of the U.S. military, 75 percent suggested that they planned to stay at the VA because it was their patriotic duty. Sally, for example, a foreign-born Indian American nurse in her early fifties, stated, "I was recruited by the U.S. [armed forces], so I joined the reserves. . . . Being in the military I learned so much. . . . I chose to go to the VA hospital because I truly believed that I could do more over there to try to help the veterans, which was my true motive, my reason for going there." Sally feels obligated to stay because of her love for veterans, a patriotic duty, and a belief that her care, like that of Carol and Missy, is special compared to others who might only see working at the VA as a job. Many other nurses I interviewed shared this belief, often making it difficult to understand the difference between the love of veterans and a patriotic duty, from an analytical perspective.

James, for example, stated, while explaining his own path to the hospital, that he was inspired by the work of the U.S. navy that was conducting medical missions in the area where he was completing his nursing degree in the Philippines. "I was so very impressed . . . I wanted to be a part of the medical mission but the other thing also was like, this country had given me so much and my family. The Philippines owes so much to the United States. So eventually I joined the military, and then worked at the VA . . . it's not always about money, it's about me being able to serve back to our country." James then suggested that this same sense of love and patriotism drives his work at the VA: "That's why I love the VA. I love to serve my fellow vets. It's another way of giving back to this great country. When I joined the military I felt like I had become a real American. Serving veterans at the VA makes me feel like a patriot. I have even taken care of WWII vets who served in the liberation of the Philippines."

James was not alone among foreign-born Filipino American nurses who mentioned the American liberation of the Philippines from Japanese occupation during WWII. In fact, this was a theme that distinguished many Filipino American understandings of patriotism from Indian Americans' or at the least provided an additional historical circumstance that they stated further compelled them to want to work at the VA.[79] Eileen, for example, a foreign-born Filipina American nurse in her early fifties who has worked at the hospital for over a decade, stated, "I always consider them [veterans] heroes. They have been involved in bringing us liberation from the Japanese or you know, looking at them, whether they fought in the Philippines or not, they are all the same to me, and I need to take care of them." However, not all foreign-born Filipino nurses feel compelled to work at the VA or make a career out of serving veterans because the United States liberated the Philippines in WWII. As Eileen points out, "I've seen many Filipinos come in and out, and you have new faces and a year later you have new faces again. I could relate this to my experience, but I don't like to generalize [about] all nurses here, but, well I hate to bring in my sister [laughs] but you asked the question." She then explained, "My younger sister came here to work in the VA, and she is also a nurse. So, she didn't last, she was just here for a year." Eileen explained that her sister's experience was different than hers and added, "I think God meant for me to serve these vets."

Interwoven in Eileen's answer, like that of many other foreign-born nurses we have seen in previous pages, Filipino or Indian American, is a belief that God called them to work at the hospital. Whether they give caring for veterans or patriotism as their top reason for staying at the VA, a deep sense of faith underlies or punctuates many of their narrative explanations for why they feel compelled to work with veterans. This should not be all that surprising given what we have learned in previous chapters about their childhood upbringing and not only the role of religion in shaping their decisions to become a nurse but the ways in which they were trained in their nursing programs to see caring for their patients as an act of faith.

Forty percent of foreign-born Filipino American nurses and 39 percent of foreign-born Indian American nurses, the overwhelming majority of both samples, stated that they intend to stay at the VA because they see working at the hospital as a calling—a direct extension of their Catholic faith in action (see figure 3.3). Explaining this belief in greater detail, Mary, a foreign-born Indian American nurse, stated rather frankly, "I came here [VA] for the pay and the benefits but stayed for the veterans. Nothing was what I thought it would be. I was really upset and then I asked God, why did you get me this job?" She then suggested, "The answer was not about pay. I could've gone elsewhere but somehow God spoke to me through these veterans. I saw his grace in their faces and knew then that I need to serve him and this country through this hospital. It was a clear calling."

Many of the foreign-born nurses I interviewed shared similar epiphanies or realizations that led to them wanting to stay at the hospital. Queenie, for example, a foreign-born Filipina American nurse in her late fifties, explained, "When I was back in the Philippines I used to work in the government, and I already had this mentality, an idea that government work is stable and based better. So I kinda already wanted to go to the VA anyway because it's a government job. When I applied I had no idea what I was getting myself into, but I quickly found out." She then added, "Veterans are not like other patients, and the VA was not all I thought it would be but who knew I would like it. I just came for the experience but stayed because I love the veterans. . . . It's like God wanted me here all along and was steering me this way."

Agreeing with Queenie, Dianne, a foreign-born Filipina American nurse who has worked at the VA for ten years and joined our conversation at a local Filipino restaurant, added a bit flippantly, "Look, many people aren't going to understand what [Queenie] said. We live in a secular society, and no one is going to believe that God actually spoke to us or is directing our lives. It's a joke to people but how else can you explain why so many of us have stayed at the VA so long if we could actually find a better job somewhere else?" She then rhetorically questioned how people might understand her decisions: "Are we just lazy immigrants that found a job and stay for the abuse knowing we could make more money elsewhere? Wake up people, we stay because there is a higher purpose calling us to serve this country." Clearly, the foreign-born nurses I interviewed not only believe that nursing is a calling but suggest that they were steered by a higher power to serve veterans. It is a unique understanding of faith and patriotism that redefines our understanding of civil religion from an immigrant perspective.

Conclusion

Foreign-born nurses appear to be an integral, if not vital part of the VA. However, due to data limitation and access, it is difficult to know exactly what percentage of the hospital's nursing staff is currently foreign born or to what extent those numbers may or may not be increasing. Perception here, again, is key. Veterans, nurses, and hospital administrators all suggest that foreign-born Filipino and Indian American nurses' presence is at the very least highly visible, and according to some, growing exponentially in recent years despite the fact that they are also part of high VA nursing-turnover rates. Although the current data does not allow for a generalizable comparison of the foreign-born nurses who are leaving the VA to those that remain and are making careers of serving veterans,[80] it is clear that those who stay may face considerable and unique challenges.

Some veterans and VA staff, as we have seen, lament their presence or raise concerns about their loyalty and ability to care for their patients. This can and does create a perception, even if not widespread, that foreign-born nurses may not be welcome. This undoubtedly complicates their work environment. At the same time, veterans are unique patients—mentally and physically—and the hospital is not exactly what many of foreign-born nurses expected when they left their previous hospitals, and it appears that better pay and opportunities may be found elsewhere. If they acknowledge this, why do they stay? As we have seen, the overwhelming majority of those I interviewed stated that they believe God brought them to the hospital for a reason. Working at the VA, despite its challenges, is described as a spiritual endeavor, one that animates foreign-born nurses' care and bridges the disconnects between how they see themselves and their care versus the ways they believe others see them.

The foreign-born nurses in this study believe that they are an invaluable part of the VA hospital. They feel empowered by the opportunities nursing has given them but also see nursing as a calling—a belief in Catholic faith in action and a patriotic duty. Rather than seeing patriotism as something independent of their faith, they see it as an essential part of being American. It is a unique understanding of patriotism and religion, a deep faith, that goes well beyond the pan-Christian understandings of civil religion that are typically celebrated by the average American at football games or on the Fourth of July.[81] Cognizant of these perceived differences, and even lamenting them, these nurses believe the average American has lost their way somewhere under the weight of modern secularizing trends. They feel compelled, like many other immigrants from the Global South, to evangelize back to the very nation that historically introduced the idea of Christian care and health to their home countries or established the nursing schools from which they graduated.[82] As such, they believe that they are uniquely equipped to care for American veterans compared to their American-born peers, as Missy described earlier in the chapter, regardless of whether their efforts are fully welcomed or recognized.

In the next chapter, I define the dimensions along which healthcare professionals, including the foreign-born nurses in this study, can and do experience racism, xenophobia, and other discriminatory behaviors. Although these problems are larger concerns that have historically impacted American healthcare, an elephant in the room no one wants to talk about, the next chapter demonstrates how it is possibly even more problematic for foreign-born nurses today—especially Asian American nurses working at the VA. It highlights the fact that these experiences are not just isolated microconcerns occurring with an occasional patient but potentially wider structural or institutional problems that can impact everything from perceptions of inequity in pay and advancement to shift preferences and scheduling for foreign-born nurses. As the United States ages and becomes increasingly dependent on foreign care to help mitigate growing needs, the problems outlined in the next chapter, as we will see, have broader implications on American healthcare beyond just a local VA hospital. Likewise, and of central concern to this study, the way in which foreign-born nurses cope with these problems further demonstrates the tensions that can exist between how they were raised and trained as Catholics nurses and the constraints of being new Americans in a secular hospital.

Chapter 4

Understanding and Coping with the Trauma of War

Not long after she got off from her shift, I spoke with Lea, a foreign-born Indian American nurse in her late thirties. Lea, like many foreign-born nurses I interviewed, described how much satisfaction she receives from caring for veterans but was also rather anxious to discuss certain problems she faces at the hospital. "A lot of times, I face major problems. . . . When they [veterans] see you, they don't know where you are from, what your background is. . . . I have a lot of patients who just based on my name alone don't want me to see them." When I asked Lea why she thought this happened, she explained, "It's not just a matter [of] war trauma. PTSD (post traumatic stress disorder) is about nightmares, it affects their work and their life and the depression that they go through with the relived trauma in their daily life. Racism is, I know your name, I know who you are, I don't want to see you." Pausing for a moment, she then added, "Inevitably, they will ask where you are from, what is your religion, what kind of nursing school did you graduate from or even question whether you love this country. Sometimes it is based on PTSD triggers, but usually you can tell by their chart. . . . Other times it's honestly hard to tell what the case is if a diagnosis is not in place in their chart."

Clearly frustrated, Lea suggested that these situations were not just her own experiences but something that happens to many other nurses and doctors, whether they are foreign born or not. "It's not about where you are born but where they think you were born or how you look. We have a doctor from Pakistan and another from India [who] face these issues every day because of their names." When I asked her where she thought these perceptions came from or how they were formed, Lea explained, "Even before they [veterans] come to the hospital they actually looked up their physicians at the Texas Medical Board's website. It tells them where they went to undergrad, what med school, and so on. But when a new patient comes in they have no idea what to make of me, because I'm not online. . . . They question my faith and my patriotism—they say, 'Oh, you must be working at the VA because you cannot get work anywhere else.'" As our conversation continued, Lea added, "It's so frustrating, but what can I do? It's not all of them, you understand. But the few cases, sometimes I don't think they know we are here for them. It's not just a job for me but a calling to serve them. I choose to work here. I could work anywhere and probably get paid much better, but it's not about the money. I wish they knew that."

On being questioned about how she deals with these challenging circumstances, she laughingly joked, "Everyone has their own challenges at work, right?" She then stated, "Look, seriously, it's a tough job. I don't know what I would do without my faith! It kind of grounds me. Every week or at least a couple times of month we come across a diagnosis of cancer or some terminal illness, and I have to tell the patient and their family. You ask how I deal with that work and how do I not bring it home and [let it] keep me down, I mean, prayer and God is the only thing that can ground me and help me through that. . . . My faith is my coping mechanism."

Later that same week, I interviewed Marcie, a foreign-born Filipina American nurse in her early forties, at her home the morning before her night shift at the hospital. Like Lea, Marcie described the joy she feels serving veterans but was also quick to highlight some of the challenges she faces at the hospital. "A Black nurse can tell a Black veteran, 'you cannot walk in.' I can't. I work in the ambulatory clinic, and they walk in when they have an issue. If I think it's not an emergency and you have walked in four times, I can try and tell him to make an appointment and not walk in, but they will get all mad." When I asked her why they get mad, she told me, "They just say they can walk in whenever they feel like it. Then they say I'm not even American. But a Black nurse can tell them they're full of shit and it's okay. So, race matters . . . sorry for cursing. Veterans sometimes want to be cared for by their own, you know. They can be rude about it. At the same time, a Black nurse might hold it against you like you're the one with the problem—like you don't belong there or like you're racist or something."

As we continued to talk, Marcie, like Lea, was clearly frustrated. "I'm sorry. I must seem like I'm really mad and bitter, but to tell you the truth, it just gets old. Sometimes they don't see me as American and other times they prefer me. Most World War II vets are older and there are fewer of them now, but with Filipinos, they like Filipinos better. They like to talk about being in the Philippines during the war or flirt with us. Most of our patients love us [Filipinos]." She then added, "Look sometimes it hurts. Every day is another battlefield and another experience. You just don't know what is going to happen or why. I just wish they knew better that I want to serve them. I choose to be at the VA." Questioned on how she deals with these challenges, she explained, "When I, how do you say it, you know how sometimes you are tempted to say something, but I bite my tongue and pray and ask God to help me to be more patient with this patient. Yeah, to give me more patience, more understanding so I can deal with him better, to not be judgmental. You know, to do God's work and not just get mad or frustrated." Marcie then added,

> This is how I cope with their trauma and everything else that hits me from day to day. I don't know if it is our Catholic upbringing or just being Filipino. We were taught all along to respect old people and be careful what you do to others because it will be done to you. . . . Our parents taught us this. Our professors, the nuns, they all taught us this. . . . I go to Mass every Wednesday before work. I lay my burdens at God's feet and ask him to make me strong for the challenges ahead. Then on Friday I go to Bible study, we pray the Rosary, and [I] learn how to better handle my stress and be a good nurse for my patients. On Sunday I go to Mass again. . . . Well, I think you get my point.

Elephant in the Room

The challenges that Lea and Marcie describe are not unique among their peers. In fact, the majority of the foreign-born nurses I surveyed and interviewed over a four-year period stated or indicated that they have all experienced similar challenges at some point while working at the VA. Although the frequency of these experiences largely depends on where any given nurse works in the hospital, what floor, and the level of contact or duration of time spent with veterans, every foreign-born nurse I spoke with stated that they were frustrated and at times emotionally hurt by some of the interactions with their patients. Whether it is the color of a nurse's skin that provokes a response or their name or even the way they pronounce the English language that leads to a series of intrusive questions, it is clear that a nurse's demographic background can matter to veterans—and not necessarily in a good way.

Veteran patients, American veterans who seek care at a VA hospital, tend to be White (77 percent) men (92 percent) ages sixty-five and older (52 percent compared to 39 percent veterans who are non-VA patients).[1] The United

States has changed demographically since many of them were first enlisted, and dramatically so. In some cases, they may simply be curious about the backgrounds of their care providers. However, the foreign-born nurses in this study believe that these inspections lead directly to discriminatory behavior and outright refusals of care. As they see it, some veterans have already prejudged them or other care providers after looking them up online. In the case of the emergency room visits, they state that these refusals may happen at first sight or contact and at critical moments in a patient's care.[2] Across these scenarios, they suggest that regardless of the circumstances, the presence of family members frequently only further complicates these interactions. Beyond the burden of harassment and discrimination that nurses and doctors may potentially face because of these situations, refusals of care also potentially create a logistical nightmare for VA administrators.

Given the reality that the VA is a unique hospital with unique patients, the challenges that Lea and Marcie describe in the opening pages of this chapter are also somewhat unique as well and are likely intensified by the fact that they are foreign-born nurses serving veterans of foreign wars. Yet, one of American medicine's well-known and open secrets is that patients across the country, veteran or not, routinely refuse or demand care based on an assigned healthcare provider's identity or appearance.[3] Although national statistics on the frequency of these refusals and demands are limited, largely due to healthcare professionals' reluctance to report incidents and the fact that many hospitals are unwilling to openly acknowledge the problem, 47 percent of healthcare professionals in one study stated that they had a patient request a different doctor or ask to be referred to someone other than the person their physician selected in the last five years.[4] Sixty percent of these same healthcare professionals also stated that they had heard an offensive remark about some personal characteristic of theirs (race, ethnicity, gender, national origin, religion, accent, etc.) at some point over the past five years. Of the one thousand and two hundred healthcare professionals of all backgrounds surveyed in the study, African American (70 percent) and Asian doctors (69 percent) were the most likely to report hearing these biased comments from their patients.[5] Without a doubt, race and identity are the proverbial elephant in the hospital room. [6] And the elephant is only getting bigger as the United States continues to become more diverse and healthcare shortages further necessitate drawing in larger numbers of foreign-born healthcare professionals.[7]

Patients often say that the best doctor or nurse is the one who looks like them.[8] Whether this is due to bias or comfort, the fact remains that race and ethnicity matter immensely to patient preferences and opinions about the quality of their care.[9] High-profile studies in medical journals and editorials in major newspapers across the country also note that nationality (nativity), religious preference, and language, specifically accents when speaking English, matter to patients as well—and in some cases equally to race and ethnicity or as a synonymous part of a healthcare professional's perceived identity.[10] As a result, foreign-born healthcare providers like Lea and Marcie state that they sometimes feel unwanted or believe that they are seen as somehow inferior to their American-born counterparts. This obviously can be frustrating, if not hurtful, and makes them feel like they constantly need to prove themselves over and over in the face of these challenging circumstances.[11]

However, research from the Foundation for Advancement of International Medical Education and Research has demonstrated, contrary to what some may believe, that accent or nationality (nativity) does not affect patient outcomes.[12] In fact, when compared directly, patients of foreign-born primary-care physicians actually fared significantly better than the patients of American-born physicians who received their medical degrees either in the United States or abroad.[13] Although comparable studies of foreign-born nurses and patient outcomes are rare, less conclusive, and hampered by poor nurse-to-patient ratios and other structural stressors associated with nursing shortages, hence a higher percentage of foreign-born nurses working in any given hospital, studies suggest that foreign-born nurses are not radically different than their American-born peers in their technical expertise nor do they hold values inconsistent with normal professional practice models.[14]

A patient's refusal of care based on a healthcare professional's identity, background, or appearance can raise a host of problematic ethical, legal, and clinical issues.[15] It can also be excruciating, painful, or emotionally confusing, as we have seen,[16] but it is important to remember that informed consent rules and common-law battery dictate that competent patients have the legal right to refuse medical care from an unwanted doctor or nurse.[17] Despite the fact that accommodation of patients' racial preferences may appear to breach antidiscrimination principles, it not only is consistent with normative commitments to racial equality but has been shown to be an effective means of alleviating race-based health disparities and improving health outcomes.[18] Veterans, for example, with PTSD who refuse treatment from a healthcare professional of the same background as their former combatants—the enemy or those who remind them of those enemies—might seek accommodations or request to have healthcare providers who look like them at their point of care. The sight of those they perceive to be the enemy may trigger past trauma and actually worsen their health.

Acknowledging PTSD issues and concerns, we must point out again that the United States has never been at war with either India or the Philippines. Americans helped to liberate the Philippines from Japanese occupation during WWII, as Marcie points out, and the United States has had fairly strong and stable peaceful relations with India since its independence (in 1947). Yet, Lea, Marcie, and the majority of their fellow Filipino and Indian American colleagues at the VA, say they have been refused by veterans or have experienced some form of discriminatory behavior at some point. Perhaps these foreign-born nurses do in fact physically look like or in some other way remind some veterans of their past combatants. Perception, as we have seen in the previous chapter, is key. However, veterans may also go into the military with their own cultural and regional biases or preconceived ideas about diverse peoples that later inform their views of these nurses when they go to the hospital. This by no means excuses veterans' behaviors and at times apparently racist or xenophobic outbursts, but it does further contextualize them. Regardless of causes, the spectrum and complexity of these situations and circumstances further demonstrate the considerable challenges foreign-born healthcare professionals can face while working with veterans at the VA. This raises several questions. What happens when a veteran's requests cannot be met because there are no medical staff at the point of care on any given shift who look like them? Likewise, what happens when the majority of these point-of-care healthcare professionals, depending on a given shift or unit, are foreign-born? Regardless of these circumstances, and a question of central importance to this study, how do foreign-born healthcare nurses cope with these challenges and the ordinary stress that come with the daily demands of their profession?

The remainder of the chapter wrestles with these questions, acknowledging that the answers are not always easy and depending on any given perspective are not necessarily in agreement with each other. It is an important exploration nonetheless, one that allows us to better understand the complexities of the relationships between veterans and foreign-born care providers. Beyond elucidating the challenges foreign-born nurses describe, this chapter reminds us that the circumstances at the VA are not necessarily unique but a possible microcosm of the broader challenges that American healthcare faces in an ever-diversifying and aging nation. In the coming pages, I further outline these challenges by defining the dimensions along which healthcare professionals say they experience discriminatory behaviors. Next, I present data on the frequency of these experiences among foreign-born nurses before contextualizing them. Moving from veteran interactions to the broader work environment of the VA hospital, the chapter analyzes the challenges foreign-born healthcare nurses say they experience with their American-born peers and administrative superiors. It demonstrates how perceived xenophobia and racism, often centered on physical appearance and language, are not just isolated microconcerns with veterans but a wider structural or institutional problem that foreign-born nurses say impacts everything from inequity in pay and advancement to shift preferences and scheduling. The chapter concludes by unpacking the important ways in which foreign-born nurses say they use their Catholic faith to cope with the challenges of working at the VA—turning the harsh realities they describe working with, the traumas of war, into what they believe is God's work.

Dimensions of Prejudice, Discrimination, and Challenge

There are a number of reasons why patients make the choices they do when it comes to selecting a doctor or making other preferences when it comes to who they want to interact with at any point of care. As we have seen, patients are often most comfortable with healthcare professionals who are of the same race or cultural backgrounds as themselves.[19] This familiarity often leads patients to be more trusting or to feel that their healthcare provider of a similar background will better promote and protect their interests when it comes to treatment or care.[20] At the other end of the spectrum, patients may have had a negative experience with someone of a particular background, which they then generalize to a larger group of people. In the case of veterans, these negative experiences might happen at war or while deployed. Regardless of when or where these experiences occur, they can lead patients to be less trusting of a particular group of people and hence more likely to reject healthcare professionals from that background.[21]

Beyond medical conditions such as PTSD or in congruence to them, when generalizations based on perceived difference become increasingly inflexible attitudes or stereotypes, and lead to negative emotions or feelings of aversion, it is considered a bias or prejudice.[22] This can occur both implicitly or unconsciously and explicitly or consciously.[23] When a bias or prejudice is acted upon—a behavior—it is considered discrimination.[24] Discrimination can take on many forms. Most of what we have seen thus far in the narratives of foreign-born nurses in previous chapters are considered isolated or microscale behaviors. Isolated discrimination occurs when a dominate-group individual, such as a White or Black veteran, intentionally does something harmful to a minority or subordinate-group individual—like rejecting a foreign-born nurse or using harsh derogatory language in a personal exchange with them at the

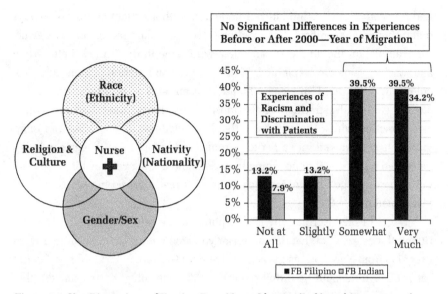

Figure 4.1 Key Dimensions of Foreign-Born Nurse Identity (Left), and Frequency of Racism and Discrimination with Patients (Right). Source: Stephen M. Cherry, Foreign-Born Nurse Survey (2015).

point of care.[25] Since such actions are variable from patient to patient as well as in frequency over time and are not supported or condoned by VA administration, they are not considered small-group discrimination.[26] Likewise, they are not considered direct institutionalized discrimination. However, when a foreign-born healthcare professional at the VA makes less money than an American-born peer or gets passed over for advancement based on where they got their education, despite the VA explicitly upholding Title VII of the 1964 Civil Rights Act and other Equal Employment Opportunity Commission regulations, it might be considered indirect institutionalized discrimination.[27] Regardless of the form, perceived and actual discrimination of any shape in the arena of healthcare can undermine individual people and the entire system of care itself.[28] It can also threaten patient safety or majorly disrupt the broader cooperation and team dynamic required to deliver the most optimal care.[29]

Figure 4.1 (left) highlights the fact that race (ethnicity), gender/sex, and nativity (nationality), among other factors of identity, are not unitary or mutually exclusive entities that can impact foreign-born nurses and other healthcare professionals but reciprocally constructed phenomena with far-reaching effects.[30] Nearly all the foreign-born nurses I interviewed who stated that they had a negative or discriminatory interaction with a patient could not always determine what specifically about themselves provoked the response. Karina, for example, an Indian American nurse who came to the United States when she was five years old, explained, "I think it is a combination of name and skin color, but that's me. [To] some others it's accent and other things. It's hard to say but God it's frustrating." Highlighting a specific incident, Karina recalled an interaction with a White veteran that happened just the week before I interviewed her. "I walked into a patient's room, and before I could even say hello, he barked out at me, 'I'm not going to understand a thing you say bitch. Just get out of here and go find an American nurse.' It really pissed me off, sorry, and just ruined my day."

When I asked Karina how she responded, she said that she simply questioned the veteran, "'What do you mean you aren't going to understand a word I say? I'm from New York, is the accent that hard to figure out?' I told him I could get another nurse, but he didn't request one." Continuing, Karina stated rather emphatically, "I guess that they think I'm a foreigner, but to be honest my mom who came to this country as an adult from Kerala [India] spoke perfectly good English too." Some combination of Karina's skin color and name led to her construction as a foreign woman before she even spoke. Perception mattered. She was judged on sight and without question. However, Karina's experience is not all that unique.

When asking foreign-born nurses whether they had personally experienced any form of racism or discrimination from their patients at the VA in the last year, over 70 percent of them indicated that they had *somewhat* to *very much* experienced these problems, as figure 4.1 (right) reflects. Roughly 40 percent of both foreign-born Filipino and Indian American nurses stated that they *somewhat* experienced these problems. Likewise, roughly 40 percent of foreign-born Filipino American nurses indicated that they experienced these problems *very much* and 34 percent of foreign-born Indian American nurses stated the same, regardless of whether they immigrated to the United States before or after 2000 as newer immigrants. In either case, it does not matter how old a nurse was/is or how long they had been in the country; the frequency of these experiences is the same.

Although the majority of foreign-born nurses I interviewed overwhelmingly stated that they believe that their patients like them, and that they even request them by name, only 13.2 percent of foreign-born Filipino American nurses and 7.9 percent of foreign-born Indian American nurses indicated that they did not experience any form of racism or discrimination with their patients at all in the last year—keep in mind that there may not be a huge difference between *not at all* (zero occurrences), and a one or two occurrences in the last year that would lead nurses to indicate *only slightly* (see figure 4.1 right).[31] Filipino Americans were significantly more likely to state *not at all*, but much of this may be attributed to where nurses work in the hospital. According to some of the nurses I interviewed, Indian Americans appear somewhat more likely to work bedside with veterans than Filipino Americans.[32] As Tess, a foreign-born Filipina American nurse, laughingly pointed out, "I hear horror stories about racism from the vets, but it's not that bad for me in the OR [operating room]. . . . By the time they see me they're either half-asleep or half-awake!" Despite the differences in experience that might exist due to hospital unit location, it is important to acknowledge that the percentage of foreign-born nurses experiencing some form of perceived racism and discrimination can obviously make their work environment challenging regardless of the causes, as Karina laments in previous pages.

Many of the foreign-born nurses I interviewed were reluctant to say whether they thought their patients were at times racist or xenophobic or whether there was a purely medical explanation for their behaviors such as PTSD. It is clearly complicated, and for a host of reasons it was not something nurses truly felt comfortable talking about. Highlighting this, Georgina, a foreign-born Indian American retired nurse who worked at the VA for over twenty years, explained, "It's just so hard to tell what's going on, and to be honest, I really don't want [to] say much about it. We all know it happens. . . . I don't want to say that it's racism that makes patients say or do these things but maybe the whole atmosphere of this country just makes their problems worse. I don't know how to say it. Maybe it's PTSD and being foreign is the trigger, but that trigger seems like it's getting cocked by the president [Trump] and the media well before they even get to the hospital. Does that make any sense?" Pausing for a moment, she then added, "If I had to pick an answer if it was racism or PTSD or some other mental [health] issue, I think I would go with all of the above!" Clarifying or perhaps qualifying her statement, Georgina questioned, "Maybe I am wrong but were we [Indians] ever the enemy or are we just foreigners? I feel for them [veterans], I really do, even pray for them, but it can be very frustrating. Let me be clear, it's not all of them. Just every once in a while, but those few cases added up across a career. I tell you, if it weren't for my faith, I am not sure I could have made it through some days. I just reminded myself that it's God's work, and I was doing something good by staying there [at the VA]."

Peers, Supervisors, and Contentious Working Conditions

Although there may be questions as to whether a veteran's negative outburst or discriminatory behavior is PTSD or xenophobia or racism or possibly all of the above as Georgina explained, there is no doubt in the minds of the majority of the foreign-born nurses I interviewed that their American-born peers and administrators treat them in discriminatory ways that are far too often clearly related, by their accounts, to xenophobia and racism. Fifty-eight percent of foreign-born Filipino American nurses and 63 percent of foreign-born Indian American nurses stated in interviews that they experienced some form of discriminatory behavior in the past year with their colleges or superiors.[33] This is obviously a clear majority in both cases and is significantly higher than what previous national studies have found. Researchers at George Washington University School of Public Health and Health Services, for example, found that roughly 40 percent of foreign-born nurses working at hospitals (non-VA) across the country stated that their wages, benefits, and shift assignments are worse than their American-born colleagues.[34] Looking at each of these domains independently, we see that 27 percent of foreign-born nurses in the study indicated that they did not receive comparable pay to their American-born peers, 16 percent said that they believed that they were not getting the same benefits, and 18 percent suggested that they received less desirable shifts.[35]

When I asked foreign-born nurses about their working relationships with their peers and supervisors/administrators, the majority of them stated that it depended on the group that a particular person was socially or racially/ethnically a member of, not necessarily the individual. Explaining this, Beth, a foreign-born Indian American nurse in her early forties, pointed out, "Most of us are kinda of cliquish. We tend to spend breaks with people from our same hometown. It's natural, I think, to want to be with them, you know what I mean? Some groups stick together, but we can still be friends and other groups just don't mix well at all. It's not about the person but like their group mentality and culture." When I asked Beth to explain this further or give me an example of her interactions with non-Indians, she quickly asserted, "We [Indians] don't get along with the Nigerians very well. They're so pushy, hard to talk to. . . . Maybe it's just my feeling, but I stay away from them if I can. I will say that we [Indians] get along with Filipinos. I have several friends that are Filipino, including my best friend. She's Catholic, like me. We go to church every morning together before work and then we see each other and our families every weekend at Mass. . . . Sometimes we do the Rosary together on breaks or lunch. That's what I mean, we share something meaningful."

Expressing a similar sentiment in another interview, Meena, a foreign-born Indian American nurse in her late forties, remarked, "There is something about Filipinos that makes them darn easy to get along with. . . . Sometimes there's tensions but I think it's a power thing. We are both the top dogs at the hospital. Those Nigerians, that's different. We cannot get along very much. Somehow, we don't have the comfort feeling that we can openly talk to them. They're kinda rough." When I asked Indian American nurses about the large number of Indian doctors working at the VA, they were quick to point out tensions. Beth, for example, emphatically stated, "We don't get along, and it's not just the doctors. I would rather have a Filipino supervisor than an Indian." Questioned why she felt this way, Beth gave me a quick lesson on caste and medicine in India today. "I thought you would know this. It's not just history. Doctors come from [the] upper caste, and nurses are looked down on as lower caste and unclean. It's been like this since the British arrived. They should know better and the ones who were educated here or have been in the United States longer are much better. Still, sometimes it comes down to us being Christian and them being Hindu. Caste is still around, even though it's illegal."

Conversely, when I spoke with foreign-born Filipino Americans about their work relations, they did not share the same sentiments as their Indian American peers about working with doctors or supervisors of their own background. Rose, for example, a foreign-born Filipino American nurse in her early forties, stated, "It's great when the doctor or manager is Filipino. We joke and there's no problem." The majority of the foreign-born Filipino American nurses I spoke with agreed with Rose. However, like Beth, Rose and others did point out the tendency of Filipino Americans to be drawn to their own group as well as some of the problems she has had with non-Filipinos because of these circumstances. [36] "We Filipinos stick together. I think it causes problems with others, but it's natural to want to be with people from your own country." She then added, without prompting, "We [Filipinos] don't always get along with Nigerians but I think it is a communication style or maybe a language issue. . . . They're so blunt. There are a lot of Indians at the hospital too, but for the most part we [Filipinos] get along with them. Sometimes I think there is some mistrust . . . a little tension." When I asked Rose why she thought this was the case, she hesitated for a minute and then said, "Filipinos are kinda of preferred by the doctors, so I think it's a little bit of competition and then there's language issues. I think it's fine to speak your own language with your peers, but maybe sometimes people think you are talking about them. But that's on them. I don't worry about that."

The VA is clearly a highly racialized environment. This is true not only in the working relations between foreign-born and American-born staff but among foreign-born nurses as well. Both Filipino and Indian American nurses, for example, appear to be at odds in some cases with foreign-born Nigerian nurses, as Beth and Rose, among others, pointed out. Some of it has to do with cultural differences. In other cases, it is racial—specifically skin color or a matter of language and communication. Regardless of the cause, it is a point of contention that these nurses say further complicates their work relations.

Pointing this out, Lani, a foreign-born Filipina American who has worked at the VA for five years, explained that she does not like to speak her native language in front of others because she thinks it causes problems. "It's okay when you're at lunch and there are only Filipinos, but if someone else is around you shouldn't do it or at least try to translate for them so no hard feelings come about. It's rude otherwise." However, not everyone I interviewed agreed. Rose, for example, emphatically stated, "It's not that big of a deal [speaking our language], and none of us would ever do it in front of a patient." Although Rose and Lani somewhat disagreed, the overwhelming majority of foreign-born nurses (roughly 95 percent of foreign-born Filipino American nurses and 84 percent of foreign-born Indian American nurses) whom I surveyed indicated that they do in fact speak their native languages on breaks or at lunch. How much of this contributes to other problems in their work environment is not clear.

As with veteran interactions, perhaps speaking a non-English language cues a sense of foreignness and hence leads to discrimination. Hinting at this possibility, Dee, a foreign-born Filipina American nurse in her early fifties, stated, "One of our Black colleagues complained just last month about us speaking Tagalog. . . . [I] remember [that] doctor] asked me if I spoke English the first day in the OR. I just wanted to slap his face, but I just said 'yes' and then he wanted to know if I could say anything other than yes. Maybe us speaking Tagalog together makes people think we are too foreign and not as capable. It's a terribly racist assumption, but maybe that's part of it."[37]

Whether it is language or a matter of racial politics and dominant group positioning, foreign-born nurses at the VA routinely complained in our interviews that they earn less than White peers, work more demanding or unpopular shifts than their American-born peers, regardless of race/ethnicity, and are passed over for promotions by Black managers and supervisors. Explaining this, Jasmin, a foreign-born Filipina American nurse in her late forties, stated, "People can be prejudice[d]. Like me and my Chinese coworker [have] to do like a double load work than my White friend or my Black coworker. Because when the workload comes, when they complain, they say no, no, don't complain, don't complain. But when a White person complains they immediately let her do whatever and we get stuck doing it . . . and I know she [White nurse] makes more than us for doing less or what's easier."

Later that week I spoke with some of Jasmin's Indian American colleagues. As we picked up on the same conversation topic, Ida, a foreign-born Indian American nurse in her early fifties, stated, "I'm not so sure it's a matter of not liking us [foreigners] but like a community nepotism. At least I'd like to think that. Maybe it's just flat out racism." Echoing this sentiment in another interview, Rebecca, the foreign-born Indian American nurse in her early forties that we met in chapter 1, stated, "I've had a problem with some managers. . . . They were Black, and when they see each other it's all fun and talk, but then they stop talking when I get around them. I try to ignore it. I wouldn't care if I didn't think it hurt my chances at a promotion. It's flat-out discrimination. They're racist. That's all."

Adding her own thoughts on the subject in a separate interview, Zoe, a foreign-born Filipina American nurse who has worked at the VA for about ten years, pointed out, "When I graduated from the leadership institute our mentor tried to find me a position in management. I got an interview, but I think it was a courtesy for my mentor. I didn't get it, and a White person from my class did. I fully understand wanting to leave [the VA]. This place discriminates against foreigners even though we're all citizens. Makes me sick. We're just as American as them! I am lead on a shift unit now but that causes its own problems." Asked to explain what she meant, she added, "You verbally complain and at first nothing is getting done so if you write it up, you turn out to be the bad guy because you wrote up this person, and so everybody turns against you because you wrote up somebody. It becomes a race war, even though you just wrote up what they did wrong out of safety for the patient or procedure."

Although I neither was able to observe any of the challenging exchanges or circumstances that foreign-born nurses described nor had access to shift schedules or their pay by unit in comparison to their American-born peers, the VA nationally has been subject to a host of allegations and lawsuits over the years that have accused the hospital of unfair treatment or inequity in pay and advancement for its racial and ethnic minority employees.[38] Perception appears to be a reality. Ironically, the majority of these cases have been raised by Black employees—the very same group of people that foreign-born nurses in this study suggest they have a hard time getting along with or believe are unfairly getting advancements over them.[39] They seem to have more in common with their Black peers than not when it comes to these grievances, but the highly racialized environment in the hospital appears to be engendered by a sense of group position versus individual motives and actions.[40] Because individuals are subject to group influence, especially the group's own sense of its relative position as dominant or subordinate, foreign-born nurses appear to see themselves as more deserving of leadership or at least believe that they should be better represented.[41] However, racial biases also appear to run both ways, further complicating these working relationships and the ways groups and individuals on either side perceive them.

When I asked foreign-born nurses how the VA tries to manage their complaints, many said that they did not say anything about it to their administrative supervisors. Most pointed out that there is policy and procedure but were not so sure how effective they were. Liezel, for example, a foreign-born Filipina American nurse in her early forties, explained, "Superficially, yes, it's effective. We have a process to make complaints, and it does work when it's so blatant that they can't ignore, but I think most of the problems are subtler and get easily lost or hard to prosecute. Then again the color of management seems like a no-brainer so I don't know." She then added, "We also have diversity training, but I think it goes in one ear and out the other for most people who need it."

Disagreeing with this sentiment in another interview, Alicia, a foreign-born Indian American nurse in her late forties, stated, "At least we have a system in place to train and address grievances. We [VA] are a magnet hospital so we are required to do cultural sensitivity, cultural competence, etcetera . . . and there are tons of online courses and resources. I think the VA tries to do a good job of stopping discrimination. The VA is very strong about that, very careful. I think it helps tremendously." Alicia was in the minority of those I interviewed. Most acknowledged that the VA has a robust legal process and diversity trainings but also added that it did not solve the inequality in pay, shifts, or promotions that many of them described.[42] This is important especially since the Houston VA is a teaching hospital that trains students from college programs in nineteen states, including Texas. How this local VA manages the racial/ethnic and nativity tensions among and between staff and their patients has far-reaching impacts not only on those employed at the VA but on those they train who go on to work at other hospitals across the country.

Regardless of the degree to which cases of discrimination and inequality are a perception versus a widespread systemic reality, these circumstances are potentially problematic on a host of levels. If we acknowledge this, it is surprising, to say the least, that the foreign-born nurses in this study are staying at the hospital. However, as we saw in chapter 3, it is their faith, a deep Catholic

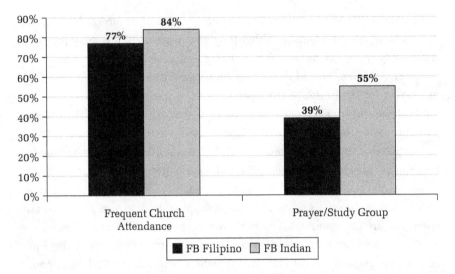

Figure 4.2 Religiosity of Foreign-Born Nurses. Source: Stephen M. Cherry, Foreign-Born Nurse Survey (2015).

devotion, that reifies their work as a religious calling and begs them to endure much. It is not legal systems or trainings that get them through the challenges they describe, whether it is with patients, coworkers, or supervisors, but their steadfast Catholic devotion and dedicated religious practice.

God Give Me Strength

It should not come as a surprise that the overwhelming majority of the foreign-born Filipino and Indian American nurses in this study say they turn to their Catholic faith for support in the face of challenge. The conversations and narratives presented in previous chapters, as well as the words of Karina, Lea, and Marcie in this chapter, for example, all point to a belief that God has not only called them to be nurses but is there for them in times of need. They are deeply religious and actively practicing or engaging their faith traditions.

As Figure 4.2 suggests, 77 percent of foreign-born Filipino Americans and 84 percent of foreign-born Indian Americans surveyed attend Mass frequently, once a week or more, not including weddings and funerals. In both cases, this is roughly twice the frequency of average American Catholics (39 percent of whom attend Mass once a week or more).[43] However, the nurses in this study are not just frequently attending Mass but participating in their churches well beyond regular Mass. Beth, earlier in this chapter stated that she goes to her church every day before going to the hospital. Additionally, 39 percent of foreign-born Filipino American nurses and 55 percent of foreign-born Indian American nurses also indicated that they are members of a weekly prayer or Bible study group that either meets at their parish church or in someone's home in the community. Beyond deepening their understanding of their own faith or praying for the health of their patients, the nurses I interviewed also told me that they use these group times as an opportunity for reflection, divine guidance, and strength to cope with the daily challenges they face at work.

Explaining this, Anju, a foreign-born Indian American nurse in her late forties, stated that she is a member of a Bible study group from her church that meets several times a week. "We encourage each other. We are mostly nurses, and it kind of boosts us up to keep the morale and when you are down and when you are disappointed. The Bible works that way. Like, if you are feeling a failure, so in spite of prejudice or the discrimination you face, the Bible shows that there is discrimination everywhere, even in the Old Testament." She then pointed out, "In spite of the challenges we face at work or in life, if you believe in God, you have the strength to keep moving. I could not do my job daily without drawing on this wisdom." Expressing a similar sentiment in another interview, Bina, a foreign-born Indian American nurse also in her late forties, reflected, "I'm a firm believer in prayer and study. I go to the same Malayan church . . . every Sunday and try to go to the Bible study often, but I also go to a local American Catholic church [Roman/Latin rite] every day before work. I need that time with God before I go to the VA. I pray for my patients, and I take my frustrations and concerns from work to him [God] personally, you know. It's how I deal with the stress at work. Sometimes when things are really bad, I take my concerns to confession and ask my priest for guidance in dealing with my patients."

Later that same week I spoke with Li, a foreign-born Filipina American nurse in her mid-thirties. Like Anju and Bina, Li described the importance of doing something religious before every shift at the hospital. "Every time I go to the hospital, I stop at the chapel and pray for my patients and my coworkers." Laughing, she explained, "I think I have more of a hard time with my coworkers than the patients. So, I pray for them too, and then I ask God to give me the strength to turn the cheek and ignore their racist discrimination against people like me." Like Bina, Anna, a foreign-born Filipina American nurse in her late thirties, added in another interview that she always seeks out opportunities to pray over work concerns. "I prefer to stop at the church in the mornings, but I also have a little prayer space in my office; it's right under my computer. It's a little picture of praying hands with a cross. Whenever I find myself in a difficult situation with a patient or my coworkers, I just take a few seconds and pray for guidance and strength. It's part of my daily thing. It's good to seek a higher power on these things, you know. God listens."

A month later, I spoke with Elsie, a foreign-born Indian American nurse who expressed a similar sentiment to the nurses in previous pages. "Our job is so stressful. Meditation on God's word and prayer help me regain my strength every day. . . . My faith is my compass to navigate life. It centers me." This is an important point that resonated across my conversations with foreign-born nurses, regardless of how old they were or what country they were from. Catholicism appears to provide a set of cultural frameworks that orients foreign-born nurses' lives by providing meaning and contextualizing the challenges they face at work. It also compels them to seek a higher power in everything they do, and in doing so they say they find resolve where others might simply leave the VA altogether.

Highlighting this, Gayla a foreign-born Filipina American nurse in her late fifties, stated, "I believe that everything happens for a reason. God has a plan." She then added, "I was called to this job even though I was not sure what I wanted to do with my life. When God closes one door, he opens a window, you know what I mean?" Asked for clarification, she added, "If a patient is acting up, I just think God is testing my resolve. If a patient dies, I know God is taking them home. Medicine can only do so much. Sometimes people who seem like they have the best chances of recovery are the very ones that end up dying with no explanation. . . . It's just their time. . . . There is always a divine reason for everything, even suffering and death. That's what I believe."

This belief in a higher purpose or divine plan apparently not only helps nurses understand death or contextualize it but seems to give them practical tools and frameworks that they can use to deal with challenging patients at the point of care or coworkers in the heat of an exchange. Emphasizing this, Irene, a foreign-born Filipina American nurse in her early forties, stated, "Nursing is so stressful. The stress can come from your patients, your coworkers, the surgeon you are with, the setting, the equipment . . . I think you get the point." Continuing, she rhetorically questioned, "You know that hormones affect your mood or stress, right? Well, you can't let it get to you. If you do, it impacts your care. Everyone says they pray, but you have to have some technique. I take a few breaths and say, 'Lord, I don't have time for this stress.' I feel his presence work its way through my body—from my head to my toes, calming me, lowering my heart rate and then the stress and everything else just melts away. That usually does the trick."[44]

Describing a similar technique, Raca, a foreign-born Indian American nurse in her late fifties, stated, "Knowing the golden rule and doing it are different things. Sometimes you're very tempted to say something to a patient who's being rude, but I grab my cross [hanging from her rosary around her neck] and count down the beads from ten backwards really quickly while I say to God, 'Please help me bite my tongue.' Then I exhale deeply. It works. I feel him steady me and I calm down. It gives me just a moment of patience enough to be more understanding and not judgmental." The techniques Irene and Raca describe, regardless of their religious framing, involve all the hallmarks of traditional stress therapy—from relaxing the body from head to toe, to counting and breathing.[45] Likewise, seeking guidance from a priest during confession as Bina described is akin to many other forms of professional counseling. However, in the context of these nurses' ardent Catholic faith, they say these techniques take on added meaning as they reify their calling to nurse and galvanize their mission to care for veterans.

Conclusion

For decades, studies have continually demonstrated that nursing is a highly stressful and emotionally demanding profession.[46] From the daily rigor of engaging complicated technical knowledge and skill in urgent situations and the added responsibility of high-stakes mistakes to the drama of competing with coworkers for limited opportunities for advancement to the frustrations of navigating institutional bureaucracy, these challenges highlight why nurses are exceptionally susceptible to burnout.[47] This is particularly true at the VA.[48] Understanding this, we should not be surprised that burnout and a general public acknowledgment that nursing is indeed a difficult profession play a vital role in American nursing shortages regardless of the type of hospital. It is not just a matter of the nation aging and thus increasing the need for more nurses that is causing the problem but the difficulty of the job and the ability of nursing programs to not only recruit but graduate enough new nurses. As a result, foreign-born nurses are likely to continue to be called on to help mitigate these perennial shortages.

Being a foreign-born nurse in the United States is not easy, as we have seen. Previous studies have clearly demonstrated that foreign-born nurses are not only more likely to report unfair treatment from their supervisors and administrators than their American-born peers but severely impacted in the long-term by this discrimination both professionally and personally.[49] Whether they are made to feel somehow lesser than their American-born peers—stereotyped as un-American, marginalized, or even passed over for promotions and advancement—foreign-born nurses in these studies consistently report feeling helpless in the face of discrimination.[50] Despite the fact that much of this discrimination does not present itself as overt institutional racism, these studies also demonstrate that more subtle forms of exclusion and racial and xenophobic hostility are pervasive and widespread enough to have a tremendous impact on foreign-born nurses' confidence and self-esteem in and of themselves, regardless of whether they are getting paid equitably or receiving promotions comparable to their American-born peers.[51]

Combined, these factors lead to increased occupational stress, which can impair performance and effectiveness, reduce productivity and job satisfaction, impact nurses' general health, increase their absenteeism and turnover, and in some cases lead to substance abuse or other destructive behaviors, including higher rates of attempted suicide.[52] All of these previous studies were conducted in public or private hospitals. At this point in this chapter, it should be obvious that nursing is stressful enough without the added challenges of being foreign born and making a career out of serving American veterans. The VA, again, is not your typical hospital, and veterans are not your typical patients.

The foreign-born nurses in this study, as we have seen, routinely complain that they earn less than their White peers, work more difficult schedules than their American-born peers, regardless of race or ethnicity, and are passed over for promotions by their Black supervisors. Despite the fact that the hospital has robust systems for reporting grievances and frequent mandatory diversity trainings, the overwhelming majority of the foreign-born nurses I interviewed stated that it is not enough to stop the harassment and discrimination they believe they face. Yet, they stay—not for the pay or opportunity, which appear to be better elsewhere, but because of their faith and an ardent belief that they are called by God to serve veterans no matter how difficult a challenge that may be.

To be clear, not all veteran interactions are problematic, as Marcie and Lea, among others, point out, but these challenging circumstances happen often enough. Even one case, as we have seen, can have a deep impact. How do they cope under such difficult circumstances? Faith and their daily religious practice. This should come as no surprise. Studies have long demonstrated that various aspect of religious practice, such as frequent church attendance and prayer, are not only strongly related to overall physical and mental well-being but especially beneficial for coping with daily stressors and specific adversities.[53] After the terrorist attacks on September 11, 2001, for example, one study in the *New England Journal of Medicine* found that 90 percent of Americans turned to religion through increased church attendance as a means to cope with their stress.[54] They also reported Americans buying more Bibles and increasing their reading of religious literature/scripture.[55] When it comes to nursing, numerous studies likewise suggest that among the top coping strategies that nurses utilize when dealing with patients, especially those who are terminally ill, is religious practice.[56] In fact, one longitudinal study of nearly fifty thousand nurses found that women who attended religious service more than once per week had a significantly lower risk of becoming depressed.[57] The foreign-born nurses in this study would agree. Going to church and praying before work is healthy.

Religion has long provided people with orienting beliefs that can contextualize suffering and provide a higher purpose in loss. As such, religion frequently serves as an individual's core schema, a set of cultural frameworks that inform beliefs about the self, the world, the universe, and our place in it. These frameworks can give form to our daily experiences and provide meaning to life's challenges.[58] Through meditation, prayer, Bible study, and spiritual reflection, for example, nurses can find various ways to cope with stress and grief.[59] Whether it is seeing something positive in a stressful situation or finding meaning in another circumstance, faith can shelter and protect nurses emotionally by adding purpose to their work. Faith can also facilitate other coping mechanisms, as we have seen, such as breathing or other therapeutic techniques.[60]

When Anju points out that she cannot deal with the challenges of her job without prayer or drawing on the wisdom of her Bible studies, she is not alone. The overwhelming majority of the foreign-born nurses in this study would agree. They believe that nursing is their calling. They see it as their God-given purpose in life, and this belief impacts everything they say they do. Clearly the nurses in this study reap tremendous benefits from their faith. It serves as a vital coping mechanism for the daily challenges they face. However, in some cases, such as Gayla's, their belief that the difficulties they face happen for a reason or are a test from God may actually lead them to underreport discrimination. When coupled with the frustrations they express with the VA system and a belief that reporting claims to administrative superiors may actually make things worse, far too many foreign-born nurses may be religiously enduring challenges, self-sacrificing, and relying on their faith when they should be reporting these incidents more frequently.

Regardless of these more social-justice concerns, religion is more than just a coping strategy or resource for foreign-born Filipino and Indian American nurses' challenges or concerns. It is, as we will see, the foundation of their care for patients. Analyzing this further, the next chapter demonstrates that the foreign-born nurses in this study see their Catholic faith and medicine as largely inseparable. This is not only how they were raised but also how they were trained as nurses. It is a holistic view of medicine, one that makes as much sense to these nurses professionally as it does religiously through the lenses of their own cultural understandings. However, as we will see, their perspectives on spiritual care can and do lead to conflict with the secular environment in which they work. How they navigate these tensions and disconnects plays an important role in shaping not only how they see themselves as Catholic nurses but their place in American healthcare.

Chapter 5

Faith and the Practice of Care

Two days after attending a seminar sponsored by the Filipino Nurses Association (FNA) on engaging best practices in nursing, I met with Cheryl, a foreign-born Filipina American nurse in her mid-fifties who attended the workshop. After Cheryl described her experiences working with veterans—both the challenges and rewards—I asked her what she thought was the single most important influence on her approach to working with her patients. "It's obviously my professional training and the experience I got in hospitals in the Philippines. If you don't know what you are doing, it's really hard to do the job right. That's why people love Filipino nurses. We know as much as the doctors, and we've seen it all a thousand times before we even immigrate." Pausing for a brief moment, she then questioned, "But you do know there is more to nursing than just medicine, right?"

Asked what she meant, Cheryl described how her faith was an important part of how she sees herself as a nurse and the way she approaches care for her patients. "I was born Catholic and we grew up Catholic, but I went to a Baptist school and I studied nursing and I studied the Bible also. . . . Religion is an important part of how I see my profession. Faith shapes how we were taught to see the body. . . . Medicine is not all. We must understand that we are physical *and* [her emphasis] spiritual, created in God's image. Nursing must grasp this holistically." She then added, "Religion and health are kinda hot right now. Everyone is starting to write about it in the big journals, but God has been telling us this all along. At least some of us were listening." Cheryl made it clear that she believes that her faith in no way diminishes her technical skills but enhances them. "I think my faith makes me a better nurse, not less or somehow backwards because I believe in God."

As we continued to talk, Cheryl stated that she sees a real disconnect between spirituality and the nursing profession today, despite its relative increase as a topic of research. She then described how she sees herself versus her American-born peers. "We [Filipinos] are more patient-oriented. The new nurses, like the Americans [native-born] that just graduated here lately are more computer oriented, and their training is more tech oriented. It's not direct patient care. They are missing that spiritual link." Clarifying this statement, Cheryl suggested, "New nurses don't ever leave their computers. I don't think they even touch their patients. . . . We learned to use the equipment too, but we never forgot that the patient is a physical *and* [her emphasis] spiritual being. That's why the vets love us. They know we care and pray for them as God would want."

A few weeks after I interviewed Cheryl, I spoke with Aly, a foreign-born Indian American nurse in her early fifties, at her home after a brief planning meeting of the Indian Nurses Association (INA). The group met that day to discuss the association's next continuing-education program. Like Cheryl, Aly was eager to share what she thought made her a good nurse. "We really are different from American [native-born] nurses. We grew up respecting faith and its importance to people in need." Expressing a bit of frustration with VA policies, Aly explained that the hospital has a chapel for contemplation and prayer but feels that it is disconnected from patient care. "It's [chapel] not where you go to help your patients or even your own faith. At any given time, if you take care of your patients, it will do more for God than going to chapel. So that's how I take it. Like Sunday, I'm obliged to go to church, but if someone else asks to take a shift, I do. . . . Being in church does not make you a Christian and it certain[ly] doesn't make you a better nurse." When I asked Aly to explain what she meant by this, she stated rather emphatically, "Faith is about works. I was called to be a nurse and to be a good nurse I must put my faith into action. I always tell God, okay, this is my thing, and this is why I'm not going to church, not to pretend I am faithful but [to] ask for guidance in the times I am actually using my faith to do his work. I work Sundays, and I feel closer to God at the hospital than at church."

Coming back to my original question, I asked Aly how she thought her approach to nursing was different than her peers, and she suggested that American-born nurses do not engage their patients spiritually. She then added that she thought that this was not due to a lack of faith but a lack of training. "Many of them are people of faith, but I don't think they get taught how to engage their faith like we did. They have beliefs but either don't know what to do with them or are afraid. . . . My patients get the best care anyone can give because it's not about the job but being a servant of care." Looking for further clarification, I asked Aly what being a servant of care meant in practice. "I always think a patient who comes to me, I will take him as a Jesus Christ. . . . I don't have to wait for Jesus Christ one day to come back. If I see a patient who is filthy, I see that's Jesus Christ. He's in front of me. I need to clean, I need to give him the best care. Each patient is a Jesus Christ to me, so that's how I take care of my patients. This is that verse from Matthew [25: 31–36]." She then added, "When you see your patients like this, they're everything to you and not just some job for pay."

Both Cheryl and Aly grew up in devout Catholic households and attended nursing programs at Christian colleges. Although Cheryl attended a Baptist university, like Aly who went to a Catholic university, she was able to find social and institutional spaces on her college campus that not only allowed her to practice her Catholic faith but engage it in new ways. As a result, both nurses, from distinctly different cultures, stated that they grew more confident in their belief that nursing was their calling throughout these years. Drawing on biblical scripture and contemplative prayer as examples, their professors, many of whom were devoutly religious themselves, if not formally clergy,[1] taught Cheryl and Aly how to further apply their Catholic faith as an instrument of care in conjunction with the more technical aspects of their training. Faith matters to these women, both personally and professionally. And they are not alone. The majority of the foreign-born nurses I interviewed stated that faith and spirituality are an integral part of their nursing care. They see themselves as different than their American-born peers. However, much of this perception is not necessarily a matter of faith, of being more religious than their American-born peers, as we have seen, but of how they were trained in another country versus the larger ongoing debates in American healthcare today over the place of religion and spiritual care, if any, in secular hospitals. As such, many foreign-born nurses may have more in common with their American-born peers than they actively perceive.

Educating the Caring Faithful

The tremendous growth of nursing migration from India and the Philippines to Western countries over the last several decades has led to a proliferation of private and for-profit nursing schools in both countries. Many of these schools continue to be run by religious institutions or provide religious instruction despite the fact that the governments in both countries increasingly regulate nursing as one of its chief exports.[2] Not too much appears to have changed since Cheryl and Aly immigrated. In the Philippines, for example, a national moratorium on opening new nursing schools[3] and a vow by the state to further crack down on underperforming schools have not diminished the role of religion in nursing schools. On the contrary, the Philippine Nursing Act of 1991 defined the scope of nursing as following four core values: (1) love of God, (2) caring as the core of nursing, (3) love of the people, and (4) love of the country—in this order.[4] Although subsequent nursing acts (in 2002 and 2015) do not explicitly define "love of God" as a core value, many of the nursing schools founded by Protestant missionaries and Catholic orders nearly a century ago remain among the most prestigious programs in the country today and hold this value as a core part of their training.

Across the four years of this study (2014–2018), four of the top six nursing programs in the Philippines, averaging fifty or more nursing students and with 100 percent or near 100 percent passing rates on the National Nursing board exam every year, are religious institutions—Silliman University (100 percent passing rate), Xavier University (100 percent), Saint Paul University–Iloilo (100 percent), and University of Santo Tomas (99.5 percent).[5] The other two programs are state institutions—West Visayas University–La Paz (100 percent passing rate) and Cebu Normal University (100 percent). It is important to note that both of these schools were founded around 1902 during American occupation and run by Thomasites, teachers who came to the Philippines on the *USS Thomas*, hence the name. In most cases these teachers were from Catholic and Protestant missionary backgrounds or devoutly religious themselves.[6] Regardless of who historically founded these universities and programs or who ran them, religion remains an ever-present part of their stated directives.

Today, Silliman University's mission statement for the College of Nursing, for example, suggests that, beyond following the aims of the revised Bachelor of Science in Nursing (BSN) curriculum that all state schools uphold, it seeks to facilitate the highest quality Christian education. "Nursing education is a holistic discipline that facilitates a person's acquisition of attitudes, knowledge, and skills towards professional nursing practice and a Christian quality of life."[7] Likewise, the mission and vision statements of Xavier University, Saint Paul University–Iloilo, and University of Santo Tomas all commit to upholding the values of Catholic nursing with an explicit emphasis on "servant leadership," the relationship between "people and God," and the goal of "strengthening one's purpose and meaning in life" through "the proclamation of the Gospel" and the integration of "faith, reason and science."[8] These values are not just hallmarks posted on a wall or website but an integral part of the core curriculum and a vital part of how these programs approach working with nursing students. It is the very foundation of their education.

Nursing students at Saint Paul University–Iloilo, for example, take the following pledge at graduation: "I solemnly pledge myself before God and in the presence of this assembly, to pass my life in purity and to practice my profession faithfully . . . and will hold in confidence all personal matters committed to my keeping and all family affairs coming to my knowledge in the practice of my calling. . . . With loyalty will I endeavor to work closely with the health team and devote myself to the welfare of those committed to my care."[9] Beyond possibly reaffirming their faith at graduation, each student is also often given a special blessing or gift before they take their nursing exams. As Minnie, a foreign-born Filipina American in her early forties who graduated from Saint Paul, explained, "When we went to Manila to take the board exams we were given a statue of the infant Jesus of Prague [by the school], and all of us carried that with us, and as soon as we sat down we were told to put that down on the front of our desks . . . so all of us from St. Paul's have that infant Jesus of Prague statue blessing us, and we all passed the boards, 100 percent! Our education, you see, is directed by the Lord's teachings and then blessed by the presence of his Holy Son." What Minnie describes is not all that unusual but rather similar to the experiences of many other foreign-born Filipino American nurses I interviewed.

By comparison, nursing is not as tightly regulated by the state in India as it is in the Philippines, nor are school performance and standards publicly posted in India, but much of this has to do with size. The number of nursing schools across the Philippines has increased roughly 175 percent since 2000, with well over four hundred and eighty-one nursing schools currently in operation.[10] Comparatively, nursing programs in India remain largely regional and concentrated in the states where nursing historically developed nearly a century ago. The state of Kerala, for example, which has been actively studying the Philippine model since 1991 as a means to inform its own policies and management strategies, has had a 187 percent increase in the number of private and government nursing colleges operating in its region.[11] However, the increase in the number of students, predominately women, seeking out nursing programs has grown so much that Kerala cannot keep up with demand, forcing many to now travel to the larger state of Karnataka to the north.

Roughly 66 percent of the nursing schools in Karnataka, which now has the largest number of nursing programs in India, were established in the last five to ten years and by some estimates upwards of 24 percent of nursing students in Karnataka are Christian despite the fact that Christians make up less than 2 percent of the overall population.[12] As in the Philippines, religious institutions remain an important part of nursing education in India, particularly in southern states such as Karnataka and Kerala. An estimated 30 percent of all nursing-degree programs in India today are run by Christian institutions, with over 30 percent of the nursing graduates being Christians from Kerala.[13] This should not be all that surprising, given the history discussed in chapter 2 nor should it shock anyone that many schools remain open about their religious affiliations and missions despite being Christian, minorities in a Hindu majority country. The Holy Cross School of Nursing and Lourdes College of Nursing, for example, both of which have historical ties to the Holy Cross nuns from Menzingen, Switzerland, who arrived in Kerala in 1906 and established four government hospitals in the state, are among the top nursing programs in the country.[14] As their mission statements reflect, both programs focus on quality nursing education from a Christian perspective with an emphasis on "holistic quality care" and a "dependence on God's healing power."[15]

Since 1977, the number of privately owned nursing schools in India, the majority of which are owned and operated by religious and charitable organizations, has grown 2,100 percent, and the number of official Christian church–run schools has increased roughly 200 percent, a stark contrast to the only three new secular government schools opened during this time.[16] Although nationally representative data does not exist, keeping in mind that the Indian government has not historically kept detailed records on nursing programs, we can conclude that Christian institutions dominate Indian nursing or at least are a high-enough percentage of the operating programs in the nation that non-Christians often complain that it is difficult for them to register or gain admission due to preferences for Christian candidates.[17] Many of the nurses in these programs, as was/is the case for those in the Philippines, started their clinical training or residencies with patients in hospital settings that were not adverse to spiritual care or in programs that did not mandate a complete separation of church and state. However, when they immigrated to the United States, many of them, both Filipinos and Indians, found the separation of church and state in American secular hospitals a challenge to how they were trained.

The remainder of the chapter explores the ways in which foreign-born nurses deal with these disconnects and tensions. It demonstrates how they see spiritual care as distinct from physical care but integral nonetheless to a more holistic understanding of well-being. Before looking at the specific ways in which foreign-born nurses say they wrestle with these issues at the point of care, I engage some of the current debates in religion and health and demonstrate how foreign-born nurses are not alone in these challenges. Despite the fact that research increasingly points to the benefits of spiritual care, American healthcare is often at odds with itself not only on how to define and teach spiritual care to healthcare professionals but also on the extent to which it should be engaged, if at all, at the point of care. What nurses do for their patients is multidimensional, rather complex, and essential. This includes evaluating how and when spiritual care is appropriate.[18] Acknowledging this, we must also recognize that the issues and concerns surrounding spiritual care can impact all nurses regardless of where they were born or trained.[19]

Debating Religion, Spirituality, and Health

Both publicly and privately, there is a debate in American healthcare today among professionals and researchers alike about the appropriate place of religion and spirituality in patient care.[20] Much of this debate, and the contention that follows, focuses on whether we know enough about the link(s) between religion/spirituality and health outcomes to institute policy changes. Questions also persist about the degree to which we can trust the scientific evidence that exists or the extent to which it truly validates the sense that religion and spirituality actually have beneficial effects on health and morbidity.[21] Despite some high-profile counterarguments and reservations,[22] every year, as Cheryl points out at the beginning of the chapter, the number of national conferences and peer-reviewed journal articles on religion and spirituality and health increases—more than doubling in the last thirty years.[23] What these works find overwhelmingly suggests that religion, religious involvement, and spirituality can have a positive effect(s) on patients' physical and mental health and well-being.[24]

The preponderance of this evidence has renewed interest in spiritual care and has increasingly led to a call for its integration into approaches to patient care. American nursing scholars have responded to these calls, with some even suggesting that spiritual care should be the cornerstone of holistic nursing practice.[25] Patients want it, and many nurses are personally interested in or at the least open to engaging in it. Nearly 90 percent of patients in one study, for example, scored themselves five or higher, *moderately* to a *large extent*, when asked to indicate how much they depend on religion to cope with illness.[26] Over 40 percent of people in the same study indicated that religion was the most important factor that kept them going when confronting their illness (ten on the scale).[27] However, despite the fact that nurses are largely aware of this research and the needs/demands of their patients—and believe that spirituality can produce emotional and physical benefits, ranging from inner peace to bodily healing[28]—many studies suggest that they are reluctant to engage in spiritual care. Much of this is due to their perceptions of their roles as professional nurses or their limited knowledge and training on how and when to engage in these practices.[29]

Contrary to the perceptions of Cheryl and Aly at the beginning of the chapter, American nursing programs do teach holistic nursing and other dimensions of religion and spiritual care. A review of one hundred and thirty-two randomly selected baccalaureate nursing programs across the United States, for example, found that the overwhelming majority included spiritual dimensions within the program's philosophy (71.4 percent) and curriculum (96.9 percent).[30] Like American medical programs more generally,[31] these nursing programs have religion and spirituality content in required courses that are not specifically about spirituality and health or have required courses dedicated to these topics. But it is important to note that much of the exposure to spirituality and healthcare topics in these programs/schools occurs during the first two years when students typically have less direct contact with patients. This potentially limits their opportunities to gain firsthand experience exploring these issues at actual points of care and implementing them in real-world situations.[32]

Across nursing textbooks, another study found that while spirituality content was largely addressed, it was either in general nursing texts for courses taken during the early years of the nursing curriculums or covered in advanced texts that students would only read if they took certain electives.[33] There was also a virtual lack of any spirituality content within broad nursing specialty texts.[34] Although curricular differences between public and private (including religious) nursing institutions/programs have led to a great deal of variation in the ways spiritual care is taught in the United States, nursing examinations and nursing accrediting agencies all expect nursing students to have a rudimentary understanding of its central concepts.[35] It is not clear, however, if this is uniformly happening across all programs. Part of the problem is actually defining spirituality and spiritual care in a way that provides a succinct and concise direction for implementation.[36] Faculty may also feel uncomfortable teaching these topics.[37] Thus, in the absence of these definitions or a concerted effort to uniformly train people accordingly, some nurses may feel ill prepared to engage in spiritual care. Likewise, and perhaps more importantly, they may struggle with the legal implication of doing so in the context of their own understanding of patients' rights and the separation of church and state.[38] This is again a potential dilemma many nurses working in the United States may face regardless of where they were born or trained.

Whether a nurse engages in spiritual care or not may have nothing to do with their own level of religiosity or spirituality. An apparent absence of engaging in spiritual care may also say nothing about the degree to which a nurse sees religion and spirituality as an integral part of what they do or their approach to care, as Aly points out at the beginning of the chapter. Roughly 70 percent of the foreign-born nurses in this study indicated that their professional training was the single most important influence on their approach to working with veterans. Seventeen percent indicated that religion was the single most important influence, followed by 9 percent who stated that their culture was the most important influence on their approach to working with patients. It should come as no surprise that these three areas emerged as the top influences. Although we might anticipate based on the narratives in previous chapters that the percentage of those who state that they were influenced by religion might be higher, many of the nurses that I interviewed explained that their answers to the survey question were too limiting to take at face value.

Karen, for example, a foreign-born Filipina American in her late forties, explained, "If you don't know how intubate a patient in an emergency or understand when and how to use a defibrillator, they might die no matter how hard you pray. God doesn't just save people when others could do it, he expects me to be a professional and do my job. When there is nothing else that can be done medically, then it is in his [God] hands. So, yes, my professional training matters the most, but like I told you before, my faith complements this training. Healing happens body, mind, and spirit." Echoing this sentiment in another interview, Bridgita, a foreign-born Indian American nurse in her late forties, stated, "Just because I said that my professional training was the single most important influence on my nursing care doesn't mean that religion isn't important too. Of course it is, but we are professionals, and we were called to learn how to heal, and when medicine needs an extra boost or fails, that's when spirituality matters. I must depend on my training to do my job correctly, but that doesn't mean I don't ask God to guide my hand. This is how we were trained—trust your knowledge, be strong and confident in your medical skills, and let God do the rest."

Looking at figure 5.1 (left side), we can see that 11 percent of foreign-born Filipino American nurses indicated that religion was the single most important influence on their approach to working with patients compared to 24 percent, more than double the Filipino percent, of foreign-born Indian Americans. Among both populations, those who had the highest rates of Mass (service) attendance in their parish churches were significantly more likely to list religion as the single most important influence on their care. Given that foreign-born Indian American nurses in this study report higher rates of Mass or church attendance (84 percent) compared to Filipinos (77 percent) (see chapter 4), we might see their higher attendance framing their responses to this question in

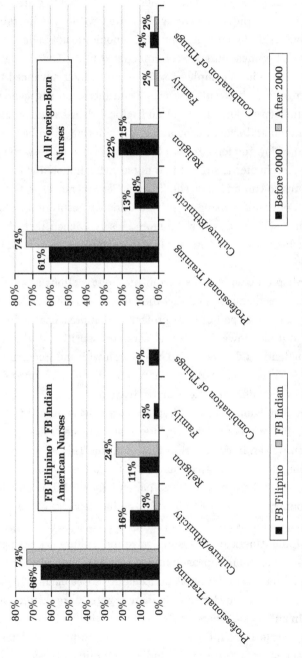

Figure 5.1 Single Most Important Influence on Patient Care for Foreign-Born Nurses. Note that Percentages may not total 100 due to rounding. Source: Stephen M. Cherry, Foreign-Born Nurse Survey (2015).

more religious terms. However, it is important to note that this may be changing with subsequent waves of nursing migration.

Those who immigrated to the United States after 2000, see figure 5.1 (right side), both Filipinos and Indians, were significantly less likely to list religion as their top influence. Although religious nursing schools are not in decline either in India or the Philippines, nurses who immigrated to the United States after 2000 are more likely to have completed some or all of their advanced training in American programs. The result, perhaps, is an increased engagement with American cultural norms and the legal and ethical debates surrounding the separation of church and state. Recognizing this shift may also be the reason that nurses such as Joy, the foreign-born Indian American nurse who spoke at the INA meeting in chapter 2, suggest that nurses who are looking to continue their education in the United States should consider programs like Grand Canyon University College of Nursing—a private Christian institution in Phoenix, Arizona. Programs such as this may be more closely aligned with the philosophical approaches to Christian nursing that these nurses experienced in India prior to migration.

How and when a nurse engages in spiritual interventions are not simple matters. Research has demonstrated that the nurses who are most effective in delivering spiritual care as part of their professional approaches are those who have favorable attitudes towards spiritual care, are sensitive to the religious needs of their patients, and have a deep connection with and understanding of their own faith.[39] These characteristics define the foreign-born nurses in this study—at least as they describe themselves. By their own accounts, many of them were raised in religious households, grew spiritually as adults, and entered a profession that they saw as a religious calling. Many attended nursing programs in which religion was an integral part of their training. This had a tremendous impact on shaping their perspectives on care. Culture may have also played a major role in shaping these perspectives, particularly for Filipinos who emigrated from a country in which Catholicism is an inescapable part of daily life, whether you are Catholic or not. It is for this reason, perhaps, that 16 percent of foreign-born Filipino American nurses indicated that culture is the single most important influence on their approach to working with patients compared to only 3 percent of foreign-born Indian American nurses (see figure 5.1)—keeping in mind that Catholicism and Christianity more generally are distinct minority faiths in India. In either case, shared perspectives on the family, as we will see, also play a major role in shaping their approaches to nursing. There is an understanding across both Filipino and Indian Catholic cultures that living a life in service to others requires not only abiding by the principles of the golden rule but expanding the family circle to include those you serve—a holistic approach to care.

Holistic Care for the Universal Catholic Family

The Catholic church pro-family. This is not to say that other religious traditions are not but a point of emphasis by which we can understand how foreign-born Catholic nurses, whether they are from the India or the Philippines, state that they do not see veterans simply as patients but as members of their own family. Through distinct cultural frameworks that promote familial obligations, a patient, the biological family, and the community are all seen as integral parts of a singular Catholic family. This constitutes the core of these foreign-born nurses' perspectives on care, whether the people within this extended family are Catholic or not.[40] Explaining this in greater depth, Gail, a foreign-born Filipina American nurse who has worked at the VA for over ten years, stated, "I am a Catholic, and my understanding of family is a little different than some. My faith helps a lot when I take care of my patients because being a Catholic we are told that whatever we do to our brothers—especially to the least of our brothers, kind of like, you know, you're helping your brothers, meaning to say that you are helping the people who need the most, so that's pretty much your approach to helping our patients. You cherish them like family. It's not enough to just do unto others, you have to make them your loved ones, literally."

Expressing a similar sentiment in another interview, Aami, the foreign-born Indian American nurse in her early forties we first met in chapter 3, stated, "It's all about the golden rule. That's the gold standard, sorry, pun intended [laughing]. Seriously, we evaluate our care not just by our technical competence but by how much the patient feels that they are loved. We often see veterans that no one ever visits. We are their family, and they need to feel like it because it helps them psychologically. When the mind and spirit are good, they get better." Many of the foreign-born nurses I interviewed, both Filipino an Indian American, shared this faith perspective on the Catholic family. However, as Aami explained, they also noted that, beyond theology or philosophical principles, nurses can actually become literal extensions of their patients' families. Giving an example of how this happens, Esther, the foreign-born Indian American nurse in her late forties we first met in chapter 3, explained, "[For] a lot of patients, especially the elderly patients, you are their only contact with the world outside of the doctors. You are their family. Others who have family that visits, you know not only them but their daughters and sons and more family. They look for you. They get to know you, and over time they become more familiar. You know some of their personal things, you become a part of what is going on in their lives and when someone passes like that I try to call the family either that week or the week after just to see how they are doing." Esther went on, like other foreign-born nurses I interviewed, to describe how this familial approach is not just religious in nature for her but part of a more holistic understanding of compassionate caregiving.[41] This was a theme that emerged throughout my interviews.

Gemma, for example, a foreign-born Filipina American nurse who has worked at the VA for over a decade, stated, "The nuns taught us so much because you have like, in dealing with the patients, you always consider looking at the person as a whole, not just in the physical [way], but you have to consider the whole being. You have to consider not only the psychological but the spiritual as well and by doing this you are giving the person respect and the dignity of being fully human." She then added, rather emphatically, "In our profession you can't ignore religion. It's fundamental to the big questions, you know, life and death. . . . The Bible gives guidance on these. In dealing with patients, you have to consider the spiritual side of the person and not just the physical. . . . It's who they are and frankly, it's how they want us to see them."

Making a similar comment, Jane, the foreign-born Filipina American nurse in her late thirties we first met in chapter 3, remarked in another interview, "I think it's not so much about religion but about being spiritual. We are spiritual beings whether we are religious or not, and understanding that means you have to look at your patients as more than physical. Sometimes it's hard to express this to everyone, but I think I have that gift for discernment." When I asked her to explain what she meant by this, she added, "You have to negotiate and pick your times and circumstances. I don't pray or ask about faith issue[s] with everyone, but there comes that time when this little voice comes in the back of my head saying you need to pray for this patient. So, I ask, and usually I'm right. I'm very careful about it, but it always works out for the betterment of my patient because you just can't split the spiritual from good medicine."

What these nurses describes is a holistic approach to medicine,[42] one that understands that spirituality can and does impact health.[43] However, despite the fact that religion and spirituality can provide perspectives that shape how people see fundamental questions about life, illness, suffering, and death as Gemma explains, they are also complicated and delicate subjects that must be approach with caution in secular settings, as Jane points out. Although the VA has changed its policy governing religious symbols and spiritual and pastoral care in recent years, effectively reversing its prior policy, serious questions remain over the separation of church and state and the best ways to implement this new policy. How and when you engage in spiritual care remain pressing questions, in addition to who should be delivering it.

Conflicts and Contradictions of Faith in Practice

The VA recognizes that religion and spirituality can play an important role in veterans' comprehensive health and well-being, as we saw in chapter 1. However, prior to its policy changes in 2019, the hospital largely relegated these duties to chaplains.[44] Chaplains are seen as an important part of care teams at the VA, but a recent study suggests that a task-oriented culture at the hospital combined with a lack of knowledge about accessing resources and an unclear organization policy on religion/spirituality present significant barriers to providing spiritual care either through chaplaincy or other members of the care team.[45] Nurse managers are especially in a unique position to facilitate appropriate approaches to integrating spiritual care, but spirituality and nursing leadership, as we have seen, remain somewhat under studied and often poorly implemented.[46] Likewise, considering the larger national legal and ethical debates over the appropriate role of religion and spirituality in health care, we should not be surprised that the VA has not only changed its policies multiple times but come under increased scrutiny for doing so from all sides.

How do you maintain patients' rights and the separation of church and state while also engaging in the spiritual care that many veterans request? Can patients legitimately expect honesty from their healthcare providers regarding their personal perspectives and beliefs on religion and spirituality—especially when these implicit or implied perspectives are being used to establish therapeutic alliances or to foster compliance with a course of treatment?[47] Does policy need to be clarified? Is more training needed? Regardless of policy and training, can spiritual care or what some people may think of as spiritual care be misplaced or even go wrong?

In 2011, Esther Garatie (actual name), a veteran who was seeking help for severe depression and suicidal thoughts, was inappropriately interrogated by a foreign-born Indian American nurse manager at a Dallas VA facility. Not only was she supposedly asked point-blank if she was a lesbian, but when she replied yes, the nurse manager reportedly suggested that she ask God into her heart because her depression was a product of guilty feelings about being a homosexual and living in sin.[48] When I asked several Indian American nurses about this case, most had not heard about it. However, Rahel, a foreign-born Indian American nurse who was about to retire from the hospital, offered a somewhat related example of what she thought was important to approaching these issues. "I was born in Kerala as a Catholic and went to nursing school at a

Catholic school. They taught us that you would bless, [and] you would baptize every patient that [would] die on your hand. And you don't even have to let the patient know, you don't have to let anybody know, you don't even do it loud enough, okay?" Continuing after a brief pause, she added, "So, this was in me ever since I [graduated] from nursing school. I've done this my entire career. . . . Someone may be even an atheist, and when he comes to know that I was baptizing him or I was praying for him, he may not like it, so it was all done anonymously while they slept." Rahel went on to explain that she never forced her faith perspectives on any of her patients during her career, but it is easy to see how praying for or baptizing patients in their sleep, even if silently, without their consent could lead to serious legal and ethical problems, if not further scrutiny and scandal, at the VA.

Although the foreign-born nurses in this study had differing opinions about how to engage their faith and when, amplifying the call for comprehensive training, policy, and procedures, most agreed that prayer is the most prevalent form of spiritual care requested by their patients. They also noted that prayer is one of the most controversial or difficult forms of care to navigate outside of the chaplaincy. Despite the fact that nearly all of the foreign-born nurses in this study indicated that they had prayed for their patients in the last year—most silently or privately—this one data point does not capture the complexity of the issue. When do you pray for a patient? Where? And even more challenging, how?[49]

Evaluating a patient's spiritual needs or well-being is difficult and is often dependent on self-reported assessments and observations. The foreign-born nurses in this study recognize this but also suggest that spiritual care is not something that should be solely relegated to the work of the chaplaincy. It should be mandated for the entire care team because, if for no other reason, it can generate hope, optimism, and hardiness in the face of illness—as research continually confirms.[50] Drawing attention to this, Pranji, a foreign-born Indian American nurse who has worked at the VA for over ten years, stated, "We have chaplains but it's different. It's not an integrated faith with health but an extra service to request. Not the same as I was taught." Further lamenting this apparent disconnect between spirituality at the point of care and using or integrating the chaplaincy, Emmy, the foreign-born Filipina American nurse we first met in chapter 2, noted, "I use to pray out loud for a patient when they asked, but now I do it silently in private and tell them that I am sorry, that it is against hospital policy, and I send in the request for a chaplain." When I asked Emmy how her patients responded, she bluntly remarked, "They're pissed, and I don't blame them."[51] This sentiment or some level of frustration was expressed by many of the foreign-born nurses I interviewed.

Orotha, for example, an Indian American nurse who has worked at the VA for over five years, pointed out, "A lot of patients come to us with no hope at all. I always tell them you have to think positive. When they ask me how I keep positive, I tell them that I personally have to pray to keep that positive energy. . . . That's what keeps me praying every day." When I asked Orotha if she had every prayed for a veteran who did not request it or openly talked to a patient about religion and spirituality without them bringing up the subject first, she responded, "Does that include when they are asleep or anesthetized? If so, yes, I see no harm in praying for them when they're unconscious. I typically do it silently, but I know many nurses that say their prayers out loud and in the room with the patient while they rest. And I don't think it's an ethical issue at all, if that's your next question?" Although Orotha did not seem to think that there were any ethical concerns or policy violations involved with praying for a patient without their consent silently or privately while they were sleeping, not all of the foreign-born nurses I interviewed agreed.

Ilah, for example, a foreign-born Filipina American who has worked at the VA for six years, insisted, "I think it really helps when we share in faith, but this is something they [patients] have to initiate. They must ask. I think it was two, twice already, where the family asked that we pray in the last few months. And we also pray when we are doing a donor. It's a truly spiritual act of compassion, but they must consent to it and that means they must be awake! Don't get me wrong, I pray for all my patients in my own head, but no one would ever know. If something comes out of my mouth, I want to be able to say it's not me but a patient request. That way I'm safe." Ilah then admitted, "Sometimes my coworkers insist on praying out loud. One nurse, my friend, she is also Filipina and very religious, said I have to because the patient is dying. So, she asked everybody to join hands and pray for the patient and we did. The veterans didn't ask for it, she initiated it, so we do it on our own. This happens a lot but personally, I'm afraid to express my faith that openly all the time. But death or dying, you know, caring for the terminally ill, that's a real exception I think."

Elaborating on this so-called exception and outlining additional exceptions, Sera, an Indian American nurse who has worked at the VA for over ten years, pointed out, "We have chaplains that they can see, but sometimes when the patient is really depressed or they are dying and know it, they say, you know, they don't know whether they are going to be all right, that kind of thing, you know, you have to reassure them with a positive attitude. So, I pray with them if they like me to pray with them, and they appreciate that." She then added, rather emphatically, "You can't deny this need, even if the chaplains should be there. You're the one there at that moment. You're there and this is just part of your care even if the VA doesn't really like you to pray for them. They want it, and if they pass out or actually die then you still pray for them. So many times, it comforts the families after the fact to know that we were there praying for their loved ones when they passed." Echoing this sentiment, Alma, the foreign-born Indian American nurse who has worked at the VA for over fifteen years that we first met in chapter 2, added in another interview, "Sometimes patients cry with the pain or are in the death process, and when you pray they feel so much more comfortable. They say that you did this and it really worked for me. You prayed and it really helped me, and they ask me to pray again. Prayer really helps them. It gives them mental comfort and satisfaction and maybe more closeness to God."

Although the foreign-born nurses in this study might not all agree on when or how to pray for their patients, they uniformly expressed a belief in the power of prayer and its importance to complete or holistic care, especially with terminally ill or dying patients.[52] Veterans want it, and the foreign-born nurses I interviewed believe that it can help in certain cases/situations. Explaining her own perspective on the power of prayer, Lani, the foreign-born Filipina American nurse in her late thirties we first met in the previous chapter, pointed out, "Sometimes you have some restless patient, and you try to tell them, 'Okay, we will take care of you and if you want to pray, we will pray for you.' And they will say, 'Oh, okay.' And sometimes the patient will ask us if they can pray for all of us at work. I'll say, 'Oh, okay. That's really nice.' They ask for prayer, and to be honest it works. I would like to think that it is the power of God, but it's psychological too. It gives them hope, a new context and belief that something more than human medicine is fighting for them. It helps to know God is with us. That's why it matters."

Sharing another example in another interview, Saba, a foreign-born Indian American nurse who has worked at the VA for a little over five years, told me about a patient she prayed with who was going through a very difficult time both physically and psychologically. "He told me he and his friend were standing in the army and they were fighting. He was crying when he was telling me this. We're not supposed talk to them about this stuff, but he was really shaking, so I didn't stop him. He said they were on the front line and they were fighting all of these people and [a] suicide bomb burst on everybody and one suicide bomb came and the friend who was standing near, all of a sudden, his head was [to] one side and his body was under this shaking. I can't imagine seeing this." Visibly upset in retelling this story, she then added, after pausing for a moment, "He doesn't know how he escaped from there. But his head is on one side, his body is one side . . . this particular young man told me, and he was like twenty-three or twenty-four. . . . He can't do anything. The Iraq War made them all sick, mentally sick. It's really sad. It's all I can do to keep them healthy. He wanted me to pray with him and I did. Nothing else was working. Really, prayer in that case is the only medicine that works."

Giving yet another example in another interview, Zoe, the foreign-born Filipina American nurse we first met in chapter 4, remarked, "I prayed for my patients all the time. Last week, I remember there was an elderly veteran [who] was brought in by his elderly wife, and briefly I came to know that they lived by themselves and they have children, yes, but they are not close by. In other words, some were in other states, and at that time looking at how fragile he was and how sick he was, and eventually he died." As Zoe continued to talk, she explained with tears in her eyes, "I could not imagine how the wife would be able to handle it, and when she was just standing by next to him, even though there was a protocol for us not to let them see how, what's the course of care that we are doing in order to save the life, I still let her stand by because I still honored him. I started to pray. If this were my parents and if that was their last wish to make them happy, then let them be together until their last breath. So, we prayed together and he passed. She was sad but at peace because he passed as he wanted, holding hands and in prayer." Pausing for a moment, Zoe rhetorically questioned what I thought would happen if she refused to pray with her patient and then added, "It's not a matter of should we pray, it was demanded, needed in the moment. They needed it and I needed it!"

This is an important point. Nurses grieve too. We often forget or at least take it for granted that when a patient dies, nurses can also be emotionally distraught.[53] They have a personal investment in each and every one of their patients. Thus, whether a prayer or spiritual intervention is private or public, for oneself or patients, it is clear that it can provide solace to those who are restless and distressed, or even comfort to those haunted by the horrors of war. Explaining this further, Elena, a foreign-born Filipina American nurse who has worked at the VA for over five years, pointed out with a bit of emotion in her voice, "It's hard to lose a patient. You can't imagine. They become our family, and we lose them as their families do. Prayer is important for the patients, and their family—and I consider myself as a part of that need. It works for them and us [nurses]." Good care, as these nurses describe it, includes sensitivity and attentiveness to the cultural and religious beliefs of their patients, but how and when these beliefs should be addressed, as we have seen, have no easy answers.[54] Clearly prayer can be an important part of this approach. Prayer matters, as Zoe and Elena point out, for both oneself and others; however, in a country such as the United States, where the separation of church and state is the law, prayer in federally-owned hospitals such as the VA is complicated legally and ethically, especially if it is engaged out loud—even by patient request rather than silently and in private or with a chaplain.

Conclusion

Spiritual care is essential to holistic or whole-person healthcare. Just as no person is simply their body or mind, any form of physical or mental healing, or even the long-term management of a terminal illness when there is no cure, requires an integrated understanding of what it truly means to be human. This includes the spirit. Spiritual care matters to healthcare, as research and the impassioned words of the foreign-born nurses in this study demonstrate throughout this chapter. However, as we have seen, it is not easy to implement, particularly in a secular hospital such as the VA. There are several complicated ethical and legal matters to consider. Spiritual care and interventions can be misplaced or even go horribly wrong, as we have seen. As a result, individual nurses and larger care teams may be reluctant to integrate spiritual interventions into their daily interactions with patients or incorporate it as a more comprehensive part of their approach to patient well-being. Although I was not able to observe how the Houston VA addresses spiritual care in training students and those in residency, it is important to note once again that it is a teaching hospital—providing clinical training for healthcare professionals through one of the largest VA residency programs in the country. As noted in chapter 1, each academic year, almost two thousand students are trained through one hundred and forty affiliation agreements with institutions of higher learning in nineteen states. How this local VA trains healthcare professionals to negotiate between church and state and deliver spiritual care at the point of care, if at all, likely has far-reaching impacts on those they train and who go on to work at other hospitals across the country.

At the center of these complex debates over the utility and application of spiritual interventions is prayer. Despite the fact that a growing body of research documents the potential positive relationships between praying and various indicators of psychological well-being,[55] including its use as a favored coping strategy for patients,[56] considerably less research exists on how nurses think about and engage in prayer with or for their patients every day.[57] What is known largely focuses on nurses working in hospice, oncology, and critical care. Among these studies, findings indicate that only 2 to 23 percent of these nurses reported praying often or very often with a patient.[58] However, most nurses do report praying for patients privately (53 percent *often* and 66 percent *very often*.[59] Clearly prayer is used in nursing practice, but it appears to rarely involve an overtly shared experience with patients. There are several reasons why this may be the case, including a lack of time, personal discomfort, lack of knowledge or experience, lack of private space, and the more pressing concern of ascertaining whether or not it is appropriate to pray with or for a patient in any given situation.[60]

Although the majority of these barriers do not appear to completely prevent the foreign-born nurses in this study from doing what they believe is best for their patients in terms of spiritual care, they lament the degree to which VA policy and procedure is either poorly defined or constantly changing. They are looking for direction or clarification because they see themselves as part of a larger care team. Whereas some American-trained nurses report that assessing and addressing patients' spiritual needs, as it relates to their medical care, is not how they see their role as professionals or is perhaps done better by others,[61] many foreign-born Filipino and Indian American nurses, especially those who immigrated prior to 2000, were largely trained to think differently. They believe delivering spiritual care is an important part of being a good nurse both morally and professionally. They also believe that these needs are not the sole responsibility of the chaplaincy. Chaplains are important, but, as Pranji, among others, points out, they cannot always be there when needed. Add to this the fact that patients often request prayer from nurses who have been their most consistent points of interaction, and it is easy to see why these nurses, like many of their American-born peers who may also want to or are asked to engage in spiritual care, face considerable professional dilemmas.

Many veterans, like other American patients more generally, want spiritual care, and many nurses want to provide it. They have seen it work firsthand, and they believe that the research supports it. In fact, failing to address a patient's spiritual needs has been shown to not only lessen patients' ability to cope with illness but actually increase their healthcare costs.[62] Understanding this, however, does not make the implementation any easier. Whose religion? What if the patient's spiritual or religious beliefs are different from the nurse's? What happens if the patient is offended by a nurse offering to pray? Can a nurse abuse the vulnerability of a patient if they pray with them? And how can a nurse support a patient's prayer practices without actually praying with them or for them? These are all important questions that must be addressed very differently when working in a pluralistic environment.[63]

The foreign-born nurses in this study see themselves as servants of care, but many, as we have seen, struggle with the disconnects between how they were trained as Catholic nurses in another country—learning to see spiritual care as an integral part of who they are and how they should best serve their patients—and the larger ethical and legal tensions that exist in an American secular hospital over the separation of church and state. Although they construct an image of themselves as different than their American-born peers, the issues and concerns surrounding spiritual care, especially prayer, can impact all nurses regardless of where they were born or trained. Many nurses want to pray with or for their patients. The foreign-born nurses in this study suggest that they do so because they are comfortable with their own spirituality and confident in their faith and training. They believe that they have a gift for discernment, as Jane puts it, knowing when it is most appropriate to engage in spiritual care and how best to carry it out. However, how well they are able to do this was not observed, is not clear, and begs for further research.

Regardless of these professional dilemmas, it is important remember that whether a nurse engages in spiritual care or not says nothing about their own personal faith. An apparent absence of engaging in spiritual care also says nothing about the degree to which a nurse sees religion and spirituality as an integral part of how they approach caring for their patients. The foreign-born nurses in this study acknowledge this, citing their professional training as the most important part of their care approaches. They also suggest that their Catholic faith frames not only how they engage in these approaches but the ways in which they see their patients. These distinctive cultural frameworks promote familial obligations to a singular Catholic family that includes nurses' patients, their biological family, and the community. This constitutes the core of their perspectives on care as they describe it, whether the people within this extended family are Catholic or not. They also believe, as we will see, that their care for veterans, their hospital family, does not stop at the VA. Exploring this in greater detail, the next chapter moves from the confines of the Houston VA hospital into the wider community. It demonstrates how Catholic cultural frameworks compel foreign-born nurses to voluntarily engage larger issues confronting veterans and the broader community, on their own time and away from their paid jobs. This, as will become more apparent, not only furthers our understanding of how these nurses extend their care to others by enlarging the family circle but also has tremendous implications for how we understand the civic lives of new Catholic immigrants today.

Chapter 6

Extending Health and Care to Community

Every December for the last twelve years, members of the Filipino Nurses Association (FNA) and the Indian Nurses Association (INA) have visited Star of Hope Mission (actual name), a homeless shelter, either as an organization or individually on separate occasions. Star of Hope provides food, shelter, counseling, and education for over one thousand homeless men, women, and children across the city every day—including an estimated two hundred veterans of the U.S. military.[1] Although these staggering numbers, particularly the number of homeless veterans, may come as a shock to the general public, the enormity of the problem is one of the reasons that the foreign-born nurses in this study say they volunteer at the shelter so frequently. Gabby, the foreign-born Filipina American nurse who has worked at the VA for over ten years that we first met in chapter 3, stated after serving food one night in December, "When you talk to veterans you realize that even though they are a veteran, they don't get anything from the government when discharged. They don't get paid anymore, so no wonder they end up not knowing what to do because they don't have any skills and they end up living on the street, you know, it's pitiful. No one wants to talk about it, but God knows that's why we are here [Star of Hope]. We come as often as we can."

Expressing a similar sentiment in another interview, Janie, a foreign-born Filipina American nurse in her early fifties, added how frustrated she is with the VA system. "Look, I talk all the time to fellow nurses from the VA, and some of them have been there forever, and one of them is a case manager and the other one is a regular unit nurse, and they were saying that how can you possibly discharge a patient when you know they don't have any place to go? The hospital is sending them to the streets! What is the sense in releasing them? I know they [VA] have programs to help but so many fall through the cracks. . . . If the VA can't provide a safety net that catches them before they fall, then we have to extend our care to the community to make sure we catch them. You can't call yourself a good Catholic and do nothing." She then added, "When I'm not [at the shelter], I'm out somewhere else in the community giving all I can to help keep this city healthy. I like to spread the love around." Other foreign-born Filipino American nurses I interviewed shared this sentiment in one way or another. Rose, for example, the foreign-born Filipina American nurse we first met in chapter 4 suggested, "Our faith demands that we do what we can with the talents and opportunities God has given us. . . . It's not like in the Philippines where there is more help for veterans and their families. Here you need volunteers, the government isn't doing enough."

The following week, members of INA held another Christmas event at Star of Hope. When I asked them how or if they coordinate their efforts with FNA, Adina, a foreign-born Indian American nurse in her early fifties, stated, "It doesn't matter when we come to volunteer as long as we are here and continue to help those in need. It's about serving God's children wherever they are. We are all supposed to be family, right?" When I asked her why volunteering at Star of Hope or other places was so important to her, she stated, "In the community there are a lot of needy people. Especially like the people who don't have any insurance or [have] no home. I mean, we get the help from the hospitals during the day to sponsor the programs here, but it is not enough. So that kind of thing I think is really important now, especially for veterans." She then added, "We have worked with the [VA] hospital to improve this. Actually, I think they are now implementing a lot of plans for the homeless veterans. They are trying to help, and all those things are working, but they miss people, and I would think it would be nice if also their family could be treated. Like back home in India, our veterans' wives and children, they get treatment too. The United States is better than this. If India can do it, you know? So frustrating . . . that's why we are here to pick up where the VA can't."

After the event, I asked Sarah, the foreign-born Indian American nurse in her early fifties we first met in chapter 3, what she hopes to get out of volunteering at the shelter. "I have been doing this for four years now. Every year I'm going and finding new ways to get them [veterans] help. What we do at the hospital is not enough. You have to be more active in the community." Sarah then explained,

The nurses' association [INA] has always helped the Star of Hope because they care for the people who need God's love and compassion. It's also near the VA Hospital. So, we help them with food and donate gifts during the holidays. . . . We sing with them, we dance with them. . . . I feel good when I go. And I know it makes a difference. We have resources and talents, so why not spread it around the community? It's a waste if we don't do more. That's what God expects of us, and right now it's Christmas too. You know [singing], "Good tidings we bring to you and your kin. Good tidings for Christmas and a happy New Year."

Civically Engaged Catholic Immigrants?

The considerable joy Sarah and other foreign-born Filipino and Indian American nurses express in serving or helping the homeless at Star of Hope Mission is obvious. It echoes throughout their narratives. However, volunteering at the shelter is not only important to them as Catholics during Christmas or special religious holidays but something they do throughout the year. They believe that the shelter needs them. They also suggest that they know the problems and challenges veterans face and have special insights into how to best serve them. Because of this knowledge and their experiences, they state that they are concerned that too many veterans are getting lost in the red tape and bureaucracy at the VA or sadly not even making it to the hospital to receive care to begin with. And they are right.

Roughly 11 percent of the current adult homeless population in the United States are veterans who served in the U.S. military.[2] It is a shocking statistic. In light of this, it is also clear that the VA system, despite its best efforts and intentions, has much work to do reaching those among the homeless that might be facing physical or mental health issues or both. It is also clear that veterans' issues and challenges are not isolated to the hospitals. As a result, the foreign-born nurses in this study see volunteering at the shelter, among other places, as an important extension of their care for veterans, even though the majority of the veterans at the shelter are not, nor have ever been, their direct patients. Volunteering, according to these nurses, is a spiritual act and a patriotic duty—something they state that they take very seriously as American Catholics. If India and the Philippines can do more for their veterans and families, foreign-born nurses such as Rose and Adina question why the United States, their adopted country, cannot at least match these efforts. They believe American veterans deserve better, and they are willing to freely give their time to help make it happen.

The opening narratives of this chapter are just a brief snapshot of foreign-born Filipino and Indian Americans' larger active community lives. The same cultural forces that motivate them to extend their understandings of family to include their patients are the same forces that structure their entire perspective on community. These forces not only shape how they see community but compel them to act. Over 90 percent of the foreign-born nurses in this study indicated on surveys that they had volunteered at least once in the last twelve months, not including programs or required events at the VA hospital. It is an astonishing percentage, one that far exceeds the national American volunteering rate (roughly 25 percent). It is even more remarkable when you consider that previous studies have largely found that new immigrants do not volunteer much beyond their own communities or are typically seen as being on the receiving end of volunteerism.[3]

The reason that new immigrants in general may not volunteer as much as the wider population can be partly attributed to the fact that they do not get asked to volunteer at the same rates as American-born Whites.[4] Since being personally asked to volunteer is among the top reasons people participate in their communities and the wider cities in which they live, not being asked has clear implications on their opportunities to get involved. Although racism and xenophobia play an important role in limiting these opportunities, as we might imagine, these forces have a smaller impact on the foreign-born nurses in this study because of their unique socioeconomic circumstances.[5] Unlike previous studies that have largely focused on the presumed negative effects of lower-skilled immigrants with poor English proficiencies on the metropolitan areas to which they migrate,[6] the foreign-born Filipino and Indian American nurses who work at the VA are clearly not lower-skilled, nor do they have poor English proficiencies.

The majority of previous studies on new immigrant volunteerism and civic engagement has largely ignored the so-called other side of immigration—high socioeconomic and upwardly mobile foreign-born professionals. Although the relevance of this socioeconomic context has been recognized in previous studies of immigrant assimilation, few have studied the volunteerism of foreign-born professionals, especially those working in healthcare.[7] Being a nurse and working at the VA can be advantageous for people who are motivated and looking for ways to get involved in their community. As Rose and Sarah point out in the opening pages of this chapter, foreign-born nurses, at least those they personally know and with whom they associate, have skills, talents, and resources that they say they do not want to waste. This is not a surprise, given what previous research has demonstrated.

Studies of American civic engagement consistently suggest that education is the most consistent predictor of volunteering.[8] It can facilitate volunteering by heightening awareness of social or community problems such as homelessness, increasing empathy for those—such as veterans—experiencing these issues, and building the self-confidence generally needed to get involved.[9] More importantly, education can impact leisure time and the extensive social networks and resources that not only increase the likelihood that people volunteer but encourage them to do so.[10] Although working at the VA has its challenges, as we have seen, it also has its clear advantages in terms of resources and connections.

Beyond the workplace, education impacts where people live and the types of communities they engage with.[11] For new immigrants, this can moderate their likelihood of interacting with American-born members of their community and hence the time it takes to structurally and civically assimilate or incorporate.[12] Understanding this, we find that the foreign-born nurses in this study are not assimilating into the Houston metropolitan area over time as a process of migrant upward mobility but are largely able to move into communities and make an immediate impact because of their relatively high socioeconomic status when they arrive in the United States. They do not need time, in the classical sense, to linearly assimilate.[13] Their high income is a relative manifestation of the professional education they received in their country of origin, which they brought with them. They may go on to attain additional education and degrees in the United States, as we have seen, but are entering nonetheless as socioeconomically mobile professionals. By the time they get to the VA hospital, with most having worked at least five to ten years at another hospital, they are also American citizens.

Status matters. However, it only explains or contextualizes the more resource-mobilization aspects of how the foreign-born nurses in this study are connected and able to do what they do in the community. It does not necessarily explain their motivations, which, as we have seen, are driven by their culturally defined faith perspectives—what they believe God asks them to do for others. And they are not alone. Faith and religiosity actually play an important role in volunteerism, particularly in the United States.[14] By some estimates, half of all American volunteerism occurs in a religious context, if not directly through a place of worship or religiously affiliated institution.[15] Research also suggests that frequent religious attendance can increase the likelihood of volunteering regardless of where actual volunteering occurs.[16] Only education rivals frequent church attendance as a predictor of volunteerism.[17] As a form of social capital, religiosity can also provide opportunities to cross socioeconomic boundaries, forge ties with people from other groups and their concerns, and bridge individuals to the communities in which they live.[18] Beyond promoting these extensive networks and the resources they present for volunteering to occur, religious institutions can also mobilize more intrinsic forms of capital that motivate volunteers by instilling a sense of duty to serve or care for others in their community. This process can draw on religious texts as well as the words and messages delivered by or exchanged with clergy, fellow parishioners, and religious media. Whatever the format or context, these messages not only motivate the faithful to volunteer, particularly those who are religiously active, but also help to further establish the cultural frameworks that encourage community engagement. [19] This is an important point, one that has clear implications for understanding the civic lives of the foreign-born Catholic nurses in this study. Yet, many scholars have suggested that American Catholic civic life, including that of new Catholic immigrants, is a puzzle.[20]

Although Catholic institutions and teachings continue to foster an expressly communitarian ethic[21] and American Catholics, including immigrants, appear, for the most part, to be receiving these messages, some studies suggest that there is little difference between the way Catholics and people of other religious traditions participate in American civic life today.[22] In other words, the messages are no more or less impactful. Other studies suggest that as Catholics become more middle-class or assimilate into American culture over time, in the case of immigrants, they tend to give up what is distinctive about their Catholic faith and adopt more Protestant traits and practices.[23] As this occurs, they are no longer all that distinguishable from other Christians.

In studies that hold that Catholic culture, particularly parish structure and practices, remain somewhat intact, scholars have found that the average size of most Catholic parishes and the church's administrative hierarchy actually inhibit the generation of social capital needed for civic engagement, compared to other Christian denominations. If true—and further study is greatly needed—the historical characterization of American Catholicism as a so-called friend of the poor or exemplifying a community-centered ethic appears to be in decline. Being Catholic may thus actually discourage civic participation and community engagement because of the hierarchical and less democratic structure of the Catholic church.[24] What does this mean for the foreign-born Catholic nurses in this study? How do we explain their active civic lives?

The remainder of this chapter addresses these questions. The chapter demonstrates how cultural forces not only shape the parish and community life of the foreign-born nurses in this study, both Filipino and Indian American, but compel them to act on issues such as poverty, community health, and homelessness that extend well beyond any one parish or any one ethnic community.[25] Although there are clear cultural differences between these nursing populations, they are united in their Catholic faith and a universal belief in serving others as one family—God's family. As we will see, the shared belief they describe is not limited to their care of veterans at the VA hospital, but much like their work at Star of Hope Mission, it extends into the communities in which they live and the wider city. I argue that this has clear implications on the ways in which we think about and understand new immigrant civic lives, their connections to community, and the deeply held Catholic beliefs that motivate them to give back to the country they believe has given them so much.

Enlarging the Family Circle Even Wider

As we saw in the last chapter, the foreign-born nurses in this study, regardless of whether they were from India or the Philippines, do not see the veterans they serve at the hospital simply as patients but as members of their own extended family—a singular and universal Catholic family. This constitutes the core of their perspectives on care.[26] It also frames the way in which they say they understand their place in society, their connections to others, and hence their perspectives on civic responsibility. Through distinct Catholic cultural frameworks that promote universal familial obligations, the health of this extended family becomes relative—pun intended. Patient needs are not restricted to official paid care in the hospital but extend to wherever they may be in the community, regardless of time or personal costs. Family is family. Explaining this in greater detail, Carol, the foreign-born Indian American nurse in her mid-forties we first met in chapter 3, pointed out, "We take the oath. This is the field you enter into primarily to really care [for] the patient. I treat them as one of my own, I see them as one of my family members, especially when you consider they have served the country, and to me it's just fair that they get, at the very least, the service that you know how best to give."

Carol then added with a bit of frustration, "The [VA] system is quite tedious sometimes, you know, the process. There is a lot of red tape also. People get lost in the system. That's why we end up working in the community so much. If you can't do everything you know you can for veterans at the hospital, you have to take the fight to the streets." When I asked Carol what she meant by this last statement, she answered with a series of rhetorical questions. "If you only visited your sick family in the hospital but didn't help them when they got home, or heaven forbid they lose their home, what kind of Christian would you be? Jesus calls us to serve others as we would serve our own, no matter where they are or who they are. . . . That's how family works, right?"

What Carol describes is a universal understanding of family, not in theory but practice. Despite the challenges of working with veterans, she sees herself as freely giving of her own time to help those she considers to be her extended family. However, this universal perspective is not restricted to veterans but applied consciously to an entire community of others that these nurses state are their extended kin.

Attempting to explain this shared familial perspective, Lettie, the foreign-born Filipina American nurse in her late forties we first met in chapter 3, added in another interview, "The community needs us. I sensed that since I was new to America. Just like back home [Philippines], we used to go to communities to visit, you know, door to door, other nurses . . . it's called, what is it called? Community health nursing. You would do home visits and also do like a clinic, you know, like in common places, health fairs. This is how to engage your faith for others. You treat them like family. They're your kin." Lettie then pointed out, "We do the same here. We're so busy in the community and not just with veterans. . . . Think about it, when your family is healthy, you're happy. That's why I volunteer so much on my free time. It makes me happy. And I think it makes God happy too."

As noted earlier, 91.2 percent of the foreign-born nurses in this study,[27] both Filipino and Indian American, indicated on surveys that they volunteered at least once in the last twelve months outside of hospital events or required programs. This, again, far exceeds the average American volunteering rate (roughly 26 percent), which should be noted has been trending downward in recent years.[28] In philanthropy, 89.1 percent of these nurses[29] also stated that they donated money to charitable causes in the last twelve months, not including to their local churches (tithing). This, too, is an astonishing percentage considering that only roughly 53 percent of Americans donated to charitable causes in the last year—part of a growing downward trend since 2002.[30] Whereas Americans in general are volunteering less and giving less, largely a symptom of a fluctuating economy, the foreign-born nurses in this study report volunteering and giving at a surprisingly high rate for a host of different causes and issues.

In looking at figure 6.1, we can see that the top three domains in which foreign-born Filipino and Indian American nurses volunteered are the same— community projects (77 percent Filipinos and 97 percent Indians), professional organizations such as FNA or INA (71 percent Filipinos and 84 percent Indians), and charity organizations such as Star of Hope Mission (62 percent Filipinos and 82 percent Indians). Although foreign-born Indian American nurses tend to volunteer at a higher rate than Filipino Americans in each of these top three

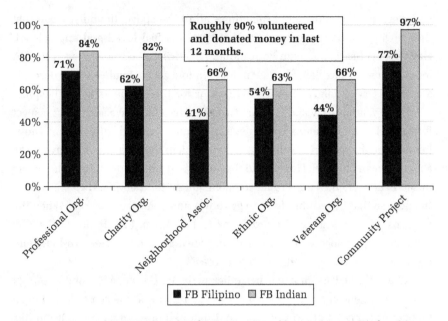

Figure 6.1 Areas of Civic Engagement for Foreign-Born Nurses. Source: Stephen M. Cherry, Foreign-Born Nurse Survey (2015).

domains, Filipinos tend to volunteer across more domains on average, including smaller domains such as sports and fraternal organizations that are not charted in figure 6.1. On average, both populations indicated that they volunteered in a minimum of five domains in the last year. When Janie states in the opening narrative to this chapter that she likes to spread the volunteering love around, she is clearly not alone. Although veterans' organizations were the fourth largest domain in which both groups volunteered, this is a bit misleading considering that both professional and charity organizations are involved in serving populations that include veterans. As such, veteran causes may be seen as an important part of many of the domains or areas that the nurses volunteer in but not an exclusive interest. Community health in general is a larger concern. This includes, as we might expect, mental, physical, and spiritual health—together comprising a holistic understanding of well-being that draws the nurses into many community projects and even the political sphere.

Every Day Is Veterans Day

Across this study, the foreign-born nurses I interviewed stated that they always did something special for their patients on Veterans Day beyond the official events scheduled at the hospital. Whether it was bringing them a small present, balloons, or a box lunch, and sometimes all of the above, the nurses said that they always found a way to make their patients feel loved and appreciated. However, as Baara, a foreign-born Indian American who has worked at the VA for over a decade, explained, these not-so-random acts of kindness they describe are not reserved solely for Veterans Day or for their patients at the hospital. "Today is Veterans Day and I visited two veterans. Oh, I have such great respect for them. I brought them something, a little note card and balloon, you know, I even brought some lunch for them. I appreciate their service. I always think about my own children. How would they deal with war?" Continuing, but visibly upset, Baara added, "I am so glad someone fought for their [her own children's] freedom so that they didn't have to go to war and come back broken. When the veterans come to see me as a provider I feel for them. I really do. That's why I did something special for two of them today. They might not live long, and I wanted them to feel loved, like true heroes."

When I asked Baara about her other patients, she quickly pointed out, "I treat them like every day is Veterans Day. You know, at the age of forty I even thought of going into the navy. And so, I inquired of some people, but I'm like too old for that. You know your patriotism really increases when you take care of these veterans. You just feel like you need to do more every day." Baara was not alone in stating she feels this way. Many of the foreign-born nurses I interviewed described how they felt compelled by their faith to do what they described as God's work in the community, but they also stated that their active civic lives started as an extension of their care for veterans at the hospital and then moved in directions that they could not have originally imagined.

Sabrina, for example, a foreign-born Filipina American nurse in her late forties, explained, "I had no idea where my life was going to take me in the community. You just get involved, wanting to do more for the veterans you serve, and next thing you know you are . . . organizing project after project after project. Have you seen our [FNA] schedule? I don't know how we keep it under control, but God looks after us because we are doing his work." When I asked Sabrina if she could recall some of the first nonhospital projects she worked on either alone or with nurses in her association, she noted, "I have no idea, but I am sure it was a health clinic at one our local parish churches. I do remember my first project to lead. I spearheaded the Project Iraq Christmas Care packages program. We sent a total of twelve huge packages of assorted clothes, toiletries, candies, and other personal necessities and treats for Christmas for our troops fighting in Iraq. I had a step son-in-law there during those times, and he confirmed receiving the packages, which were distributed to his marine troop members. It was not much, but he said it meant a great deal to them."

Sabrina was not alone in finding a familial connection to veterans. In fact, as we have seen, many of the foreign-born Filipino American nurses I interviewed had relatives who were either currently serving in the military or served specifically during World War II. However, in the case of the latter, this was a bit of a sore point. Highlighting this, Melody, a foreign-born Filipina American nurse whose father served in the U.S. military, emphatically stated, "The situation of Filipino veterans from World War II is truly sad! Just sad. They were robbed of honor and deserve our recognition. Unfortunately, all that has been done is too little and too late, you know what I mean? We don't really know anyone alive from that war now in Houston [who] would need our support, but we remember them on Veterans Day and try to educate people on their circumstance. We keep their memory alive by telling their story and demanding what is right even if their numbers are dying out. We want justice. I write my congresswoman every year." What Melody alludes to is the fact that over two hundred and fifty thousand Filipinos volunteered to fight alongside U.S. troops during World War II but were largely denied the benefits they were promised by President Roosevelt. Among the veterans of the sixty-six countries that allied and fought with the United States during WWII, only Filipinos were denied these benefits.[31]

Although the majority of the foreign-born Indian Americans I interviewed did not share the same familial connections to the U.S. military as Filipino Americans, they also suggested, as Sabrina and her Filipino American peers did, that helping veterans in the community was what kick-started their civic lives. Bev, for example, a foreign-born Indian American nurse who has worked at the VA for thirteen years, stated, "When you work at the VA you quickly learn that if the government can find a way to fail its veterans, it does. This is why you see so many of us working in the community. We have to go and pick up the pieces that get left behind. . . . Once you get started helping them you realize the work is endless. Then you realize they are not alone. One project leads to another. Before you realize it, you're always doing something in the community."

Community Health and Education

Perhaps the greatest impact foreign-born nurses in this study have on their communities is through health fairs and community health projects/programs across the Houston metropolitan area. Given the narrative of Lettie in this chapter, this should come as no surprise. Community health truly matters to these nurses. In fact, a quick perusal of FNA's calendar posted on their website reveals that Filipino American nurses typically have at least one community health clinic planned for every other week of the month throughout the year, excluding the summer when many nurses travel home to the Philippines and major holidays such as Christmas, which they typically spend volunteering at places such as Star of Hope Mission. Although INA is a smaller association with fewer members and resources than FNA, Indian American nurses have a similarly busy calendar providing healthcare to communities throughout the year.

When I asked nurses how they make time to do all that they do in the community, most could not provide an explanation. Dianne, for example, a foreign-born Filipina American nurse in her late fifties, simply stated, "I really don't know. It just gets done by the sheer power of God. People just call us [FNA] if they need a health fair and we do it. The thing about Filipinos is that we drag each other [in], you know, even if there is only like one person involved with a group. I mean, you will drag your friends. And that's how we always go. . . . Before you know it, it's done and we're off to the next project. We do a lot of health fairs and clinics just as needed but sometimes for an emergency. We actually did a big health fair when [hurricane] Ike hit Houston and Galveston."

Adding a similar sentiment in another interview, Alma, a foreign-born Indian American nurse in her early forties, acknowledged, "It's mind-blowing how this all comes together. We are so busy it's often more than I can keep up with, but I have several goals when I work in the community. Number one would be to share my blessings with others, especially my knowledge. I want to motivate others, and like for the [INA], we have to show to the community, and not just to the Indian community, that wherever we are, we have to show that we are hardworking and we make a difference in the lives of other people." She then pointed out, "Not for show but so they know we are there for them, someone they can count on, someone doing good for them, you know. . . . When that's the goal, it just works out."

Sharing a similar sentiment in another interview, Joy, the foreign-born Indian American nurse we first met in chapter 2, explained, "You know, I like giving back to the community because America has really been good to me. Nursing feeds my family. I'm fortunate to have this job, and most people have accepted me. I have so many blessings in my life." Pausing, Joy then added, "I think sometimes, I mean [hesitating], sometimes I feel like I love America more than those people who were born here because it's really a land of opportunity and it has opportunities for you. It's there, you just have to grab it and stuff. I guess it's just one way for me to give back. Just a way of saying like, 'thank you.' I think the people born here take this for granted."

Many of the numerous health fairs and clinics (figure 6.2) that both nursing associations facilitate throughout the year are at local churches. Explaining why this is the case, Sharon, a foreign-born Indian nurse who has worked at the VA for over a decade, pointed out, "It's a natural extension of our parish

FNA (Oct. to Nov.)	INA (Oct. to Nov.)
[St. John's] Catholic Church Fair	Project Houston ISD
Picnic & Health Fair	Center Health Fair
[St. Justine's] Fall Festival Health Fair (twice during this time)	Community Health Fair
Annual Health and Community Resource Fair (twice during this time)	Houston Heart Walk & Blood Drive
Houston Boot Walk & Blood Drive	Nepali & Bhutanese Health Clinic

Figure 6.2 Filipino and Indian American Nursing Association Activities. Source: FNA and INA (pseudonyms) official associational calendars.

ministries. We learn about needs from our priest and then act on it, particularly through the lady's ministry.[32] We are all nurses. We do home visits to all the sick people, we go to their houses and pray for them, and when there is a larger problem or a need for screenings then we get [INA] to set something up at the church. We also try to do education programs, you know, for more preventative health."

Adding to this conversation in another interview, Lis, a foreign-born Indian American nurse who has also worked at the VA for over ten years, stated, "Last year we had a health seminar, and actually one of the doctors came from VA hospital, and he had a talk about the men's health issues with prostate problems and all. The previous year we had a gynecology doctor come and talk to the ladies. At the health fair we had blood draws. [The] cancer center, the blood bank, they all came to our church, but it wasn't just for Indians but other folks too, yeah." When I asked who else comes, Lis stated, "We advertise, and older people or just anybody who wants to have their blood pressure checked or glucose [come]. If we diagnose them for diabetes or high blood pressure then we send them on to a clinic, even without insurance. It's a diverse group, yeah, from the surrounding area. [INA] also raised like $110,000 to host the fair annually. We do a lot of good through this and the retirement home we sponsor." Ironically, the retirement home for Indian American Catholics that Lis mentioned is next door to a local Veterans of Foreign Wars meeting hall. When asked if the veterans knew that the nurses hosting the health fairs worked at the VA, she stated with a big smile, "Of course, we have a great relationship. We share parking space for events. It's a small world, right?"

Like foreign-born Indian American nurses, foreign-born Filipino nurses also conduct many of their FNA community health fairs through their local parish churches. Explaining this, Gail, a foreign-born Filipina American nurse in her mid-fifties, pointed out in an interview after working at a blood pressure booth at a local health fair, "In addition to being in [FNA], I'm the pastoral council president of [my church], so I'm very involved in the church. Whatever the church or the community needs, I'm in the right position to hear it and then do something about it through the nurses association [FNA]. My fellow nurses are always ready to help."

Explaining FNA activities further, Zoe, a foreign-born Filipina American nurse in her late forties, added in another interview, "In the church we try to offer free blood pressure check-ups, glucose monitoring, and the bike helmet activity for young kids, and we let them see a video to help. For those who are not able to buy helmets, we [also] try to provide as much as we can from the supply that we get. We have to set up this program through affiliations with different organizations. Some schools get involved, and the hospital, we get a lot of help, but it's mostly us Filipinos working the event. This is pretty much how it goes everywhere we put on one of these fairs. Some are bigger than others, but the churches always offer the best spaces and opportunities." Like members of INA, foreign-born Filipina American nurses have found a great deal of success addressing broad community health needs by working through their local parish churches. However, given that many Indian American Catholic churches are largely ethnic parishes, specifically of Syro-Malabar and Syro-Malankara East Syriac rite churches, they tend to be smaller in their reach compared to the larger multiethnic Roman Catholic churches many Filipino Americans attend. Due to these circumstances, the health fairs that FNA sponsors tend to be much larger and draw in both a larger and more diverse group of people.

The Alief Health and Civic Resources Fair, for example, is one of the largest annual health fairs in the Houston metropolitan area. It started out rather small, but with the aid and mobilization of foreign-born Filipino American nurses and of parishioners of their local Catholic church, it has grown immensely over the last decade.[33] In 1997, a local outreach forum for community and parish problems called SAVE (Stand Against Violence Everyone) grew into a broad coalition of groups and individuals that aimed to hold a community health fair in Alief, which is a suburb in the southwestern Houston metropolitan area.[34] The first fair was held in 2002 with a modest attendance of one thousand attendees and nearly sixty providers and sponsors, including FNA. By 2005 the fair had nearly tripled in attendance, with over five hundred people receiving some form of health screening, one hundred and thirty-five children receiving close to four hundred and fifty immunizations, and nineteen pints of blood donated. At least two hundred underprivileged families received nearly fourteen thousand fresh produce items, and over six hundred children received backpacks and school supplies.[35]

Today, the fair has grown so large that it is no longer held in the parking lot of a local parish church. It is now held in larger school facilities in the Alief Independent School District (ISD) school district but is still sponsored and staffed by foreign-born Filipino American nurses, among others. The fair continues to serve largely lower-income families in the Houston metropolitan area and in several languages. Health fair literature, for example, is often printed in Cantonese, Mandarin, Spanish, Filipino (Tagalog), and Vietnamese. It is a diverse group the nurses serve. Obviously, they cannot do it alone. There are too many people of various linguistic backgrounds to serve, and the sheer size of the event requires multiple groups and community sponsorships. However, it should be noted that since the Filipino language employs grammar similar to Spanish grammar, foreign-born Filipino American nurses are actually able to rudimentarily converse in more than just English and Tagalog. This allows them to work with many other groups.

The difference here is not necessarily impact but scope. Foreign-born Indian Americans are making a broader impact on the community through their parish health fairs. However, it is happening with a significantly smaller scope and in parish churches that largely do not serve a diverse population outside of Christians from Kerala or other Indian American Christian immigrants. This is not to say that foreign-born Indian American nurses are not making an impact outside of their parish health fairs. They are. As we have seen, they are drawn into projects and volunteering opportunities well beyond their own churches, including working with or coordinating events and projects with others. In some cases, this may mean bringing the health fair to the community rather than the community to the fair.

On one occasion, for example, INA found out through one of their members that Nepali and Bhutanese refugees who had just arrived in Houston were in dire need of medical assistance. After a few quick calls and an emergency drive for supplies, the nurses put together a health clinic for the refugees at the apartments that they had been assigned. Describing how it all came together, Sheila, a foreign-born Indian American nurse in her mid-fifties, pointed out, "They don't have anything. . . . You know, they have some kind of help through the government, but they don't have insurance, so we go, we have to help. Our providers, like nurse practitioners, PAs [physician assistants], some doctors from the VA went. It was a rush, but we are going to do it again next year." Pausing for a moment, she then added, "We gave them medications, we did the health check, the doctors check them. The nurses do the initial screening, and we give them medications. We give some money, not a lot, but we give them some things, like they collected used clothes, and we gave [the clothes] to them. Whatever it takes, wherever the need, we make it happen. I mean, God really is the one that makes it happen. We just need to do the work, continue to fight for people's health when the government is not there to do it." And fight they do, not just through their health projects but wherever they see that their voices and actions are needed most.

Righteous Indignation

Volunteering and philanthropy are not the only ways in which the foreign-born nurses in this study try to make a difference in their communities. Unusual circumstances such as the VA scandal (of 2014) in which patients died waiting to get appointments at the VA,[36] also compel them to take unlikely actions, including engaging in various forms of political activism that they would not ordinarily consider. The emergence of details and circumstances surrounding the scandal, even several years after the fact, changed the nature and tone of the conversations foreign-born nurses had with me, as well as the places we met to talk. These conversations were angry, fueled by what could only be described as righteous indignation, and the nurses were looking for an outlet to express their frustrations. For better or worse, I became that outlet.

After answering an unidentified call on my cell phone, one nurse, for example, stated, "Forgive me for interrupting your day, my name is [Agnes]. I am a nurse at the VA, and one of my fellow nurses said that you were looking to talk to people about the hospital. I would like to talk to you. I'm so angry. . . . I can't stand silent. God as my witness, someone needs to hear what I have to say. When can you meet me?" Although I explained that the main focus of my study was not the scandal, Agnes, a foreign-born Indian American nurse, said she still wanted to talk and agreed to meet me at her home the next morning, after her night shift at the hospital.

After I arrived at the home, Agnes invited me in, offered me a cup of hot chai (tea) and then sat down to talk. "Before you ask me any questions, I need to say something." She then blurted out "I think I am known for standing up. Maybe when something happens, but a lot of time, I was looked upon as, oh yeah, she's the whistleblower, she's the bad guy, okay, and so that shuts people [off] from doing anything further. So, it's time that they did something, uh, something [is] wrong with the VA. So, if you want to call it bad press or call it a scandal it's time that somebody did something. . . . You don't understand how much I pray over this."

Agnes was visibly upset. Asked if she wanted to end the interview, she stated "no," and then apologized for displaying her emotions. "I'm pretty stoic at work. So, I'm sorry. You see, so all this mess [the scandal], it's not our fault. God knows we do our best for these veterans. It's the system." After calming down a bit and taking a few more sips of chai, Agnes tried to articulate her frustrations more clearly. "Unfortunately, the veterans themselves want to continue to keep the VA system because they want to call something their own, which I can understand. I personally would give them health insurance so they can go to any hospital, but if they want to keep the VA for themselves, the least we can do is fix it so that it's the best care anywhere." As Agnes continued to explain her personal vison for a better VA system, she pointed out, "We are morally obligated to do better, but either way the nurses will remain. . . . I try to do all I can at the hospital, but I also understand that it is not enough. That's why I'm so involved in the community. Somewhere between working inside and outside the system, I pray things will change."

Two weeks or so after speaking to Agnes, I received a call from another foreign-born Filipina American nurse who works at the VA. Like Agnes, Tess, a foreign-born Filipina American, sought me out after talking to other foreign-born nurses who had spoken to me. Agreeing to meet at a local bakery, Tess, like Agnes, was concerned about talking publicly about her experiences at the hospital. When I arrived at the bakery, Tess was already sitting and waiting for me at a table next to the kitchen. "Thank you for meeting with me. I apologize for meeting you here," Tess stated. I had never conducted an interview in a bakery or near a noisy kitchen before, but I told Tess that I was happy that she agreed to talk with me and made the best I could out of the unusual circumstances.

"I know you have many questions, but I need to get something off my chest before we begin," Tess stated. She then explained, "Everything you read and see [about the VA] is true, so true. It's not just Phoenix, it's the whole damn system nationwide. Held together by a thread and now it's finally out for all to see what we already knew." As in my conversation with Agnes, I explained to Tess that my study was not about the scandal, to which she emphatically suggested, "Well, it should be. If you are a God-fearing person you will tell the world what I am telling you. I can't say anything, I'm too afraid, but you must speak for us. It's your moral duty. I want everyone to know that it's not us that's the problem. It's the system. . . . It's the way the hospital does things."

When I asked Tess to explain what she meant by this statement, she suggested, "We [VA hospital] wouldn't stay open if we were like [another hospital] or something but it's the government. Maybe they should just give the veterans the option to go public with their own insurance? Something has to change.

For example, they hire nurses, they hire doctors, and they hire more doctors who just stay there for a few years and leave because they start their own practice." Questioned about why this was a problem, Tess explained, "The VA has a lot of funding, that's why doctors are getting everything that they want. They get millions and millions of dollars that they can use for equipment, and that's why there is a lot of equipment that is ordered and sometimes they don't even use it." Tess was visibly angry.

Apologizing for her outbursts, Tess then attempted to explain why she was so angry. "If we are going to keep making wars, then we will keep having veterans who need care. So, you can't do this. I am so sick [of this]." Summarizing her concerns, Tess added, "Look, I'm sorry. We nurses can do all we can, but in the end the system needs to change. As much as I love the VA, maybe it's time to give veterans freedom to go to other hospitals? They fight to protect us and then come home to subpar care. Is that right? I ask you, is that right? I don't think so. Half these wars are not even worth fighting but [are] about oil and egos. Working at the VA has really changed the way I see our country at war." After apologizing again, Tess, exclaimed,

> Yes, I'm angry. That doesn't mean I'm any less of a Christian. Ask yourself, when did Jesus get angry? Remember when he went after the money changers in the temple? That's what we need to do at the VA, but we are afraid to speak up too much. So yes, I'm so thankful to talk to you, but to be honest, this is why you see us [nurses] doing so much in the community. . . . We do what we can in the hospital and then take it to the streets. If I have to knock on the front door of the White House, I will. . . . You realize that our healthcare system is not even as good as what we have back in the Philippines? And we're [the Philippines] supposed to be a third-world country. Think about that the next time you go vote."

Agnes and Tess were not alone in expressing their frustration. Most of the foreign-born nurses I interviewed shared their views in one way or another, but many were also afraid to talk to an outsider, and perhaps rightfully so. The VA nationally leads all federal agencies in the number of whistleblowers who say they have been retaliated against—up to 40 percent annually, according to federal testimony.[37] For this reason, many nurses were not as blunt as Agnes or Tess, even two or more years after the scandal.

However, what they did share demonstrated a clear and compelling concern for veterans and others, a concern driven by a stated belief that God expects them to not only be angry in the face of perceived injustices but do something about it.[38] Coco, for example, a foreign-born Indian American nurse who has worked at the VA for over five years, explained, "God understands our [nurses] rage, but he expects us to do something about [it]. The VA survives because of us. We need the government to help us, but until that day comes, this country and its veterans must depend on our care. When we can't get what we need done in the hospital, there's always a way in the community with some project or at the ballot box. . . . [pausing] I don't understand why so few Americans vote. It's a privilege you really shouldn't waste, you know? I am surprised, but looking back it also shocks me, some of the things I've done to make it right! I don't really think of myself as one of those activists." Expressing a similar sentiment, Dali, a foreign-born Filipina American nurse who has worked at the VA for over ten years, added in another interview, "The politicians don't see what we do, and they aren't the ones fighting [wars] either. If you don't vote, you let them dictate things, and they don't know anything about veterans or community health. Healthcare in this country is a mess."

Although politics was often the last thing foreign-born nurses in this study wanted to talk about, much of their community action might be seen as political or having political ramifications. From Melody and other foreign-born Filipina American nurses who write to their congressional representatives about veteran concerns, with some even supporting marches for the recognition of Filipino veterans of WWII, to Agnes and other foreign-born Indian American nurses who have spoken out about veteran concerns, all are fully aware of their voices and rights as American citizens. Whether it is through an act of protest and defiance or through simply voting by their conscience, they say they feel obligated to act not only as citizens but good Catholics. This is what they believe God asks them to do. They also state that they believe it is their patriotic duty to give back to the country that they believe has given so much to them.

An overwhelming majority of the foreign-born nurses in this study (89.4 percent) indicated on surveys that they voted in the 2012 presidential election.[39] As in volunteerism and philanthropy, this percentage far exceeds the national average. In the 2016 presidential election, for example, roughly 61 percent of eligible adult Americans voted.[40] Add to this the fact that only 49 percent of eligible adult Asian Americans voted in that same election, and it becomes clear that the foreign-born nurses in this study, the majority of whom identified as Asian on their last U.S. census questionnaire are doing more than just talking about the community problems that concern them the most.[41] The question is, Why? By now, it should come as no surprise that it is their Catholic faith that compels them, whether it is at the ballot box or, as we have seen, in working on numerous community projects.

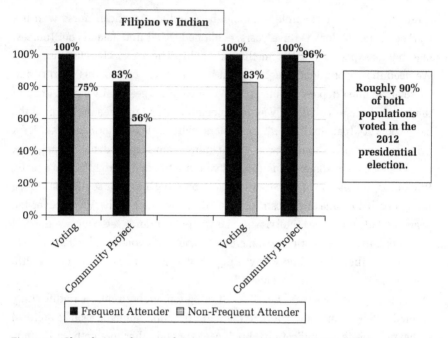

Figure 6.3 Church Attendance and Civic Engagement for Foreign-Born Nurses. Source: Stephen M. Cherry, Foreign-Born Nurse Survey (2015).

As figure 6.3 suggests, foreign-born Filipino and Indian American nurses who are frequent attendees of Mass at their parish churches (weekly or more, not including weddings and funerals) are significantly more likely to vote (100 percent) compared to their peers who only attend a few times a year or less (75 percent of Filipinos and 83 percent of Indians). They are also more likely to work on a community project, the top domain of their volunteerism—and significantly more so in the case of Filipino Americans (83 percent versus 56 percent). Indian Americans who attend Mass more frequently were more likely to work on a community project (100 percent frequent attenders versus 96 percent who are not frequent attenders, although this is not a statistically significant difference). The fact that foreign-born Indian American church attendance does not have a significant impact may be attributed to several factors. First, foreign-born Indian American church attendance is actually higher than foreign-born Filipino Americans' attendance (84 percent versus 77 percent), and thus there is less variance. Second, this could be a product of the size of their ethnic churches and the number of health fairs that their parishes are able to host. No significant differences between Filipino and Indian American nurses' other reported top domains—professional and charitable organizations—were found. Mass attendance also does not appear to impact these other domains. Although this is not charted in figure 6.3, it is important to note that being a member of a prayer group or Bible study group, either one affiliated with their church or an independent group, did have an impact on foreign-born nurses' civic engagement. Foreign-born Filipino Americans who are members of these groups are significantly more likely to vote than those who aren't members (100 percent versus 75 percent), and foreign-born Indian American members are likewise slightly more likely to vote (100 percent versus 94 percent, not a statistically significant difference). However, being a member of these groups did not impact foreign-born nurses' likelihood of working on a community project.[42]

Taken in the context of the more qualitative and ethnographic data presented throughout this chapter, these findings seem to further indicate that getting involved in their parish churches is actually beneficial to foreign-born nurses' civic life. This is despite the findings of other studies, which suggest that messages of community service may not be conveyed well to Asian Americans by the Catholic church.[43] Far from being sequestered to ethnic enclaves or absorbed in their own community concerns, foreign-born Filipino and Indian American nurses are engaged in a host of community projects and concerns beyond their own, because they believe their faith calls on them as a part of the Catholic family to do so. They say they are morally bound not just as Catholics but as American Catholics and believe they that have a responsibility to act on their faith.

Conclusion

Over the last decade both scholars and social pundits alike have increasingly questioned how immigrants will contribute or give back to the United States. The answer, at least for the foreign-born Filipino and Indian American nurses in this study, is quite clear. They not only report giving back but do so at rates that far exceed those of the average American. Likewise, their nursing associations are actively and visibly present in helping people across the Houston metropolitan area. Amid an alarming rise in xenophobic sentiments and attitudes, the foreign-born nurses in this study have built rather robust civic lives that impact the wider communities in which they live, including in some cases the very people who may question their increasing presence in the country. These nurses see themselves not only as good citizens but as good Catholics. And they are acting on it. However, as we have seen, this is somewhat puzzling given that some studies suggest that American Catholics, especially immigrants, participate less in civic life or no differently than people of other religious traditions even though Catholic institutions and teachings appear to support a very communitarian ethic.

Echoing classic arguments that the Catholic church actually inhibits the ability of American Catholics to acquire civic skills, many scholars of religion and civic life continue to suggest that despite changes in Catholic culture since the Second Vatican Council, the locus of moral authority within the Church remains highly centralized and does not allow Catholics to get democratically involved in their local parishes.[44] They suggest that this explains why Catholics reportedly have a lower sense of civic efficacy compared to Protestants that may negatively impact their ability and desire to work in the wider community. Looking specifically at the case of Asian American Catholics, some scholars have also suggested that Asian American Catholics, including those who are foreign born, not only participate less in their communities compared to Asian American Protestants but are faced with other internal concerns or barriers that limit their community life.[45] But if this is indeed the case, what are we to make of the foreign-born Filipino and Indian American nurses in this study? Although comparative Protestant analyses lie beyond the scope of my current data, this study suggests that foreign-born nurses are getting involved in the wider community, and it is because of their Catholic faith, not in spite of it.

The parish churches that many foreign-born Indian American nurses in this study attend are largely ethnic churches, and hence smaller in scope and reach compared to the larger, more multi-ethnic Roman Catholic churches that most foreign-born Filipino American nurses attend. As a result, much of their community volunteerism is for their fellow coethnics from Kerala or other Syro-Malabar and Syro-Malankara East Syriac rite Catholics. However, this has clearly not prevented them from getting involved in a host of community projects that are outside of their community, including health fairs for Nepali and Bhutanese refugees and the homeless at Star of Hope Mission. Like their fellow foreign-born Filipino American nursing peers, foreign-born Indian American nurses are compelled by their Catholic faith to act and help those in need—extending care to the community wherever they can.

Starting with the messages of divine love and stewardship they receive from their priest in weekly homilies or in discussions during Bible study, the foreign-born nurses in this study, as we have seen, say that they take these words to heart and use them as a guide for how they believe all Americans should care for one another. When Carol says that she has taken an oath to give care to all she can and then questions what kind of Christian she would be if she did not act on that oath, she is not alone in expressing these views. The overwhelming majority of the nurses I interviewed share this sentiment in one way or another. They have a unique understanding of community, one that they say is driven by a belief in faith in action. Inspired and motivated by this, they always seem to find the time and the resources to help others, regardless of public sentiment about new immigrants or any other barriers that might get in the way of their community goals.

The majority of the foreign-born nurses I interviewed, while fully cognizant of increasing anti-immigrant attitudes or fears, including those held by some of their patients and coworkers, are not necessarily trying to prove fears wrong. Their impetus, as they describe it, comes from a higher power. They state that they are doing what they believe is right—God's will—with no stated expectations or reported desire for recognition. Although this (a pious person) may be how they want to consciously be seen, they are actively and visibly present in their communities regardless of how they describe their motivations. The majority of them, as we have seen, are not even all that aware of all that they have accomplished in the community until they are asked to sit down and think about it. When they do acknowledge it in interviews, listing one community project after another from the active community calendars of their nursing associations, they often admit to being perplexed by how they have managed to find the time and resources.

In the decades since political scientists such as Robert Putnam first questioned what killed American civic engagement in the last third of the twentieth century, the civic engagement of the foreign-born Filipino and Indian American nurses described in this chapter reminds us that immigrants are a vital and active part of American civil society today.[46] Given the fact that many Americans, even a majority depending on the racial or ethnic group you specify, do not vote in national elections, do not volunteer, and do not give money to charitable causes, the civic engagement of foreign-born Filipino and Indian American nurses in this study is vibrant by comparison. It is also clearly connected to the traditional social structures such as voluntary associations and the church that some scholars once feared were in atrophy.[47]

Being a nurse, a degreed professional, and working at the VA also play a significant role in bridging resources to the wider community, as Rose and Sarah point out in the opening pages of this chapter. Foreign-born nurses have numerous skills, talents, and resources that they say they do not want to waste. As such, their education and resources are an equally powerful predictor of their volunteerism, but, as we have also seen, this does not account for their motivations to act, which they state are driven by their ardent Catholic faith.

For all the public and political contention surrounding immigration today, foreign-born nurses, at least in this study, not only are helping to mitigate perennial American nursing shortages but also appear to be more involved in their communities than the average American. Although the present data do not allow for a comparison between the civic lives of foreign-born nurses and their American-born peers—perhaps all nurses regardless of nativity are more engaged than the average American—it is clear that foreign-born Filipino and Indian American nurses in this study not only want to be seen as patriotic nurses and good Catholics but are attempting to carve out a place for themselves in the new American story.[48] In doing so, they seek to change or at least challenge any xenophobic fears or concerns some people may have of them in the process.

The next chapter explores the implications of this study in the context of political and popular concerns over the ongoing American healthcare crisis. By all indications, nursing shortages are not coming to an end anytime soon. As these shortages remain or worsen, and as the nation continues to age, further increasing the need for more nurses, foreign-born nurses appear to have a role to play, but their recruitment and increasing presence often runs contrary to many popular sentiments and concerns over immigration. Engaging this contradiction, the conclusion of the book summarizes the major arguments and evidence presented in previous chapters and weighs in on what a study of foreign-born Filipino and Indian American Catholic nurses working at a VA hospital tells us not only about the future of American healthcare and the roles that immigrants might play but about the ways in which these nurses are helping to shape an ever-changing country.

Chapter 7

Who Will Care for America?

Once a month for the last several years, an unlikely group of nurses and nurse managers from the VA, some retired, and many nearing retirement, gather at a local restaurant to eat lunch, celebrate birthdays, and talk about everything from family to the latest happenings at the hospital. Regardless of where they meet, the small group that gathers changes from month to month depending on who is available. Most nurse retirees tend to make every lunch. On the one occasion that I joined, the group was held at a local barbeque joint. I had already interviewed many of those who gathered that day. People smiled with nods of acknowledgment or greetings and handshakes as I took a seat at the end of the large table. "I see many of you know Dr. Cherry," Susana, a retired foreign-born Indian American nurse manager, stated from the head of the table. She continued, "I hope you all don't mind that I invited him to join us. He's studying foreign-born nurses at the VA, and I thought our little group might give him something to think about."

Looking around the table, I watched people seated closely together make room for each other, twelve including me. I sat at the only open seat, which was next to two foreign-born Filipina American nurses. Turning to my left, I asked Janel, a foreign-born Filipina American nurse who was about to retire from the hospital, how the lunch group got started. "It was [Susana]. You know she use[d] to be our manager, right? When she retired she started this group." When I asked Janel how she joined the group, she stated, "To be honest, I don't remember. I think someone dragged me here. You know I didn't really get along well with [Susana]. She was really harsh with me, but then I figured out that's just how she is." Janel then added rather emphatically, "It made me a better nurse. However, at the time I didn't care for her at all. Not at all! I thought maybe she didn't like Filipinos. I couldn't have been more wrong. She just wanted the best of me, and I ended up giving it to her. Then the first time I came to the lunch group, she gave me a cake for my birthday. I couldn't believe she remembered. You see, she really does love us."

As Janel excused herself to go to the restroom, Darcy, a retired White nurse who was sitting across from us, added in a near whisper, "That's funny what [Janel] said. I felt the same way at one time, but I got to tell you, I always thought [Susana] favored the Filipinos. . . . They can be so cliquish. So, I didn't really like [Susana] for that, and if I'm being honest I didn't really get along that much with [Janel] either, not that she wasn't a damn good nurse. Still is. Well, I guess you can see we all got over that." In an interview the next day, Eliza, the foreign-born Indian American nurse who still works at the hospital that we met in chapter 3, confessed that Janel and Darcy were not alone in the feelings they expressed. "I think we all originally fought over turf and who was the best, you know, issues of pride and place, but in the end, I think we all wanted the same thing. I like to think of it as if we're answering God's call or some higher purpose. That's why we serve American veterans to the best of our ability. I think that's what we've done, and that's why it matters so much."

Many of those who gathered at the restaurant shared these sentiments with me either in front of those they were sitting next to or later in private interviews. Susana was well aware of our conversations. Tapping her fork on the side of her water glass to get our attention, Susana stated with a commanding yet compassionate tone,

> You see Dr. Cherry, I started this group because I missed my hospital extended family when I retired. We have our differences, as I'm sure you've heard [laughing from my end of the table], but we are family now. When my husband passed away, they were there for me. When my mom passed away, they were there for me. When I was sick, they were there for me. We have been through so much together. Remember the night of Hurricane Rita? [everyone moaning in acknowledgment] We have shared so much of our lives while at work that I wanted to keep us together. I wanted to celebrate birthdays, celebrate our lives, and enjoy a meal without having to rush back to work, well for most of us anyhow [laughing]. It's also good to just talk about the hospital. God knows it's always on my mind or in the news!

"You can say that again," Rosie, a foreign-born Filipina American nurse in her late fifties who still works at the VA, added to me as others continued their own conversations. She then exclaimed, "[Susana] is right, we're family. I don't know what we would do without each other. I look forward to retiring, but I'm sad to say that I'm not real[ly] sure I should. Who is going to care for our veterans when we leave? Maybe I should just put in a few more years until the VA can figure this mess out?" Later that day, Darcy commented on her own recent retirement during an interview at her home. "I get why so many people at lunch are worried about retiring. I felt guilty too. Who's going to replace us?"

Back at the restaurant, Lucy, the foreign-born Filipina American nurse who still works at the VA that we met in chapter 1, pulled on my arm and stated, "I know we've talked so much already, but you need to hear this again . . . what happens when I retire in the next five to ten years? We nurses can do all we can, but in the end the system needs to change. I love the VA, but maybe it's time to give veterans freedom to go to other hospitals?" As words of agreement that changes were desperately needed at the VA echoed around the table that day in one conversation after another, Rosie interjected on the side, "But when they [veterans] get there [non-VA hospitals and clinics] they will still find that those hospitals need more nurses, and we [foreign-born] are the ones who will be taking the jobs because no one else will. The shortages [nursing] aren't ending. It's all about demand and no supply, so it's an immigration issue . . . and don't get me started on that messy politics. No one wants us but everyone needs us!"

The conversations at lunch never got too heated. Many chose to ignore the debates and talk about family or simply eat their food. Susana also did her best to bring the conversation back to lighter topics. Despite the seriousness of some discussions, all of the nurses genuinely seemed to enjoy being together. As the cakes and other desserts to celebrate birthdays arrived at the table, singing and a real jovial spirit spread among the nurses. I knew they had their differences—many had bluntly made sure I was aware of these—but, in this moment, they seemed like a family.

The following week I sat down with Sally, the foreign-born Indian American nurse in her early fifties we met in chapter 3, at her home and asked her if she had anything to add to our conversation from lunch. Visibly more serious than at lunch, she stated, "Let me say this. God as my witness, we [foreign-born] nurses are not the problem at the VA. We are the solution. They all know this, but that doesn't mean they like it. Nurses are the only ones who will defend these veterans. We were the first whistleblowers. Through all the bureaucratic lies and failures, we stand with the veterans. Not once did you see a foreign-born nurse [make] the news for not doing her job." Pausing for a moment, Sally rhetorically asked, "If we [foreign-born nurses] did not work there, who would?" Answering her own question with another question, she remarked, "You have to ask yourself who stays and who goes. . . . Seriously, ask yourself, after all we experience and go through at the VA, who in their right mind would stay if they didn't flat out love these veterans? Truth is, we love them and this country. We were called to this. That's the real story you need to get out in your research."

The Future of American Veteran Care

Sally was clearly not alone in expressing concerns about the future of veteran care, nor was she the only nurse in the "lunch bunch" to suggest that the VA continues to face considerable challenges. Her concerns resonated across most of the discussions I had with the lunch bunch nurses, both foreign born and American born, and were overwhelmingly echoed throughout my interviews with their peers in one form or another. It was and is a seemingly universal concern but one not without historical precedent. As we saw in chapter 3, scandal, controversy, and veterans care have gone hand in hand since the founding of this country. The 2014 scandal was not the last incident in this trend. In the last several years, the VA has improperly canceled tens of thousands of orders for veterans' diagnostic medical tests without explanation, required thousands of unwarranted reexaminations for veterans receiving disability benefits, and seen its secretary fired for supposedly getting the federal government to arrange and pay for his personal summer vacation to Europe with his wife.[1] And these are just a few examples. When Susana suggested that the hospital was always in the news, she was not exaggerating.

After each new incident or scandal, a period of highly publicized outrage is typically followed by new leadership and a promise to do better. Since President Trump took office in 2016, the Department of Veterans Affairs has had five secretaries, including the current secretary, who has served twice, first as the acting head amid a scathing audit of veterans care and now as the full-time head of the VA. Although the current secretary has vowed to make changes and introduce further reform, he readily admits that the VA currently faces a number of daunting and complex challenges. Among the most pressing of these challenges is a severe staffing shortage. There are currently over forty-nine thousand vacant VA staff openings across the country, the majority of which are nursing vacancies.[2] Like private and public hospitals, the VA desperately needs more nurses, especially experienced nurses with advanced degrees and training. It is a seemingly endless problem, further complicated, as we have seen, by the fact that the VA is not your typical hospital and veterans are not your average patients. However, beyond this reality, the VA's nursing shortages are not due solely to a lack of qualified applicants but to competition with the private and public sector. There is a widening understanding, one acknowledged by the Government Accountability Office (GAO), that many nurses may be able to find more satisfying jobs elsewhere and get paid better or at the least, find better opportunities to advance in their careers in an environment that is less stressful and more supportive than the VA.

Despite these compounding barriers to nursing recruitment and retention, the foreign-born nurses in this study are making the VA their carrier, and service to American veterans their life's work. They believe that they are an invaluable part of the VA hospital. They feel empowered by the opportunities nursing has given them but also see nursing as a calling, a belief in Catholic faith in action and a patriotic duty to serve their adopted country. This is the so-called real story Sally alludes to during her interview. She, like her fellow foreign-born nurses, do not see themselves as part of the larger problems facing the VA but the solution—an impassioned last line of defense for veterans care and larger veteran concerns. They love their patients and embrace them as extensions of their own family, but, as so many nurses in the lunch bunch lamented, what happens when they retire? Who will replace them? These are good questions with no simple answers.

According to the GAO, roughly 30 percent of VA employees who were on staff as of 2017 will approach retirement age by 2022.[3] This does not mean that they will actually retire. Some, like Lucy and Rosie, might stay on longer, but if they do retire en masse they will add to an already growing staffing crisis. Since the GAO started tracking staffing shortages in 2018, nothing the government or the Veterans Administration has done—and it has attempted to do a lot—has solved the problem. All indications suggest that the problem is going to get worse, much worse, and very soon. What is the long-term solution? To this point, the government has explored or enacted two options: changing the VA system and the way it approaches and manages veterans care, and providing additional incentives to recruit new nurses.

In 2018, President Trump signed the VA Mission Act into law in an attempt to help veterans receive healthcare faster and closer to their homes. It replaced the often poorly funded Veterans' Choice Program (VCP) with the new Veteran Community Care program.[4] According to the VA Secretary, the new program will make it easier for veterans to get care through an expanded list of private-sector healthcare providers.[5] Critics of the legislation, including former VA secretary David Shulkin, worry about privatizing veterans care not only because of its effect on comprehensive care at the VA but also because community providers are "ill-prepared to treat the high volume of veterans expected to be pushed to the private sector."[6] Part of the reason that the private sector is so ill prepared is that, like the VA, it is under staffed. The nursing shortage crisis is universal. As such, the Veteran Community Care program is not necessarily an improvement nor is it what Lucy and her fellow lunch bunch nurses had in mind when they suggested that veterans be given the freedom to go to other hospitals.

According to the U.S. Bureau of Labor Statistics, American healthcare will need over two hundred and three thousand new nurses each year through 2026 to fill its current vacancies—and this does not include emerging needs with COVID-19, the privatization of veteran care, or the projected one million nurses expected to retire by 2030.[7] It also does not account for the nearly eighty thousand nurses expected to leave healthcare in the next few years for non-nursing jobs or those who are not retiring but expected to leave the paid workforce altogether.[8] California is expected to face the largest shortage, followed by Texas.[9] As we might expect, understaffed hospitals often create higher patient loads, reduce the amount of time a nurse can spend with any given patient, and, most importantly, can increase patient readmission rates and mortality.[10] All of these are outcomes the VA is desperately trying to avoid. The VA cannot afford another scandal. Any new scandals would not only further tarnish the hospital's reputation but negatively impact its ongoing attempts to recruit new nurses.[11]

Thus far, nursing incentives have done very little to solve the VA's recruitment and retention problems. At the same time, the VA, like the public sector in general, is increasingly aware that American nursing school enrollment has begun to level off. Although it remains to be seen how interest in nursing as a profession will be fully impacted by the COVID-19 pandemic or how the pandemic will force changes in federal support for nursing programs,[12] there is little doubt that healthcare workers are leaving their jobs at alarming rates. As we saw in chapter 1, about one in five healthcare workers has left their job since the pandemic started.[13] The U.S. Bureau of Labor Statistics estimates that American healthcare has lost roughly half-a-million workers since February 2020. This includes nurses.[14] If staffing shortages continue as projected or even worsen, it should come as no surprise that many healthcare policy leaders today are once again encouraging Congress to look at new ways of changing or amending American immigration laws to import more care to help mitigate these shortages.

In a rare moment of bipartisan agreement, the House of Representatives passed (365–65) the Fairness for Higher-Skilled Immigration Act (H.R. 1044, 2020).[15] Recognizing that the current 7 percent per-country rule for granting green cards does not consider that different countries obviously have different populations with different skill sets, the House bill sought to remove per-country caps for family-based green cards by increasing the numeric limitation to 15 percent. It also sought to completely eliminate caps from employment-based green cards.[16] This ostensibly would reduce backlogs for many foreign nationals who have just become eligible to apply for green cards after initiating the process some ten to twelve years ago. As such, the legislation appears to be an improvement over the current system. However, there is one exception: nurses—especially Filipino nurses.

The Fairness for Higher-Skilled Immigration Act potentially disadvantages nurses because it is often difficult for nurses to obtain H-1B visas. In addition to the suspension of or added obstacles created for H-1B visas by President Trump, H-1Bs are contingent on a bachelor's or higher degree, and many countries do not require these degrees for a typical registered nurse position. Consequently, a nurse may not be able to get employment sponsorship where they are most needed because they are overqualified. Even when this is not the case, the House bill, as originally written, would increase green-card wait times for many foreign-born nurses to over eight years. Since the House legislation is largely aimed at relieving green-card backlogs, it would essentially allow Chinese and Indian citizens seeking to immigrate to move to the front of the line, given that they are the top applicants. Eight-five percent of available green cards, for example, would go to Chinese and Indian applicants in the first year, and then 90 percent would go to them in the second and third years.[17] This would effectively lock out Filipino nurses, although the Philippines, as we have seen, is by far the largest source of nursing immigration to the United States.

Concerned with these potential barriers, several senators urged that the bill be amended to include a provision that would allow five thousand foreign-born nurses to immigrate to the United States per year for the next decade on temporary visas.[18] The amendment did not receive much support, and subsequent amendments that included provisions for occupations such as nursing that are experiencing shortages later failed. No new bills have moved forward. Although many in Congress acknowledge the need for foreign-born nurses or see the bill as a viable means to mitigate perennial shortages, immigration remains a highly contentious and divisive issue.[19] How much traction any future bill makes remains to be seen. In the meantime, what should the country do? More importantly, and beyond our immediate crisis and current political climate, what should be done that is in the best long-term interests of American healthcare?

Although there is considerable debate about the causes of the current American nursing shortage and the degree to which the international recruitment of nurses is the solution or even part of the solution, it is clear that foreign-born nurses' presence, despite these debates, continues to grow. Foreign-born nurse recruitment has not slowed, and this does not look like it will change anytime soon. However, many nursing leaders, as we saw in chapter 1, continue to suggest that importing foreign-born nurses does not address larger and more serious workplace problems that are driving native-born Americans away from nursing. They also fear that continually drawing nurses away from foreign countries will create staffing shortages in their home communities. This might temporarily provide a short-term solution that serves the interest of the American hospital industry but does not necessarily serve the long-term interest of patients or create better incentives and work conditions for all nurses in the United States or in the countries that foreign-born nurses leave. It is a complicated problem, one that is not just about needs and economics but ethics as well.

Historically, foreign-born nurses appear to have played an important role in helping to mitigate American nursing shortages over the last several decades, but many still ask, At what cost? Immigrants currently make up roughly 14 percent of the American population, but 16 percent of all registered nurses and 22 percent of all nursing assistants are foreign born. Despite popular sentiments to the contrary, as we saw in chapter 4, they do not appear to negatively impact long-term American nursing wages and employment but in fact report making less than their American-born peers and are a part of the VA's high employment turnover.[20] They are also not radically different than their American-born peers in terms of their technical ability and their larger values of normative professional practices. Rather than only evaluating the costs of imported care—an important issue that demands further research—this study has also pointed to the case for evaluating the potential benefits. As the United States continues to change demographically, foreign-born nurses are not just filling jobs but dedicating themselves to meaningful careers that increasingly serve American healthcare's diverse needs.[21]

Changing Nation Made Better by Importing Care?

The United States is in the midst of one of its greatest demographic revolutions. By 2050, if not sooner, the United States is expected to become a majority-minority population with no single racial or ethnic group constituting the clear majority of the country. Evidence of this change can already be seen across the country. From 2000 to 2018, for example, one hundred and nine counties in twenty-two states, representing roughly 99 percent of the American population, went from majority White to majority non-White.[22] Although Whites remain the single largest racial or ethnic group in the country, and likely will be for some time, it is clear that the face of America is literally and rapidly chang-ing.[23] Much of this expected demographic change is a direct result of increased immigration since 1965. New immigrants come from a greater variety of coun-tries than previous eras and thus have significantly increased the number of non-White racial and ethnic minorities in the United States.[24]

By 2060, the percentage of the American population that is foreign born is projected to rise from where it is today, from roughly 14 percent to at least 17 percent—higher than the record percentage of immigrants set in 1890.[25] One of the groups propelling this change is Asian Americans.[26] From 2000 to 2015, the Asian American population grew 72 percent, a net gain of roughly eight million people, largely due to continued migration.[27] Asians now account for roughly one quarter of all immigrants who have arrived in the United States since 1965.[28] If this growth continues as projected, Asian Americans will even-tually become the country's largest immigrant group. Among the groups respon-sible for these gains are Filipino and Indian Americans who already represent the fourth- and third-largest immigrant populations in the country, respectively.[29] One of the major reasons for their increasing presence in the country, as we have seen, is the perennial American healthcare staffing shortage.

This trend, and our increasing reliance on foreign-born nurses to meet grow-ing healthcare needs, may have several possible long-term consequences, none of which appear to threaten the employment of American-born healthcare workers or those hoping to go into the field.[30] Obviously, the United States needs to educate, recruit, and retain more American-born healthcare profes-sionals, but the overall impact of foreign-born healthcare workers on wages is rather short-term at worst. Although the arrival of foreign-born nurses during any given staffing shortage initially reduces wages for all nurses because foreign-born nurses are often willing to work for less than American-born nurses, the repeated cycle of shortages over the long-term typically drives wages up because there are not enough foreign-born nurses to meet American needs and higher wages are often the only way to incentivize Americans to go into nurs-ing.[31] Foreign-born nurses are not the problem but their impact on nursing in America is more important than just wages. In the long term, an increasingly diverse country will produce a growing number of diverse patients who in turn will have increasingly diverse needs.[32] In light of this, the increased presence of foreign-born doctors and nurses in the country may allow American health-care to better serve these diverse populations in several important ways.

First, research suggests, as we saw in chapter 4, that patients prefer health-care providers who look like them or come from the same communities and cultural backgrounds. The demographic characteristics of a primary doctor or nurse, particularly their race and ethnicity, matter a great deal to patients at the point of care. It also shapes their overall perception and satisfaction with that care. Although these preferences can complicate the interactions between foreign-born nurses and American veterans, we must keep in mind that the majority of the problems that patients raised in this study were in cases where a lack of racial concordance occurred because there were no American-born, White nurses to address the complaints of White veterans. This circumstance of not having enough White nurses is the inverse of most cases in the literature where the key problem has been presented as not having enough diverse healthcare workers, including nurses, to meet the needs of racial and ethnic minority patients. Too few White nurses, in the case of the VA is still a problem, as we have seen from veteran complaints in previous chapters, but it is a challenge that is lessening as the country becomes more diverse.

A diverse country increasingly has a more diverse military. In 2004, roughly 36 percent of active-duty military were Black, Hispanic, Asian, or some other non-White racial or ethnic group.[33] By 2017, the share of active-duty military who were non-Hispanic White had fallen, while racial and ethnic minorities grew to roughly 43 percent of those serving.[34] This does not address the problem of a lack of White nurses available to serve White veterans if requested, but it does point to a time when White veterans, and hence White VA patients, may no longer be the majority. This is obviously not unique to the VA hospital but something that will impact all of American healthcare as the country becomes more racially and ethnically diverse.

Second, greater racial concordance between patients and their care providers in an increasingly diverse country may promote greater understanding of the social, cultural, and economic factors that influence patients, as well as the health concerns and diseases that are more prevalent in their communities. In turn, this may also foster greater trust and thus improve communication.[35] Obviously, the growing presence of foreign-born Filipino and Indian American nurses and other coethnic healthcare providers will not increase racial concordance for Black and Hispanic patients. However, research suggests that these populations are more trusting of racial- and ethnic-minority care providers than those who are White.[36] Therefore, communication should potentially get better, not worse, with an increase in the number of foreign-born healthcare providers serving them over time. We should also note, however, that the nurses in this study suggest that any problematic circumstances that arise as a result of their race or nativity are a rare occurrence, not the daily norm. They say that their patients overwhelmingly love them, and studies suggest that foreign-born nurses from India and the Philippines are in general sincere, patient centered, caring, and compassionate in their approaches.[37] Although more research is needed, foreign-born Filipino and Indian American nurses appear to be more than capable of serving all patients, regardless of their background. Racial concordance may be the ideal but not always possible.

Third, and related to the previous points, 22 percent of Americans, roughly sixty-seven million people, now speak a language other than English at home.[38] From 2010 to 2017 the largest percentage increases of people speaking a foreign language were seen among those using Indian languages—Gujarati (up 22 percent), Hindi (up 42 percent) and Telugu (up 86 percent), followed by Chinese (up 23 percent) and Arabic (up 42 percent).[39] The largest numerical increases were seen among people speaking Spanish (up four million), Chinese (up 653,000), Arabic (up 363,000), Hindi (up 254,000), Telugu (up 192,000) and Tagalog (up 173,000), also known as Filipino.[40] And the percentage or numerical increases in major metropolitan areas are even greater. Nearly half of all residents in the five largest cities in the country, for example, now speak a foreign language at home. This includes Houston, Texas, the site of this study, and the most racial and ethnically diverse, rapidly growing metropolitan area in the United States. Roughly 49 percent of Houstonians currently speak a language other than English at home, and of those, 82 percent speak Spanish and roughly 9 percent speak an Asian language.[41] What Houston looks like today is the model of what the larger country is expected to look like demographically in the next thirty years.[42]

The ability of American healthcare to serve these populations increasingly hinges on its ability to communicate with patients effectively. Regardless of a patient's English proficiency, illness and emergency may complicate point-of-care interactions, thus necessitating a need for bilingual healthcare professionals or those with the cultural proficiencies to better understand their patients.[43] When people are in distress, speaking in their native language is not only more direct and hence more effective but also a source of comfort. Obviously foreign-born Indian American nurses may not speak all Indian languages, but the probability of them finding greater common linguistic and cultural ground with an Indian patient than with a non-Indian care provider is higher, even if the exchange is in English. Conversely, all foreign-born Filipino American nurses speak Filipino (Tagalog) to some degree, in addition to their own regional dialect and English. Although this may allow them to speak with and thus serve fellow Filipinos better, it is important to remember that roughly 40 percent of the Filipino language comes from Spanish. Thus, many Filipinos, as we saw in chapter 6, can understand and converse with Spanish-speaking patients at a basic level. Beyond this, it is also important to note that many foreign-born

Filipino and Indian American nurses also worked in other countries, including Arabic-speaking countries in the Persian Gulf, before coming to the United States. Understanding this, we might speculate that many of these nurses have at least a cursory understanding of several languages in addition to English. They also have considerable cultural experience in a host of diverse settings. This is clearly an asset in an increasingly diverse America.

As the United States continues to grow ever more diverse, we must not forget that it also continues to age. The percentage of Americans ages sixty-five and older is increasing at a historic pace. By 2050, Americans ages sixty-five and older are predicted to outnumber those who are younger than eighteen.[44] Straining under the weight of these dramatic changes is American healthcare. An aging population often requires more care and thus needs more healthcare providers. American healthcare, as we have seen, also needs people to replace those who are retiring. Understanding this, the country desperately needs to educate more American-born healthcare professionals, but this is only part of the problem. It also needs to find a way to encourage people to take the vacant jobs in nursing that so many are apparently unwilling to fill and remain in for the duration of their career.

Most American patients, I imagine, would prefer healthcare providers who do not simply want to fill these positions merely as jobs to meet financial ends, but instead want to find people who make caring for others their passion and career. Throughout this book, foreign-born Filipino and Indian American nurses such as Rebecca and Lani to name a few, have suggested that they have this passion. Not only do foreign-born nurses want to be here, they are often highly qualified and experienced, and in many cases more so than the average American-born recent nursing-school graduate. They also have a great deal of experience caring for their own aging families in their home countries.

Unlike the United States, India and the Philippines do not have expansive retirement-home systems. Families are largely expected to care for their sick and aging relatives in their own homes.[45] Caring is a cultural norm, one in which Filipinos and Indians are socialized to think about others before themselves. This not only draws them to care for the immediate needs of their own families but frames their wider understandings of what it means to support others by extending the family circle to include everyone in their community. Many nurses in this study, as we have seen, found their initial interest in nursing either by caring for someone in their own family or, after graduating from nursing school, by taking their new skills back into their communities to care for their extended family and neighbors who were aging. Understanding this, foreign-born Filipino and Indian American nurses say they are more than prepared to take care of an aging America. They say they want to do it. More importantly, they believe that they were called as Catholics to do it.[46]

Like the Calvinist Puritans whom Max Weber describes, the foreign-born nurses in this study, although Catholic and not Protestant, do not see nursing simply as a job but a calling—a career that has deep religious meaning and purpose. They did not necessarily choose nursing of their own volition but rather, as Emmy, Joy, and others describe in chapter 2, say that God chose it for them. Approaching nursing from this perspective they believe that serving others is a natural extension of their devout Catholic faith and ardent devotion to God. At the same time, they do not believe that their migration to the United States was some chance happening or something driven purely by economic necessity and opportunity but suggest that this is where God called them to serve. Most, as we have seen, would go as far as to say that God eventually directed them specifically to the VA hospital to care for American veterans.

Although the foreign-born nurses in this study see themselves as unique compared to their American-born peers—more patient oriented, less computer driven, and willing to engage in spiritual care—they are not necessarily all that different. As Aly points out in chapter 5, whether a nurse engages in spiritual care or not says nothing about their own personal faith nor does it say anything about how a nurse may see religion and spirituality as an integral part of patient care. These are potential professional dilemmas all nurses may face, regardless of nativity. Many nurses, for example, want to pray with or for their patients but may struggle with the legal and ethical implications of doing so in the context of their secular hospital settings, their understanding of patients' rights, and the separation of church and state. The debates over the place of religion and spirituality at the point of care, if they transpire at all, in American hospitals is not unique to foreign-born nurses. However, understanding these broader issues, we must also recognize that in many ways the nurses in this study, as we have seen, find themselves foreign in more ways than just their nativity. This can and does further complicate these dilemmas. They were raised and taught in another country to think differently about nursing and spiritual care. How they cope with these tensions and disconnects plays an important role in not only shaping how they see themselves as Catholic nurses but the ways in which they navigate their places, as immigrants, in the new American story.

Devoutly Catholic and Decidedly American

From the late nineteenth through the early twentieth century, successive waves of new immigrants elevated the American Catholic church to become the single largest religious denomination in the United States.[47] Today, Catholic immigrants are once again transforming the American religious landscape. In the last several decades, immigration has accounted for roughly three-quarters of American population growth, and much of this change has been a direct result of Catholic migration—especially of foreign-born nurses from Asia.[48] Even though Catholics from Kerala represent a considerably small proportion of larger Indian migration to the United States, Catholics from the region represent a disproportionately large number within the profession of nursing. By comparison, the Philippines is the second-largest source of Catholic immigration to the country today, and Catholics, by all accounts, are well represented within the nursing profession.[49]

Both populations, as we have seen, are potentially playing a significant role in transforming the American racial and ethnic landscape. They are also moving the American Catholic church further from its historical European roots in the process. This should come as no surprise. Racial and ethnic diversity has always been a hallmark of American Catholicism. This was true of the great immigration era of the late nineteenth and early twentieth centuries, but, as scholars such as Jay P. Dolan have pointed out, such diversity may be even more pronounced today.[50] Like Catholic immigrants of the past, new Catholic immigrants enter the country at a time when the American social and political climate is once again increasingly unwelcoming to many of them as immigrants. Although the widespread anti-Catholic fervor of the Know Nothings party of the mid-nineteenth century is largely—if not completely—absent from today's xenophobic rhetoric, increasing anti-immigrant sentiment and threats leave many Catholic immigrants today struggling to find their place and acceptance in American society. The impassioned words and narratives of the foreign-born nurses in this study are a testament to this. As Rosie points out at the beginning of this chapter, "No one wants us but everyone needs us!"

This sentiment of feeling unwanted, unwelcomed, or distrusted—somehow not fully American—despite being citizens and passionately serving American veterans at the VA, resonated across my discussions with foreign-born nurses throughout this book. How they navigate these tensions and disconnects, not only reveals how they see themselves but exposes the challenges and predicaments they face. They do not believe that they are any less American because of the color of their skin, the way they pronounce the English language, or their devotion to their Catholic faith. In fact, as we have seen, they believe that it is their unique cultural perspectives, their upbringing, and nursing training in another country that distinguishes them from their American-born nursing peers and makes them better. For these nurses, being Catholic is American.

They believe that they were called by God to serve American veterans but also state that it is their patriotic duty to do so—giving back to the country they believe has given them and their families so much. They say that they treat veterans like their own biological family with a care and compassion that is befitting the best ideals of their faith. Yet, as we saw in chapters 3 and 4, they also report considerable scrutiny and harassment—if not flat-out discrimination—from both their patients and peers. Although they are quick to point out that this is not the daily norm, at least with patients, the agony of these experiences has clearly made a deep impact on them personally and the ways they see their social location as immigrants in American society. Despite this, they continue to work at the VA and in their communities with great joy, which suggests that they find more reward than challenge in their efforts. When things get difficult, they turn to their faith to cope or state that God is testing them. This is how they feel. More importantly, this is how they want to be seen by their fellow Americans.

We must recognize that national political sentiment has done little to create a more positive image of immigrants in the minds of many Americans in recent years, despite foreign-born nurses' efforts and hard work in helping to care for the country. In fact, as many nurses alluded to throughout our discussions, perception has gotten worse in recent years, especially for Asians. From the beginning of the outbreak of the coronavirus, President Trump insisted on calling COVID-19 the "Chinese virus" or "kung flu," echoing anti-Asian and xenophobic sentiments from over a century ago. Far from benign, the former President's labels and subsequent comments by numerous others, both those in elected office and not, fueled hate crimes against Asian Americans.[51] Between January and February of 2020, there were reports of over one thousand xenophobic and racist cases of violence against Asian Americans in thirty-two states.[52] In sixteen of the largest, most populous cities in the United States, hate crimes against Asian Americans has increased nearly 150 percent from 2019 to 2020, according to an analysis of official preliminary police data by the Center for the Study of Hate and Extremism at California State University, San Bernardino.[53] As these cases continue to rise, this hate has impacted people of all Asian and Pacific Island heritages and across all socioeconomic and demographic backgrounds, including Asian American healthcare workers.[54] An American-born Korean American doctor, for example, was kicked out of a Marathon Petroleum gas station in Martinsville, Indiana, without being allowed to buy anything or use the bathroom after being mistakenly identified as Chinese. He was repeatedly verbally harassed, called the cause of the coronavirus, and told to never come back.[55] And this is but one example.[56] Like Asian immigrants in previous eras, new Asian immigrants face considerable challenges today.

While these cases, in and of themselves, create enormous problems for foreign-born nurses and the environments in which they live and work today, especially in VA hospitals serving American veterans, they are nothing new. They are part of a much longer historical narrative in which Americans have seemingly always feared or raised concerns about immigrants, including foreign-born nurses. As historian Erika Lee has brilliantly explained, xenophobia has been neither an aberration nor a contradiction in American history.[57] Today, as in previous eras, xenophobia has become good politics. And this, as we might expect, has major implications for American healthcare and foreign-born nurses who state that they want to do their part to help the country meet its pressing healthcare needs.

As the United States continues to search for solutions to its growing healthcare staffing crisis amid a global pandemic, while simultaneously debating the place of immigrants in the country, we should not take for granted that foreign-born nurses will always be there en masse, as in past decades, when we call on them.[58] As noted previously, we often forget that the rest of the world is facing its own nursing shortages, including the very countries that these nurses are leaving.[59] Understanding this, we must ask, How much longer will the United States continue to be their migration destination of choice as such an increasingly unwelcoming, if not outright hostile, environment? It is an important question, one that is sure to shape renewed debates and concerns over the United States's seemingly perennial dependence on imported care.

Despite the complexity of these debates and ongoing concerns about future nursing shortages, the foreign-born nurses in this study state emphatically that they want to be here—that they are called to be and serve Americans. They also suggest that they have much to offer American society that extends well outside their work at the VA. This is not just an expressed sentiment but something demonstrated in action. They have raised and built families in their new American homes, and have attempted to bridge divides with their American-born peers in retirement. At least in the case of the lunch bunch described in this chapter, once-perceived adversaries now form an important part of nurses' extended family. Throughout their careers as American nurses, and in the process of extending their care to a more universal understanding of family, they have also built and bridged communities in the process of making this country their own.

Foreign-born Filipino and Indian American nurses, as we saw in chapter 6, report volunteering and donating money to charitable causes at rates that far exceed those of the average American (roughly 90 percent versus 26 percent of Americans in general). They also report voting in presidential elections at rates that are overwhelmingly higher than the average American (roughly 90 percent versus an estimated 61 percent of all Americans in the 2016). Amid rising xenophobic fears and hostilities, the foreign-born nurses in this study have managed to build rather robust civic lives. Whether it is volunteering at homeless shelters, cooking meals for veterans, conducting free health clinics for those without insurance, or advocating for veterans' rights, and even calling out as whistleblowers about problems they see at the VA, just to name a few examples, their actions show that they are making a tremendous impact on people across the Houston metropolitan area and beyond. This includes people who not only might question their increasing presence in the country but are rallying against them. Although far too many people may see them as foreign, unwanted, or even a threat amid increasing anti-Asian sentiments, these nurses see themselves as good Catholics and good Americans—as Asian Americans. And they are acting on it. Perhaps it is they, like immigrants of previous eras, who hold some of the greatest potential to make America great again? That is, if we let them.

Methodological Appendix

This study developed out of a multinational project initiated by the Kinder Institute for Urban Research at Rice University. Metropolises' Responses to Migration and Urban Growth (MR MUG) studied six key topics/themes in two cities—Houston, Texas, and Shanghai, China. I studied the social and economic integration of various immigrant populations to Houston through the Texas Medical Center (TMC) with my colleague Amy Lucas. Among the hospitals that encompassed the original MR MUG pilot study, the local VA hospital produced the most distinctive data. With every new visit and meeting, the VA appeared to be a unique hospital and its patients, American veterans, appeared to be unique as well.

Site Selection and Limitations

Houston, Texas, was selected as the site of study for MR MUG and my subsequent VA study for several reasons. First, Houston is the most racially and ethnically diverse, rapidly growing metropolitan area in the United States. Much of this diversity and growth has occurred as a result of immigration.[1] As an emerging, major immigrant-gateway city, and a model of what the country is expected to look like demographically in the next thirty years, Houston poses a unique and important case for study. Second, the TMC, of which the Michael E. DeBakey VA Medical Center (Houston VA) is a part, is the largest medical complex in the world and the largest single employer in the city. The TMC serves over eight million patients a year through the care of over one hundred and six thousand healthcare workers.[2] Although the nativity of its employees is not fully known,[3] like other medical centers and hospitals across the country, the TMC depends heavily on foreign-born workers to maintain its steady institutional growth and meet the needs of an increasingly diverse and aging population.[4] Third, Texas has the second-largest veteran population in the country, roughly 1.5 million veterans, and the Houston VA is in the top twenty largest veterans hospitals in the country by number of staffed beds.[5]

The Houston VA was originally opened by the U.S. navy in 1946 on one hundred and eighteen acres of land adjacent to the TMC in Houston.[6] President Harry Truman then transferred operation of the hospital from the U.S. navy to the Veterans Administration by executive order in 1949. It is at this point that the hospital officially became the Houston VA hospital.[7] In 1978, all VA hospitals across the country, including Houston's, were given the designation "Medical Center" to reflect the broad range of healthcare they provided to veterans.[8] In 1985, the Houston VA officially joined the TMC.[9] Finally, in 2003, President George W. Bush signed Public Law 108–170 to officially change the name of the Houston VA to the Michael E. DeBakey VA Medical Center in recognition of Dr. DeBakey's well-documented efforts on behalf of American veterans.[10]

I quickly discovered that immigrant healthcare professionals had always played a vital role serving American veterans within this history. I also discovered that the VA has typically magnified broader American sentiments about new immigrants. It was a puzzle I could not ignore. In the fall of 2013, I applied to the hospital to become a Without Compensation (WOC) researcher.[11] After being officially processed by the hospital, I began setting up the protocol that I hoped to use for a unique ethnographic study of the VA and its foreign-born nurses. Many people cautioned my optimism. I quickly found that I was an outsider in more than one way. Recalling the discussion of Charles Bosk's perspectives on medical research in Wendy Cadge's seminal work *Paging God*,[12] a book on religion in hospital settings that inspired many of my aspirations, I came to the realization that I was an uninvited intruder. Charles Bosk distinguishes between researchers, in his case sociologists who are invited by medical staff to study them as welcome guests, and those who are uninvited intruders.[13] I was not completely welcomed by many administrators whom I initially spoke with, and my focus on foreign-born employees appeared to arouse suspicion. When I finally submitted my protocol to BRAIN (Biomedical Research and Assurance Information Network),[14] I was afraid it would not get approved. I lacked real internal support.

In June of 2014, five months after I formally started working at the VA hospital as a WOC researcher, the federal government opened a criminal investigation into the VA system. The scandal was not the only problem to draw attention to the VA system in recent years, but the investigation was the largest in over a decade. Since my protocol had not yet been approved and was still

working its way through the BRAIN review process, my WOC status was revoked, and I was asked to leave the hospital. Even as the investigation ended,
I was never able to get back into the VA system and use the hospitals' administration and the BRAIN protocol to help legitimize and manage the study. This
lack of access posed several obstacles to the study, some of which actually
ended up being strengths rather than weaknesses—and all of which fundamen-
tally shaped the stories I am able to tell. I was disappointed that I could not
directly observe foreign-born nurses working with and caring for American
veterans. I wanted to see these interactions for myself through participant ob-
servation. Knowing that this was not possible, I began to search for new ways
to interview veterans. This had limited success.

As the scandal gained wider publicity, many veterans I initially spoke with
only wanted to discuss problems with the VA. Rather than committing to formal
interviews, many directed me to veteran blogs and other resources online. Beyond the small sample of veterans who did give formal interviews (see discussion in this appendix), these online sources proved to be valuable voices but
perhaps not representative ones. This is a clear limitation. Nevertheless, the silence of veterans and their families in this study, outside of the ways foreign-
born Filipino and Indian American nurses describe them, enabled me to focus
more centrally on the ways in which these nurses not only see the place of religion and spirituality in healthcare but negotiate the tensions between trying to
be good nurses, Catholics, and patriotic Americans—doing what they think and
feel is best for veterans according to their faith and training while working within
the constraints and policies of a secular government hospital. This strengthened
my research by placing greater emphasis on the understudied voices, perceptions, and subjective experiences of foreign-born nurses.

Despite some of the emergent limitations that these unusual circumstances
presented, the scandal did not deter foreign-born nurses from participating in
the study outside of the hospital. On the contrary, it seemed to embolden their
desire to talk about their nursing experiences. Although the original project had
nothing to do with larger systemic VA problems or any scandal per se, it was
an unavoidable subject moving forward as the study shifted from the hospital
to a snowball sample drawn largely from the members of associations that
represented the two largest groups of foreign-born nurses working at the VA
hospital—the Filipino Nurses Association (FNA, pseudonym) and the Indian
Nurses Association (INA, pseudonym).

FNA was established in 1980 and is a much larger organization than INA
both in membership and reach. Much of this has to do with the fact that Filipino Americans have a larger presence in the TMC. FNA also represents part of

the mass national mobilization of Filipino American nurses in response to the 1975 Narciso and Perez case discussed in chapter 1.[15] Although INA was not officially formed until 2014, the core group of nurses who make up its most active membership had been together for over fifteen years prior to this. The association serves much of the same functions for the Indian American nursing community in Houston as FNA does for Filipino American nurses but, again, is smaller and typically holds its monthly meetings in member homes, in contrast to FNA, which meets in larger auditoriums in local hospitals.

When the scandal broke, I already had several contacts in FNA, including the president at the time. Many also knew me from my previous research in the Filipino American community, and most knew that I was married to a foreign-born Filipina American. This gave me unprecedented access. The overwhelming majority of nurses treated me like an insider, despite the fact that I am a White man. Because I also know some basic conversational Filipino (Tagalog), many foreign-born Filipino American nurses often spoke to me in Taglish—a mixture of Filipino and English. As both an insider and outsider, I found myself conducting research over a four-year period in a community that was very familiar but one that is not my own by birth or upbringing.

Conversely, I did not personally know anyone in INA nor had I ever conducted research in the Indian American community. I also do not have any immediate family who are Indian. However, my father lived in India for seven years as a young child (roughly 1952–1959), and I grew up with him telling me stories about India, teaching me its history, and introducing me to Indian food. It may seem funny at first, but this initially meant a great deal to the foreign-born Indian American nurses in this study. When I first emailed the president of INA and then spoke with her briefly on the phone, for example, she suggested that we meet at a local Indian restaurant to discuss the study. When I arrived, I discovered that she had invited several additional members of INA to join us. After introducing ourselves to each other, the owner of the restaurant, a family friend of the president, brought over a menu and told us we could order from it or suggest other dishes that were not on the menu. I inquired about several dishes I did not see on the menu, and the mouths of everyone at the table literally dropped open. As they each asked me how I knew so much about Indian food, our discussions shifted from talking about my research to talking about my father. From that point forward, word spread, and I was less of an outsider than I had initially anticipated.

Foreign-born Filipino and Indian Americans nurses readily welcomed me into their homes and lives. They spoke freely with me and never seemed to hold back their emotions or opinions. I never fully felt like an outsider personally, despite the fact that I was in many ways. I am not a nurse, nor am I a medical sociologist. This presented a host of challenges to the conversations I had with those I interviewed. It was rather apparent, for example, that I did not speak like a medical doctor or nurse, nor was I familiar with terms and circumstances that everyone else understood as commonplace. Nurses largely laughed off my lack of medical knowledge or were exceptionally patient with me as they explained certain specific details. The acronyms alone signaled to me that we did not speak the same technical language. I was an outsider, but my lack of knowledge actually helped to focus foreign-born nurses' interview responses on their subjective experiences over some of the more technical aspects of medicine. This was an unexpected strength of my outsider status. However, later in the analysis phase, it became more obvious that there were a host of orienting assumptions and medical epistemologies that I was not familiar with and needed to read/study in order to properly contextualize the highly nuanced conversations I had with nurses.[16]

Foreign-Born Nurse Interviews and Analysis

Building on the original MR MUG protocol and securing institutional human subjects' approval through my own institution, over a four-year period (2014– 2018) I interviewed one hundred and sixteen healthcare providers, of which eighty-seven are foreign-born nurses originally from India (N=39) and the Philippines (N=48), and are currently or formerly employed at the local Houston VA. I also conducted several focus groups and panel discussions at the general meetings of both their nursing associations, some of which included doctors and second-generation Filipino and Indian American nurses. The snowball sample was built after the 2014 VA scandal, as noted earlier. After I relaunched the project outside of the hospital, the sample grew largely through nurses who worked at the VA and were/are members of FNA and INA or knew someone who was. Others reached out independently to me as word about the study spread in friend and community circles. The majority of nurses in the sample had worked at the VA over five years (see figure A.1), are first-generation immigrants, and tended to be not only very religious but active in their communities. Sample selection was an issue. None of the samples were randomly gathered. I also was not able to interview a large enough sample of foreign-born nurses who left the VA to make any true analytical comparisons with those who stayed or retired. Many of those who left the VA were also unwilling to commit to an interview or were suspicious of who/how I was given their contact information by their peers. Hence, the focus of the study is on those who remain at the hospital or have retired. This was/is a clear limitation to the

	Filipino American n = 48	Indian American n = 39
Age (years, mean)	52	47
Gender (% women)	90%	100%
Education (degree mean)	Master's	Master's
Income (household mean)	$75K–100K	$75K–100K
Years at Houston VA (mean)*	13	12
Marital status (mean)	Married	Married
Number of children (mean)	2	2
Roman Catholic (%)	95%	45%
Other rite Catholic (%)	0%	43%
Protestant (%)	5%	7%
Hindu (%)	0%	5%

*Includes retirees

Figure A.1 VA Foreign-Born Nurse Interview Sample Demographics.

study. Had my BRAIN protocol been approved or had the scandal not occurred when it did, a more generalizable sample of foreign-born nurses, not just a subset of Filipino and Indian Americans, would have likely emerged across all work units/floors in the hospital and across wider demographics—including length of employment at the hospital. This hindered my ability to fully compare nurses and their subjective experiences along these lines. However, the emergent snowball samples are fairly representative of the demographic profile of other foreign-born Filipino and Indian American nurses across the county with a few notable exceptions.[17]

All of the nurses in this study are U.S. citizens, which is not the case nationally.[18] This is largely a function of site selection. The VA requires all of its staff, with the exception of doctors in residence, to be citizens before they can be employed at the hospital. In order to gain eligibility for employment at the VA, the overwhelming majority of the foreign-born nurses in this study worked at a public or private hospital before joining the VA. During their time at these other hospitals, which is typically five or more years, they became U.S. citizens. Because of this, the age of the foreign-born nurse interview sample is a bit older than the national average. The average age of foreign-born Filipino American nurses in the interview sample is fifty-two, compared to forty-five on average nationally.[19] The average age of foreign-born Indian American nurses in the interview sample is forty-seven compared to forty-three on average nationally.[20] The difference in average age, roughly five years, is largely again a function of site selection; otherwise, the foreign-born nurses in this study demographically look like other foreign-born nurses across the country.

As figure A.1 reflects, roughly 10 percent of the foreign-born Filipino American nursing interview sample is male (and 90 percent female) versus 0 percent of the foreign-born Indian American sample. This mirrors national estimates and is largely a function of cultural and historical circumstance in India and the Philippines.[21] Nursing remains a gendered profession globally, as women's work, but men are significantly more likely to become nurses in the Philippines because of American geopolitical ties to the country and the saliency of nursing as a source of economic opportunity. See discussion in chapter 2. On average, foreign-born Filipino American nurses in the interview sample have worked at the VA for thirteen years compared to twelve years for foreign-born Indian American nurses. This includes the number of years worked by retirees of both groups. In terms of other demographic characteristics, the foreign-born Filipino and Indian American nurses in the interview sample have an average education of a master's degree with an average household income between $75,000 and $100,000. They also on average are married with two children. This again is fairly representative of larger national estimates.[22]

In terms of religious affiliation, 95 percent of the foreign-born Filipino American nurses in the interview sample identify as Roman Catholic and 5 percent identify as Protestant of some variety. By contrast, 45 percent of foreign-born Indian American nurses identify as Roman Catholic (Latin rite), 43 percent identify as Syro-Malabar/Malankara or East Syriac rite Catholic (with a total of 88 percent Catholic), 7 percent identify as Protestant of some variety, and 5 percent identify as Hindu. Despite significant differences in the rites that they practice at Mass, both sample populations are overwhelmingly Catholic. In the case of Filipino Americans this is a higher percentage of Catholics than the U.S. national average (65 percent) but is closer to the percentage of Filipinos in the Philippines who are Catholic (81 percent).[23] The percentage of Indian American Catholics—Roman Catholic (Latin rite), Syro-Malabar/Malankara or East Syriac rite—is significantly higher than the U.S. national average for Indian Americans in general (5 percent) but is indicative of what we know about Indians going into nursing from the Indian states of Kerala and Karnataka.[24] The majority of Indian American nurses in the interview sample were from these two regions. See further the historical discussion in chapter 2.

The majority of interviews were conducted in peoples' homes, but in many cases I also interviewed people on the phone, at restaurants/bakeries, banquet halls during special events, and celebrations at other locations. Face-to-face and phone-recorded interviews typically lasted anywhere from one to four hours, after I first described the study and secured informed consent. Many interviews were often followed up with by email or phone conversations. This was particularly true during the transcription and analysis phase of the project. Any lingering questions were often returned to and addressed in subsequent conversations with those I had already interviewed.

Although my primary interest in the interviews was structured around foreign-born nurses' subjective experiences working at the VA—why they said they chose to work at the hospital, why they said they stayed, and how they described working with veterans as patients, religion and faith, as noted earlier, quickly emerged as a central topic of discussion. This led to my focus on Catholics and the role of Catholicism in informing and shaping their professional and civic lives. Despite the fact that foreign-born Filipino and Indian American nurses spoke at length about their parish churches and despite the fact that I did some participant observations at these churches, the focus of this study was always centered on faith in practice rather than institutional or organized religion. Churches, priests, and fellow parishioners all have a tremendous impact on the foreign-born nurses' spirituality in this study, but these influences played a lesser role in my interview questioning than the ways in which they engage their faith at work and in their community.

I started each interview by asking people to describe their life in India and the Philippines, their upbringing, how they got into nursing, where they went to school/college, how they were trained, and the general importance of religion and faith to them. I then asked what the circumstances were surrounding their immigration and why they left. From here, I asked people about what it was like immigrating to the United States, any hardships they faced, and the ways they went about trying to establish a sense of community in their new American homes. These questions provided a rich context and life histories to better understand peoples' answers to subsequent topics of interest and further illuminated the ways they described their nursing careers and experiences at the VA.[25] Since I was not able to actually observe the nurses firsthand at the hospital, it was important first to listen to what they were trying to tell me, repeat it, and then engage it by asking for further clarification—questioning both the intent and meaning—while also allowing them to vividly paint their own picture of their work and community lives.[26]

The approach I took to analyzing these interviews was informed and shaped by previous scholarship in a host of areas and disciplines. Understanding the subjectivity that comes with doing qualitative interviews and the various perspectives that both the interviewer and interviewee can bring to any given exchange—my own made as transparent as possible in this appendix—I initially analyzed (1) what each nurse was trying to convey about themselves, their lives, and experiences; (2) how they constructed certain images of themselves and others based on repeated questions or in the context of survey analyses (where possible); and (3) how these intersubjective dynamics influenced their individual perspectives.[27] Drawing on hermeneutic strategies, I then sought to draw out the commonalities and differences among the nurses' interviews, moving beyond representations of their specific subjective views to locating patterns across and within them.[28]

I first coded the data by question and then deductively developed more codes by key themes. It was not until certain patterns began to emerge from the transcriptions and subsequent analyses highlighting the role of religion in their nursing care—and the belief that they were called by God to serve veterans—that I began to see the larger story of this book. Once these patterns emerged, I retested my original assumptions by returning to the interviews and recoding them along these theoretical lines following a grounded theory approach.[29] The names of all individuals interviewed in the study were changed to maintain anonymity and confidentiality. In some cases, I changed more-identifiable demographics (not nationality) or in a few cases created composite characteristics to further protect their identity where needed. This was an important measure since the hospital where the nurses work is identifiable.

Foreign-Born Nurse Surveys and Analysis

Beyond the interviews, I also surveyed foreign-born Filipino and Indian American nurses who currently or formerly worked at the VA. I first asked questions to best assess their demographic profile—about age, race/ethnicity, education, nativity, income, and other factors. I then asked questions on issues ranging from their work life and experiences to their religious and community engagement. The response rate was 73 percent—considerably lower than I anticipated.[30] Part of the lower response was a result of timing. Many foreign-born Filipino and Indian American nurses later explained to me in interviews that the VA scandal and the scrutiny that came with it made them reluctant to answer the survey or at least certain questions.

Survey analyses were restricted to Catholics—Roman Catholic (Latin rite) and Syro-Malabar/Malankara or East Syriac rite. Survey data presented throughout the book are based on seventy valid cases, all foreign-born Filipino and Indian American Catholic nurses working (or retired) at the VA. Although this is a small sample, it mirrors the demographic profile of the larger interview

	Filipino American n = 38	Indian American n = 32
Age (years, mean)	52	47
Sex (% women)	90%	100%
Education (degree mean)	Master's	Master's
Income (household mean)	$75K–100K	$75K–100K
Marital status (mean)	Married	Married
Number of children (mean)	2	2

Figure A.2 VA Foreign-Born Catholic Nurse Survey Sample Demographics.

sample described in previous pages and is thus fairly representative of foreign-born Filipino and Indian American nurses nationally with exception of age, citizenship, and religious affiliation.[31] See figure A.2. It should be noted that it is difficult to know how representative the interview or survey samples are of foreign-born Filipino and Indian American nurses working at the VA, especially since the hospital does not keep records on the nativity or religiosity of its employees. Comparative data along other demographic characteristics are also not publicly available. See the discussion in chapter 3.

Other Samples and Methods

In addition to interviewing and surveying foreign-born Filipino and Indian American nurses, I interviewed thirty-five U.S. veterans, the majority of whom are White (77 percent) men (94 percent), ages twenty-three to forty-eight (with the average age being thirty-four), with an average education of a college (bachelor's) degree, and with an average household income of $50,000 to $74,000. They are also, on average, married (70 percent). See figure A.3. This is not completely representative of the average demographic profile of American veterans nationally nor does it fully represent the average veteran patient at a VA hospital. The average American veteran is a white (77 percent) man (91 percent), married (68 percent), ages fifty-five years and older (68 percent) with some college, whether an associate's degree (36.7 percent) or a bachelor's degree (28.4 percent) (with a total of 65 with either), and an average household income of $88,000.[32] See discussion in chapter 3. The average VA patient is a White (77 percent) man (92 percent), ages sixty-five and older (52 percent compared to 39 percent of veterans who are non-VA patients), a higher percentage of whom have less than a high school education (9 percent compared to roughly 6 percent of veterans who are non-VA patients), and who on average have a household income that is

n = 35	
White (%)	77%
Black (%)	14%
Hispanic (%)	9%
Age (years, mean)	34
Sex (% men)	94%
Education (degree mean)	Bachelor's
Income (household mean)	$50K–$74K
Marital status (mean)	Married
Number of children (mean)	1

Figure A.3 Veteran Patient Sample Demographics.

roughly $10,000 less than non-VA patients.[33] The sample is thus not generaliz-able in terms of age, education, or income. See discussion in chapter 4. This is largely a result of the sample frame and temporal circumstances. The snowball sample was drawn largely from veterans' organizations and veteran students—hence a sample that is younger and more educated. The wider range in ages has also likely impacted the average household incomes relative to the national averages.

Recorded interviews lasted an hour on average. After first describing the study, exploring the relationship between veterans and nurses/doctors at the VA, and securing informed consent, I simply asked veterans if they had been a patient at the local VA and if so, to describe what it was like visiting the hospi-tal. I then asked them about their experiences as patients. I did not initially prompt them to address my underlying interest in the specific relationship be-tween veterans and foreign-born care providers, but one by one, the veterans in the sample uniformly wanted to discuss two issues, the VA scandal and the presence of foreign-born workers at the hospital. The approach I took to analyz-ing these interviews follows the same general investigative guidelines de-scribed in previous pages for the foreign-born Filipino and Indian American samples.

In addition to the methods described above, I also monitored and engaged with foreign-born Filipino and Indian American nursing blogs, veterans' blogs, and other relevant online groups. I found these spaces important venues for bet-ter situating the ways in which foreign-born Filipino and Indian American nurses think about their profession, their patients, and the way they build and engage community.[34] The same was true of veterans blogs and groups. Although questions remain about how representative these voices may be, these data provided yet another means to observe patterns of perspectives and opinions in nursing and patient relations that I did not otherwise have access to. In some ways people were more honest or blunt online than in person. This provided a sounding board for ideas and perspectives that I then carried into qualitative interviews. It also allowed to me to stay better informed and engaged with a host of so-called hot issues as they made news on these posts.

Triangulating this unique and original data collection, I situated the central arguments of this book within an exhaustive exploration of the current literature on race, gender and nursing, immigrant religious life, and the ongoing debates over the role of spirituality and religion in American healthcare. Drawing heavily on previous scholarship across several fields, I placed these data in a wider historical context. This allowed me to better explain not only why these countries remain the top sources of nursing migration to the United States but also why the majority of these nurses have historically been and continue to be from Catholic communities. Many scholars have alluded to these cross-national contexts, but to this point a comprehensive comparative history of nursing in India and the Philippines has yet to be fully written from a more sociological perspective. This is obviously beyond the scope of this study, but it is my hope that outlining these shared contexts and themes comparatively allows people to gain a larger understanding of the historical circumstances that still impact the lives of foreign-born nurses today.

Acknowledgments

This book would not have been possible without the love, dedication, and support of many people. First and foremost, I owe a great debt of gratitude to the Filipino and Indian American nurses in the Houston metropolitan area who participated in this study. I am thankful to all the individuals who graciously welcomed me into their associations and homes and took the time out of their busy schedules to share their lives with me. They continually inspired me with their words and stories. Beyond research and academics, I am grateful to these nurses not only for their dedication to serving American veterans, often in the most difficult of circumstances, but their tireless commitment to humanity on the front lines of the Coronavirus. Amidst the chaos and uncertainty of a global pandemic, they exemplify the best of us. It is my hope that this book further illuminates their lives and concerns as they describe them, the often unseen side of healthcare, and allows scholars and the general public alike to better understand their motivations to care and the full depth and breadth of that care.

Research for this book started while I was a scholar (affiliated fellow) at the Kinder Institute at Rice University. I am grateful to the Kinder Institute and its affiliated faculty and staff, particularly Michael Emerson, without whom the seeds of this project would not have been planted. I would also like to thank Sharmila Rudrappa and Bob Woodberry for their suggestions and sage advice during the early stages of forming this project. Beyond helping to shape the eventual direction and research for this book, I am indebted to them for their continued support and mentoring. Tricia Bruce made invaluable suggestions during later iteration of the manuscript. I am thankful for her keen insights and continued friendship. I am also thankful for the support of Helen Rose Ebaugh, who has always been a true colleague, friend, and mentor over the years.

A number of other people helped to shape this book. I benefitted greatly from the anonymous reviewers solicited by Rutgers University Press as well as from the encouraging feedback and editorial suggestions of Peter Mickulas. My colleague Amy Lucas helped manage and run the survey analyses. I am thankful for her assistance and support both as a colleague and friend. Another colleague and friend, Stuart Larson, helped transform the original charts and figures for the book into their current high-resolution form. Graduate student Kemal Budak also provided invaluable help with several aspects of data management and collection throughout the project. Special thanks go to Jenifer K Wofford for graciously providing the cover art for the book.

Above and beyond all those acknowledged here, this book ultimately would not have been possible without my wife, Emily. In everything, she is my foundation and inspiration. For our children, Amelie and Wesley, thank you for always believing in me and helping each other, and me, deal with all the craziness while we were quarantined together throughout the pandemic. In many odd and difficult ways, we wrote this book together. Last, but not least, I would like to thank my Mom (1940–1998), my Dad, and my Dad's partner in life, Howard, without whom none of this would have been possible. I cannot thank them enough for all their love and support.

Abbreviations

ANA	American Nursing Association
BRAIN	Biomedical Research and Assurance Information Network
BSN	Bachelor of Science in Nursing
CLF	civil labor force
EVP	Exchange Visitor Program
FBI	Federal Bureau of Investigations
FNA	Filipino Nurses Association (pseudonym)
GAO	Government Accountability Office
GDP	gross domestic product
INA	Indian Nurses Association (pseudonym)
MAVNI	Military Accessions Vital to the National Interests program
MOAA	Military Officer's Association of America
MR MUG	Metropolises' Responses to Migration and Urban Growth
OECD	Organization for Economic Co-operation and Development
OIG	Office of the Inspector General
OR	operating room
PA	physician assistant
PTSD	post-traumatic stress disorder
SBTPE	State Board Test Pool Examination
TBI	traumatic brain injury
TMC	Texas Medical Center
VA	Veterans Administration hospital
VACAA	Veterans Access, Choice, and Accountability Act
VCP	Veterans' Choice Program
WOC	Without Compensation (research status)

Notes

1. Veterans and a Crisis of Care

1. The names of all individuals interviewed in the study have been changed in the text to maintain anonymity and confidentiality. In some cases, I changed more-identifiable demographics (not nationality) or in a few cases created composite characteristics to further protect their identity where needed. This was an important measure since the hospital the nurses work at is identifiable. All quotations come from field notes and interviews. Note that I use the terms "Filipino American" and "Indian American" throughout the book despite the fact that a host of terms can be used to describe these populations. See methodological appendix.

2. Note that I use Filipino to describe people from the Philippines or their descent but use Filipina to specify a woman of Filipino descent. Although non-binary terms such as Filipinx are appropriate in this context, I used the term my respondents used to describe themselves.

3. Country names are listed alphabetically throughout the book.

4. Where appropriate, Filipino and Indian American are listed alphabetically.

5. Throughout this book, I refer to Catholics, whether from India or the Philippines, in the broadest, most universalist understanding of the global Catholic church. As I describe in chapter 1, a large percentage of the foreign-born Indian American nurses in this study practice the East Syriac Rite in either the Syro-Malabar or Syro-Malankara church. Both of these churches are under the auspices of the larger Catholic church, and hence the pope, but practice their own rites at Mass rather than the Latin rite many people may be more familiar with in the Roman Catholic tradition. A rite simply represents an ecclesiastical tradition about how the sacraments are to be celebrated. As vicar of the universal church, the pope is the sole authority and shepherd of the rites of the West and the East. However, each rite and church also have their own fairly autonomous system of authority and governance despite being under this larger institutional umbrella. Understanding this, I note that a significant percentage of the foreign-born Indian American nurses who attend Syro-Malabar or Syro-Malankara churches on the weekend during normal Mass times also attend Roman Catholic (Latin Rite) churches throughout the week, typically in the morning before they go to work at the VA. The universal understanding of Catholicism that I adopt in simply labeling foreign-born Filipino and Indian Americans as Catholics is not my invention but something foreign-born Indian American nurses carry out in their daily understandings of their faith. Conversely, most foreign-born Filipino American nurses in this study do not attend East-Syriac rite churches, although they do see them as part of the same Catholic family.

6. Andy J. Semotiuk, "COVID-19 Crisis Will Require More Foreign Health Care Workers," *Forbes*, March 31, 2020, https://www.forbes.com/sites/andyjsemotiuk/2020/03/31/solving-the-covid-19-crisis-will-require-more-foreign-health-care-workers/#67e4b59e5a62.

7. Leodoro Labrague, Denise McEnroe-Petitte, Romero H. Achaso, Geifsonne S. Cachero, and Mary Rose A. Mohammad, "Filipino Nurses' Spirituality and Provision of Spiritual Nursing Care," *Clinical Nursing Research* 25, no. 6 (2015): 607–625.

8. See discussion in Wendy Cadge, *Paging God: Religion in the Halls of Medicine* (Chicago: University of Chicago Press, 2012). Also see Wendy Cadge and Mary Ellen Konieczny, "Hidden in Plain Sight: The Significance of Religion and Spirituality in Secular Organizations," *Sociology of Religion* 75, no. 4 (2014): 551–563.

9. David J. Bier, "Immigrants Aid America during COVID-19 Crisis," *CATO at Liberty*, March 23, 2020, https://www.cato.org/blog/immigrants-aid-america-during-covid-19-crisis.

10. Throughout this book I will refer to registered nurses simply as nurses, unless otherwise specified.

11. For research on nursing need trends, see Patricia Cortes and Jessica Pan, "Foreign-Nurse Importation to the United States and the Supply of Native Registered Nurses," *Journal of Health Economics* 37, issue C (September 2014): 164–180; Stephen P. Jurascheck et al., "United States Registered Nurse Workforce Report Card and Shortage Forecast," *American Journal of Quality Medicine* 23, no. 3 (2012): 241–249; Gavin Yamey, "Obama's Giant Step towards Universal Health Insurance," *British Medical Journal* 340, 7748 (2010): 663–664.

12. See Jeanne Batalova and Michael Fix, *Uneven Progress: The Employment Pathways of Skilled Immigrants in the United States* (Washington, DC: Migration Policy Institute, October 2008; Kristen McCabe, *Foreign-born Health Care Workers in the United States* (Washington, DC: Migration Policy Institute, June 2012), http://www.migrationpolicy.org/article/foreign-born-health-care-workers-united-states; Joanne Spetz, Michael Gates, and Cheryl B. Jones, "Internationally Educated Nurses in the United States: Their Origins and Roles," *Nursing Outlook* 62 (2014): 8–15; Allison Squires and Hiram Beltrán-Sánchez, *Strengthening Health Systems in North and Central America: What Role for Migration?* (Washington, DC: Migration Policy Institute, February 2013), https://www.migrationpolicy.org/research/strengthening-health-systems-north-and-central-america-what-role-migration?pdf=RMSG-HealthCare.pdf; Amani Siyam and Mario Roberto dal Poz, eds., *Migration of Health Workers: WHO Code of Practice and the Global Economic Crisis* (Washington, DC: Migration Policy Institute, May 2014), https://www.migrationpolicy.org/research/migration-health-workers-who-code-practice-and-global-economic-crisis.

13. See data analysis "Occupational Outlook Handbook, Registered Nurses," U.S. Bureau of Labor Statistics, accessed April 2020, https://www.bls.gov/ooh/healthcare/registered-nurses.htm#:~:text=in%20May%202019.-,Job%20Outlook,the%20average%20for%20all%20occupations. Also see Christopher J. Goodman and Steven M. Mance, "Employment Loss and the 2007–09 Recession: An Overview," *Monthly Labor Review*, April 2011, 3–12, http://www.bls.gov/opub/mlr/2011/04/art1full.pdf; Siyam and dal Poz, eds., *Migration of Health Workers*; Catherine A. Wood, "Employment in Health Care: A Crutch for the Ailing Economy during the 2007–09 Recession," *Monthly Labor Review*, April 2011, 13–18, http://www.bls.gov/opub/mlr/2011/04/art2full.pdf.

14. Linda H. Aiken, Robyn B. Cheung, and Danielle M. Olds, "Education Policy Initiatives to Address the Nurse Shortage in the United States," *Health Affairs* 28, no. 4 (2009): w646–w656.

15. Healthcare accounts for roughly 18 percent of the United States gross domestic product (GDP). The United States also spends more on healthcare than any other Organization for Economic Co-operation and Development (OECD) country. See David I. Auerbach, Peter I. Buerhaus, and Douglas O. Staiger, "Will the RN Workforce Weather the Retirement of the Baby Boomers?," *Medical Care* 53, no. 10 (2015): 850–856;

Cortes and Pan, "Foreign-Nurse Importation"; C. Brett Lockhard and Michael Wolf, "Occupational Employment Projections to 2020," *Monthly Labor Review*, January 2012, 84–108, http://www.bls.gov/opub/mlr/2012/01/art5full.pdf; Siyam and dal Poz, eds., *Migration of Health Workers*; U.S. Department of Health and Human Services Health Resources and Services Administration (HHS), *The Registered Nurse Population: Findings from the 2008 National Sample Survey of Registered Nurses* (Washington, DC: U.S. Department of Health and Human Services, 2010), http://bhpr.hrsa.gov /healthworkforce/rnsurveys/rnsurveyfinal.pdf; U.S. Bureau of Labor Statistics, "Occupations with the Largest Predicted Number of Job Openings due to Growth and Replacement Needs, 2012 and Projected 2022," *Economic News Release*, 2013, http://www .bls.gov/news.release/ecopro.t08.htm.

16. See data at U.S. Bureau of Labor Statistics, "Projections of Occupational Employment, 2016–26," October 2017, https://www.bls.gov/careeroutlook/2017/article/occupational -projections-charts.htm; Peter I Buerhaus, Lucy E. Skinner, David I. Auerbach and Douglas O. Staiger, "Four Challenges Facing the Nursing Workforce," *Journal of Nursing Regulation* 8, no. 3 (July 2017): 40–46; Jurascheck et al., "United States Registered Nurse"; Richard A. Smiley et al., "The 2017 National Nursing Workforce Survey," *Journal of Nursing Regulation* 9, no. 3 (October 2018): s1–s88.

17. John D. Daigh, Jr., *OIG Determination of Veterans Health Administration's Occupational Staffing Shortages FY 2019*, report #19-000346-241 (Washington DC: Department of Veterans Affairs, Office of Inspector General, Office of Healthcare Inspections Online, September 30, 2019), https://www.va.gov/oig/pubs/VAOIG-19 -00346-241.pdf.

18. See data at U.S. Bureau of Labor Statistics, "Projections of Occupational Employment."

19. Peter Buerhaus, "Health Care Payment Reform: Implications for Nurses," *Nursing Economics* 28, no. 1 (2010): 49–54; Jurascheck et al., "United States Registered Nurse"; Lynn Y. Unruh and Myron D. Fottler, "Projections and Trends in RN Supply: What Do They Tell Us about the Nursing Shortage?," *Policy Politics and Nursing Practice* 6, no. 3 (2005): 171–182.

20. U.S Bureau of Labor and Statistics estimates that 203,700 additional registered nurses will be needed per year from 2016–2026. As of 2020, these estimates have proven to be fairly accurate. With the same base rate of need (203,700 per year) the minimum projected need over the next ten years (2020–2030) is over two million nurses; see Elka Torpey, "Employment Outlook for Bachelor's-Level Occupations," *U.S Bureau of Labor and Statistics*, April 2018, https://www.bls.gov/careeroutlook/2018/article /bachelors-degree-outlook.htm#Healthcare%20and%20science. For the estimated 28 percent increase in demand, see U.S. Department of Health and Human Services, Health Resources and Services Administration, Bureau of Health Workforce, National Center for Health Workforce Analysis, "Supply and Demand Projections of the Nursing Workforce: 2014–2030," *HRSA Health Workforce* (Washington, DC: U.S. Department of Health and Human Services, 2017), https://bhw.hrsa.gov/sites/default/files /bhw/nchwa/projections/NCHWA_HRSA_Nursing_Report.pdf.

21. U.S. Department of Health and Human Services, "Supply and Demand Projections."

22. Rob Elgie, "Politics, Economics and Nursing Shortages: A Critical Look at United States Government Policies," *Nursing Economics* 25, no. 5 (2007): 285–292; Jurascheck et al., "United States Registered Nurse."

23. Cheryl A. Peterson, "Nursing Shortage: Not a Simple Problem—No Easy Answers," *Online Journal of Issues in Nursing* 6, no. 1 (2001), https://ojin.nursingworld.org

/MainMenuCategories/ANAMarketplace/ANAPeriodicals/OJIN/TableofContents
/Volume62001/No1Jan01/ShortageProblemAnswers.html.

24. American Association of Colleges of Nursing, *2018–2019 Enrollment and Gradua-tions in Baccalaureate and Graduate Programs in Nursing* (Washington, DC: AACN, 2019); Douglas O. Staiger, David A. Auerbach, and Peter I. Buerhaus, "Registered Nurse Labor Supply and the Recession: Are We in a Bubble?," *New England Journal of Medicine* 366, no. 16 (2012): 1463–1465.

25. Auerbach et al., "Will the RN Workforce"; James R. Knickman and Emily K. Snell, "The 2030 Problem: Caring for Aging Baby Boomers," *Heath Service Research* 37, no. 4 (August 2002): 849–884.

26. See previous note. Also see Grayson K. Vincent and Victoria A. Velkoff, "The Next Four Decades: The Older Population in the United States: 2010 to 2050," *2010 US Census Report*, May 2010, https://www.census.gov/prod/2010pubs/p25-1138.pdf.

27. A. Christine Delucas, "Foreign Nurse Recruitment: Global Risk," *Nursing Ethics* 21, no. 1 (2014): 76–85; Meghan Hoyer, "Nation's Sickest Seniors Reshape Health Care," *USA Today*, June 5, 2015, http://www.usatoday.com/story/news/2015/06/05/medicare -costs-seniors-sick-chronic-conditions/27390925/.

28. See reviews Buerhaus et al., "Four Challenges"; Cortes and Pan, "Foreign-Nurse Importation"; Chiara Dall'Ora et al., "Association of 12 H Shifts and Nurses' Job Sat-isfaction, Burnout and Intention to Leave: Findings from a Cross-Sectional Study of 12 European Countries," *BMJ Open* 5 (2015): 1–7; Baoyue Li et al., "Group-Level Impact of Work Environment Dimensions on Burnout Experiences among Nurses: A Multivariate Multilevel Probit Model," *International Journal of Nursing Studies* 50, no. 2 (2013): 1–91; Katie Tulenko, *Insourced: How Importing Jobs Impacts the Healthcare Crisis Here and Abroad* (Hanover, NH: Dartmouth College Press, 2012); Jean Whelan, *Nursing the Nation: Building the Nurse Labor Force* (New Brunswick, NJ: Rutgers University Press, 2021).

29. See previous note.

30. Jurascheck et al., "United States Registered Nurse"; Smiley et al., "2017 National Nursing Workforce Survey."

31. See previous note.

32. The largest cohort of registered nurses to join the American workforce was before the 1970s when women's career choices were more limited. See interview with American Nursing Association president, Pam Cipriano, in the *Atlantic*: Rebecca Grant, "The U.S. Is Running Out of Nurses," *Atlantic*, February 2016, http://www .theatlantic.com/health/archive/2016/02/nursing-shortage/459741/.

33. See discussion in Brent Robert MacWilliams, Bonnie Schmidt, and Michael R. Ble-ich, "Men in Nursing," *American Journal of Nursing* 113, no. 1 (2013): 38–44.

34. Susan Reinhard, Donald Redfoot, and Brenda Cleary, "Health and Long-term Care: Are Immigrant Workers Indispensable?," *Generations* 32, no. 4 (2009): 24–30.

35. See data at U.S. Bureau of Labor Statistics, "Projections of Occupational Employ-ment, 2016–26"; Buerhaus et al., "Four Challenges"; Jurascheck et al., "United States Registered Nurse"; Smiley et al., "2017 National Nursing Workforce Survey."

36. Potential nursing students also struggled to find the money to attend programs. This was made even more dire when President Trump eliminated all funding to Title VIII Nursing Workforce Development programs with the exception of the Nurse Corps. On the struggles of nursing programs in general, see American Association of Col-leges of Nursing, *2018–2019 Enrollment and Graduations*.

37. The U.S. Bureau of Labor Statistics estimates that American healthcare has lost roughly half-a -million workers since February 2020. Additional data from Morning Consulting suggests that upward of 18 percent of healthcare workers have quit their jobs since the pandemic began. See Ed Yong, "Why Health-Care Workers are Quitting in Droves," *Atlantic* November 18, 2021, https://www.theatlantic.com/health/archive/2021/11/the-mass-exodus-of-americas-health-care-workers/620713/

38. I will discuss this history in chapter 2.

39. Cortes and Pan, "Foreign-Nurse Importation."

40. "Improving the Processing of 'Schedule A' Nurse Visas," Department of Homeland Security, December 5, 2008, http://www.dhs.gov/xlibrary/assets/cisomb_recommendation_36.pdf; Leah E. Masselink and Cheryl B. Jones, "Immigration Policy and Internationally Educated Nurses in the United States: A Brief History," *Nursing Outlook* 62, no. 1 (January–February 2014): 39–45.

41. Several different temporary-work and exchange-visitor visa categories are used to admit foreign-born healthcare professionals into the United States. These categories include H-1B (specialty occupations), H-2B (nonagricultural workers), H-3 (trainees), TN (Mexican and Canadian NAFTA professionals), J-1 (exchange visitors), and O-1 (persons with "extraordinary ability or achievement"). As is the case with other immigrants, foreign-born healthcare professionals can also apply for visas based on family, employment connections, and through humanitarian and other routes. See current regulation with restrictions post-COVID-19, "Health Care Worker Certification," U.S. Citizenship and Immigration Services, last updated July 30, 2021, https://www.uscis.gov/working-united-states/temporary-workers/health-care-worker-certification. In general, see McCabe, *Foreign-born Health Care Workers*; Spetz et al., "Internationally Educated Nurses"; Squires and Beltrán-Sánchez, *Strengthening Health Systems*; Siyam and dal Poz, eds., *Migration of Health Workers*.

42. Cortes and Pan, "Foreign-Nurse Importation."

43. Patricia Pittman, Catherine Davis, Franklin Shaffer, Carolina-Nicole Herrera, and Cudjoe Bennett, "Perceptions of Employment-Based Discrimination among Newly Arrived Foreign-Educated Nurses," *American Journal of Nursing* 114, no. 1 (January 2014): 26–35.

44. A. Christine Delucas, "Foreign Nurse Recruitment: Global Risk"; Nicola Yeates, *Global Care Economies and Migrant Workers: Explorations in Global Care Chains* (New York: Palgrave Macmillan, 2009).

45. See previous note.

46. Mireille Kingma, "Nurses on the Move: A Global Overview," *Health Services Research* 42, no. 3 (June 2007): 1281–1298.

47. Moira Herbst, "Herbst M. Immigration: More Foreign Nurses Needed?," *Bloomberg BusinessWeek Online*, June 22, 2009, https://www.bloomberg.com/news/articles/2009-06-21/immigration-more-foreign-nurses-needed.

48. See, for example, "It's Time for Us to Buck Up," *Truth About Nursing*, July 15, 2009, https://www.truthaboutnursing.org/news/2009/jul/15_obama.html#gsc.tab=0.

49. See, for example, "Marion Barry, Hospitalized for Blood Clot In Las Vegas, Thanks Filipino Nurses," *Huffington Post*, May 21, 2012, http://www.huffingtonpost.com/2012/05/21/marion-barry-filipino-nurses_n_1533407.html.

50. See, for example, Dartunorro Clark, "Trump Says Hire American. These Businesses Say They Can't—and Foreign Labor Limits Are Killing Them," *NBC*, August 6, 2018, https://www.nbcnews.com/politics/white-house/trump-says-hire-american-these

-businesses-say-they-can-t-n896766; Camilo Montoyo-Galvez, "Republicans Will Buck Trump on Immigration if 'They Feel the Heat,' Schumer Says," *CBS*, March 13, 2019, https://www.cbsnews.com/news/republicans-will-buck-trump-on-immigration -if-they-feel-the-heat-schumer-says/.

51. Bridget Carney, "The Ethnics of Recruiting Foreign Nurses. How Should Catholic Organizations Approach This Problem?," *Health Progress*, November–December 2005, https://www.chausa.org/publications/health-progress/article/november-december -2005/the-ethics-of-recruiting-foreign-nurses; Peterson, "Nursing Shortage."

52. See George Borjas, *Friends or Strangers: The Impact of Immigrants on the U.S. Economy* (New York: Basic Books, 1990); Peter Brimelow, *Alien Nation: Common Sense about America's Immigration Disaster* (New York: Random House, 1995); Erika Lee, *America for Americans: A History of Xenophobia in the United States* (New York: Basic Books, 2019); Wayne Lutton and John Tanton, *The Immigration Invasion* (Petosky, MI: The Social Contract Press, 1994); John Kuo Wei Tchen and Dylan Yeats, *Yellow Peril! An Archive of Anti-Asian Fear* (Brooklyn, NY: Verso Books, 2014).

53. It is beyond the scope of this book to detail the history of American xenophobia in full. See Lee, *America for Americans*. Also see Adrian de Leon, "The Long History of US Racism against Asian Americans, from 'Yellow Peril' to 'Model Minority' to the 'Chinese Virus,'" *Conversation*, April 8, 2020, https://theconversation.com/the -long-history-of-us-racism-against-asian-americans-from-yellow-peril-to-model -minority-to-the-chinese-virus-135793.

54. Lee, *America for Americans*.

55. Jay P. Dolan, *In Search of American Catholicism: A History of Religion and Culture in Tension* (New York: Oxford University Press, 2003); Jay P. Dolan, *The American Catholic Experience: A History from Colonial Times to the Present* (New York: Doubleday, 1985); John T. McGreevy, *Catholicism and American Freedom: A History* (New York: W. W. Norton & Company, 2003); Kerby A. Miller, *Emigrants and Exiles: Ireland and the Irish Exodus to North America* (New York: Oxford University Press, 1985).

56. From 1866 to 1926, Catholics, largely led by immigrant sister-nurses (nuns), established nearly five hundred hospitals in the United States. See Barbra Mann Wall, *Unlikely Entrepreneurs: Catholic Sisters and the Hospital Marketplace, 1865–1925* (Columbus: Ohio State University Press, 2005); Barbra Mann Wall and Sioban Nelson, "Our Heels Are Praying Very Hard All Day," *Holistic Nursing Practice* 17, no. 9 (2003): 320–328; also see Sioban Nelson, *Say Little, Do Much: Nursing, Nuns, and Hospitals in the Nineteenth Century* (Philadelphia: University of Pennsylvania Press, 2001).

57. Digby E. Baltzell, *The Protestant Establishment* (New York: Random House, 1964); Ray Allen Billington, *The Protestant Crusade, 1800–1960: A Study of the Origins of American Nativism* (New York: Quadrangle Books, 1964); M. Jeffrey Burns, Ellen Skerrett, and Joseph M. White, eds., *Keeping Faith: European and Asian Catholic Immigrants* (New York: Orbis Books, 2006),; James D. Davidson and Mark McCormick, "Catholics and Civic Engagement: Empirical Findings at the Individual Level," in *Civil Society, Civic Engagement and Catholicism in the U.S.*, ed. Antonius Liedhegener and Werner Kremp (Germany: WVT Wissenschaftlicher Verlag Trier, 2007), 119–134; John Higham, *Strangers in the Land: Patterns in the American Nativism, 1860–1925* (New Brunswick, NJ: Rutgers University Press, 2002).

58. Tyler G. Anbinder, *Nativism and Slavery: The Northern Know Nothings and the Politics of the 1850s* (New York: Oxford University Press, 1994).

59. Anbinder, *Nativism and Slavery*.

60. Ronald Formisano, *The Transformation of Political Culture: Massachusetts Parties, 1790s–1840s* (New York: Oxford University Press, 1983).

61. From 1929 through 1930, for example, anti-Filipino riots broke out in rural communities such as Watsonville, California, in response to Filipino men dancing with White women at local bars. On numerous occasions Filipinos were beaten by angry mobs. See Fred Cordova, *Filipinos: Forgotten Asian Americans: A Pictorial Essay* (Dubuque, IA: Kendall/Hunt Publishing Company, 1983); Ronald Takaki, *In the Heart of Filipino America: Immigrants from the Pacific Isles* (New York: Chelsea House Press, 1996).

62. See Warwick Anderson, *Colonial Pathologies: American Tropical Medicine, Race, and Hygiene in the Philippines* (Durham, NC: Duke University Press, 1987); Carol Nackenoff and Julie Novkov, "Who is Born a Citizen," *Conversation*, January 15, 2020, https://theconversation.com/who-is-born-a-us-citizen-127403.

63. Lee, *America for Americans*.

64. Dolan, *In Search of American Catholicism*.

65. This view largely overinflates their actual socioeconomic status. See Mia Tuan, *Forever Foreigners or Honorary Whites: The Asian Ethnic Experience Today* (New Brunswick, NJ: Rutgers University Press, 1998).

66. Tuan, *Forever Foreigners or Honorary Whites*.

67. ANA denied membership to Black nurses until 1950. See Daline C. Hine, *Black Women in White: Racial Conflict and Cooperation in the Nursing Profession, 1890–1950* (Bloomington: Indiana University Press, 1989).

68. Sujani Reddy, *Nursing and Empire: Gendered Labor and Migration from India to the United States* (Chapel Hill: University of North Carolina Press, 2015); Sujani Reddy, "Women on the Move: A History of Indian Nurse Migration to the United States," (PhD diss., New York University, 2008).

69. Munira Wells, "The Experience of Indian Nurses in America," (PhD diss., Seton Hall University, 2013).

70. See discussion of the EVP system and its impact on American nursing in chapter 6 of Reddy, *Nursing and Empire*.

71. Barbara Brush, "Exchangees or Employees? The Exchange Visitor Program and Foreign Nurse Migration to the United States, 1945–1990," *Nursing History Review* 1, no. 1 (1993): 171–180.

72. From 1956 to 1969, eleven thousand Filipino nurses participated in the EVP program with an unknown but estimated significantly smaller number of nurses participating from India. See Brush, "Exchangees or Employees?"; Catherine Ceniza Choy, *Empire of Care: Nursing and Migration in Filipino American History* (Durham, NC: Duke University Press, 2003); Yin Li Espiritu, "Gender, Migration, and Work: Filipina Health Care Professionals to the United States," *Revue Européenne des Migrations Internationales* 21, no. 1 (2005): 55–75; Reddy, *Nursing and Empire*; Reddy, "Women on the Move."

73. Brush, "Exchangees or Employees?"; Barbara Brush, "Sending for Nurses: Foreign Nurse Immigration to American Hospitals, 1945–1980," (PhD diss., University of Pennsylvania, 1994).

74. Beatrice J. Kalisch, Philip A. Kalisch, and Jaqueline Clinton, "Minority Nurses in the News," *Nursing Outlook* 29, no. 1 (January 1981): 49–54.

75. Kalisch, Kalisch, and Clinton, "Minority Nurses." Also see Janet Henning, "Nurses from Overseas," *Modern Healthcare* 5, no. 5 (1975): 21–28.

76. Brush, "Sending for Nurses"; Barbara Brush, "The Potent Lever of Toil: Nursing Development and Exportation in the Postcolonial Philippines," *American Journal of Public Health* 100, no. 9 (September 2010): 1572–1581; Susan Dudas and Mary T. Whalen, "Working with the Foreign Nurse in the United States," *Journal of Nursing Education* 10, no. 1 (1971): 27–31; Virginia Sweeny, "Working with Nurses from Overseas," *American Journal of Nursing* 73, no. 10 (1973): 1768–1770.

77. See previous note.

78. Choy, *Empire of Care*; Espiritu, "Gender, Migration, and Work"; Sheba George, *When Women Come First: Gender and Class in Transnational Migration* (Berkeley, CA: University of California Press, 2005); Reddy, *Nursing and Empire*; Reddy, "Women on the Move."

79. George, *When Women Come First*.

80. Brush, "Sending for Nurses"; Brush, "The Potent Lever of Toil"; Gita L. Dhillon, "Study Programs for Foreign Nurses: Special Needs of Foreign Nurses," *Nursing Outlook* 24, no. 1 (January 1976): 42–44.

81. See previous note.

82. David Boaz, "Yellow Peril Reinfects America," *CATO Institute*, originally published April 7, 1989, last updated 2015, https://www.cato.org/publications/commentary /yellow-peril-reinfects-america.

83. Brush, "Sending for Nurses"; Brush, "The Potent Lever of Toil"; Choy, *Empire of Care*; Espiritu, "Gender, Migration, and Work"; George, *When Women Come First*; Reddy, *Nursing and Empire*; Reddy, "Women on the Move."

84. I only present key themes and points of this case to better contextualize my arguments in subsequent chapters. For a detailed discussion and historical analysis of the case, see chapter 5 in Choy, *Empire of Care*.

85. Choy, *Empire of Care*. Also see the documentary film, *U.S. vs. Narciso, Perez and the Press*, directed by Andrea Raby 2013, https://usvnarcisoperezpress.wordpress .com, https://usvnarcisoperezpress.wordpress.com/.

86. Greg Stejskal, "A Retired FBI Agent's View of Mystery Deaths in Ann Arbor," *Deadline Detroit*, March 20, 2015, https://www.deadlinedetroit.com/articles/11829/a_retired _fbi_agent_s_view_of_the_mysterious_deaths_at_the_ann_arbor_va_.

87. Kirik Cheyfitz, "Nurses Convicted in Poisoning Case," *Washington Post*, July 14, 1977, https://www.washingtonpost.com/archive/politics/1977/07/14/nurses-convic ted-in-poisoning-case/391d50cd-27b7-446d-a434-27f8cf428297/; "Long Count to A Guilty Verdict," *Time*, July 25, 1977, http://content.time.com/time/magazine/article /0,9171,919117,00.html.

88. Choy, *Empire of Care*; Espiritu, "Gender, Migration, and Work."

89. Jean S. Arbeiter, "The Facts about Foreign Nurses," *RN*, September 1988, 57–73.

90. Maria Baptiste, "Workplace Discrimination: An Additional Stressor for Internationally Educated Nurses," *OJIN: Online Journal of Issues in Nursing* 20, no. 3 (August 18, 2015), http://ojin.nursingworld.org/MainMenuCategories/ANAMarketplace/ANA Periodicals/OJIN/TableofContents/Vol-20-2015/No3-Sept-2015/Articles-Previous -Topics/Workplace-Discrimination-for-Internationally-Educated-Nurses.html; M. M. Jose, "Lived Experiences of Internationally Educated Nurses in Hospitals in the United States of America," *International Nursing Review* 58, no. 1 (2011): 123–129; Pittman et al., "Perceptions of Employment-Based Discrimination."

91. Baptiste, "Workplace Discrimination"; Jessy Jose et al., "Demands of Immigration among Indian Nurses Who Immigrated to the United States," *Asian Nursing Research* 2, no. 1 (2008): 46–54.

92. Choy, *Empire of Care*; Anh Do, "Filipino Nurses Win Language Discrimination Settlement," *Los Angeles Times*, September 19, 2012, https://www.latimes.com/health/la-xpm-2012-sep-18-la-me-english-only-20120918-story.html; Naty Lopez, "The Acculturation of Selected Filipino Nurses to Nursing Practice in the United States" (PhD diss., University of Pennsylvania, 1990); PTI, "Indian-American Nurse Sues Employer, Alleges Discrimination," *Indian Express*, November 14, 2015, http://indianexpress.com/article/world/indians-abroad/indian-american-nurse-sues-employer-alleges-discrimination/. Also see Wells, "The Experience of Indian Nurses."

93. Momo Chang, "Despite Being Valued and Essential Members of the American RN Workforce, Filipino Nurses Must Still Often Challenge and Overcome Bias and Discrimination," *National Nurses United*, October 2011, 15–19.

94. Baptiste, "Workplace Discrimination"; Barbara Dicicco-Bloom, "The Racial and Gendered Experiences of Immigrant Nurses from Kerala, India," *Journal of Transcultural Nursing* 15, no. 1 (2004): 26–33; Kavitha Mediratta, "How Do You Say Your Name?," in *Struggle for Ethnic Identity: Narratives by Asian American Professionals*, eds. Pyong G. Min and Rose Kim (Walnut Creek, CA: Alta Mira, 1999), 77–86; Rebecca M. Wheeler, Jennifer W. Foster, and Kenneth W. Hepburn, "The Experience of Discrimination by US and Internationally Educated Nurses in Hospital Practice in the USA: A Qualitative Study," *Journal of Advanced Nursing* 70, no. 2 (2014): 350–359.

95. See, for example, Emilia Benton, "Should EPs Accommodate Patient Requests for a Specific Doctor? Many Do," *Emergency Medicine News* 33, no. 4 (April 2011); Vida Foubister, "Requests by Patients Can Put Doctors in Ethical Bind," *AMA Medical News*, January 22, 2001, http://www.ama-assn.org/amednews/2001/01/22/prsb0122.htm; Jacqueline Howard, "Racism in Medicine: An 'Open Secret,'" *CNN*, October 26, 2016, https://www.cnn.com/2016/10/26/health/doctors-discrimination-racism/index.html; also see Cynthia Spry, "Between Two Cultures: Foreign Nurses in the United States," *Global Perspective AORN Journal* 89, no. 3 (2009): 593–595.

96. Masselink and Jones, "Immigration Policy"; Squires and Beltrán-Sánchez, *Strengthening Health Systems*.

97. Edward J. Schumacher, "Foreign-Born Nurses in the US Labor Market," *Health Economics* 20 (2011): 362–378; Siyam and dal Poz, eds., *Migration of Health Workers*.

98. Masselink and Jones, "Immigration Policy"; Pittman et al., "Perceptions of Employment-Based Discrimination."

99. Baptiste, "Workplace Discrimination"; Megan-Jane Johnstone and Olga Kanitsaki, "The Spectrum of 'New Racism' and Discrimination in Hospital Contexts: A Reappraisal," *Collegian* 16, no. 2 (April–June 2009): 63–69; Joanne T. Moceri, "Bias in the Nursing Workplace: Implications for Latino(a) Nurses," *Journal of Cultural Diversity* 19, no. 3 (2012): 94–101.

100. See Joseph Berger, "Filipino Nurses, Healers in Trouble," *New York Times*, January 27, 2008, https://www.nytimes.com/2008/01/27/nyregion/nyregionspecial2/27Rnurses.html.

101. Lopez, "Acculturation of Selected Filipino Nurses"; Jane G. Ryan, "Adjusting to the United States Healthcare Workplace Perceptions of Internationally Born and Educated Registered Nurses" (PhD diss., Widener University, 2010).

102. Dave Holmes, Bernard Roy, and Amelie Perron, "The Use of Postcolonialism in the Nursing Domain: Colonial Patronage, Conversion and Resistance," *Advances in Nursing* 31, no.1 (2008): 42–51.

103. See, for example, Michael S. Goldstein, "The VA and Limits on Veterans' Religious Freedom," *American Thinker*, December 4, 2015, http://www.americanthinker.com /articles/2015/12/the_va_and_limits_on_veterans_religious_liberty.html.

104. See "Chaplain Says Officials Ordered Him to Cover Christian Symbols in VA Chapel-Truth!," *Truth or Fiction*, February 9, 2015, https://www.truthorfiction.com/va-covers -religious-symbols/.

105. See, for example, Olaf Eckberg, "BE _____!' Texas VA Censors Veteran's 'Overly Religious' Christmas Decorations," *American Mirror*, December 14, 2015, http:// www.theamericanmirror.com/be-_____-texas-va-censors-veterans-overly -religious-christmas-decorations/.

106. U.S. Department of Veterans Affairs, "VA Overhauls Religious and Spiritual Symbol Policies To Protect Religious Liberty," press release, July 3, 2019, https://www.va .gov/opa/pressrel/pressrelease.cfm?id=5279.

107. Eric Katz, "Citing New Supreme Court Ruling, VA to Allow Religious Displays at Hospitals and Facilities," *Government Executive*, July 3, 2019, https://www.govexec .com/management/2019/07/citing-new-supreme-court-ruling-va-allow-religious -displays-hospitals-and-facilities/158209/.

108. Cadge, *Paging God*; Cadge and Konieczny, "Hidden in Plain Sight." Also see Elaine Howard Ecklund, *Science vs. Religion: What Scientists Really Think* (New York: Oxford University Press, 2010).

109. Hugh Small, *Florence Nightingale: Avenging Angel* (New York: St. Martin's Press, 1998). Also see Nightingale's writing while traveling in Egypt, in Edward Chaney, "Egypt in England and America: The Cultural Memorials of Religion, Royalty and Revolution" in *Sites of Exchange: European Crossroads and Faultlines*, eds. Maurizio Ascari and Adriana Corrado, (New York: Rodopi, 2004), 39–74; Florence Nightingale, *Florence Nightingale to Her Nurses: A Selection from Miss Nightingale's Addresses to Probationers and Nurses of the Nightingale School at St. Thomas's Hospital* (London: Macmillan, 1914), 116.

110. See discussion of Nightingale's full break from Victorian norms and her feminist perspectives in Myrna Stark, ed., *Cassandra: Florence Nightingale's Angry Outcry against the Forced Idleness of Victorian Women* (New York: The Feminist Press, 1979).

111. Barbra Mann Wall, "American Catholic Nursing: An Historical Analysis," *Medizinhistorisches Journal* 47, no. 2–3 (September 2012): 160–175.

112. Mann Wall, "American Catholic Nursing."

113. See Lynn McDonald, ed., *Florence Nightingale's Theology: Essays, Letters and Journal Notes: Collected Works of Florence Nightingale Vol. 3* (Waterloo, Ontario: Wilfred Laurier University Press, 2002). Also see Gerard Vallee, ed., *Florence Nightingale on Mysticism and Eastern Religions: Collected Works of Florence Nightingale Vol. 4* (Waterloo, Ontario: Wilfred Laurier University Press, 2003).

114. McDonald, ed., *Florence Nightingale's Theology: Essays.*

115. Nightingale was a devout Anglican (Church of England) with a keen interest in the Bible and a personal devotion to God. However, she sought to secularize nursing because she thought religious orders could not carry the profession forward. She also thought that nursing care should not be contingent on proselytizing—care for conversion—and thought nursing schools should be open to all regardless of their religious commitment. See Lynn McDonald, ed., *Florence Nightingale's Theology.* Also see Gerard Vallee, ed., *Florence Nightingale on Mysticism*; Judith Allen Shelly and Arlene B. Miller, *Called to Care: A Christian Worldview for Nursing* (Downers Grove, IL: IVP Academic, 2006).

116. Michael J. Balboni et al., "Nurse and Physician Barriers to Spiritual Care Provision at the End of Life," *Journal of Pain & Symptom Management* 48, no. 3 (2014): 400–410. Also see Roberta Cavendish et al., "Patients' Perceptions of Spirituality and the Nurse as a Spiritual Care Provider," *Holistic Nursing Practice* 20, no. 1 (2006): 41–47; Roberta Cavendish et al., "Spiritual Perspectives of Nurses in the United States Relevant for Education and Practice," *Western Journal of Nursing Research* 26, no. 2 (2004): 219–221; Harold Koenig, "The Spiritual Care Team," *Religions* 5, 2014: 1161–1174; Koenig, *Medicine, Religion, and Health* (West Conshohocken, PA: Templeton Press, 2008); Susan Stranahan, "Spiritual Perception, Attitudes about Spiritual Care, and Spiritual Care Practices among Nurse Practitioners," *Western Journal of Nursing Research* 23, no. 1 (2001): 90–104.

117. See previous note.

118. Dalia Fahmy, "Americans Are Far More Religious than Adults in Other Wealthy Nations," *Pew Research Center*, July 31, 2018, https://www.pewresearch.org/fact -tank/2018/07/31/americans-are-far-more-religious-than-adults-in-other-wealthy -nations/; Pew Research Center, "In U.S., Decline of Christianity Continues at Rapid Pace," October 17, 2019, https://www.pewforum.org/2019/10/17/in-u-s-decline-of -christianity-continues-at-rapid-pace/.

119. See, for example, Megan Besta, Phyllis Butowb, and Ian Olverc, "Do Patients Want Doctors to Talk about Spirituality?," *Patient Education and Counseling* 98, no. 11 (November 2015): 1320–1328; John Ehman et al., "Do Patients Want Physicians to Inquire about Their Spiritual or Religious Beliefs if They Become Gravely Ill?," *Archives Internal Medicine* 159, no. 15 (1999): 1803–1806; Ronit Elk et al., "The Role of Nurses in Providing Spiritual Care to Patients: An Overview," *Journal of Nursing*, September 1, 2017, https://www.asrn.org/journal-nursing/1781-the-role-of-nurses-in-providing -spiritual-care-to-patients-an-overview.html; Don Grant, "Spiritual Intervention: How, When, and Why Nurse Use Them," *Holistic Nursing Practice* 18, no. 1 (2004): 36–41; Gary McCord et al., "Discussing Spirituality with Patients: A Rational and Ethical Approach," *Annals of Family Medicine* 2, no. 4 (July 2004): 356–361; Melanie McEwen, "Spiritual Nursing Care," *Holistic Nursing Practice* 19, no. 4 (2005): 161–168.

120. Michael J. Balboni et al., "Why Is Spiritual Care Infrequent at the End of Life? Spiritual Care Perceptions among Patients, Nurses, and Physicians and the Role of Training," *Journal of Clinical Oncology* 31, no. 4 (February 2013): 461–467; Karen A. Boutell and Frederick W. Bozett, "Nurses' Assessment of Patients' Spirituality: Continuing Education Implications," *Journal of Continuing Education* 21, no. 4 (1987): 172–176; Timothy P. Daaleman and Donald E. Nease, Jr., "Patient Attitudes Regarding Physician Inquiry into Spiritual and Religious Issues," *Journal of Family Practice* 39, no. 6 (1994): 564–568; John W. Ehman et al., "Do Patients Want Physicians to Inquire about Their Spiritual or Religious Beliefs if They Become Gravely Ill?," *Archive of Internal Medicine* 159, no. 15 (1999): 1803–1806; Grant, "Spiritual Intervention"; Aru Narayanasamy, "Nurse Awareness and Preparedness in Meeting Their Patients Spiritual Needs," *Nursing Education Today* 13, no. 3 (1992): 196–201; Dana E. King and Bruce Bushwick, "Beliefs and Attitudes of Hospital Inpatients about Faith Healing and Prayer," *Journal of Family Practice* 39 (1994): 349–352; Gary McCord et al., "Discussing Spirituality with Patients: A Rational and Ethical Approach," *Annals of Family Medicine* 2, no. 4 (July 2004): 356–361; Aru Narayanasamy, "Recognizing Spiritual Needs," in *Spiritual Assessment in Healthcare Practice*, eds. Linda Ross and Wilfred McSherry (Keswick, England: M&K Update Ltd., 2010): 37–55.

121. Koenig, "The Spiritual Care Team"; Mary Elizabeth O'Brien, *Spirituality in Nursing* (Burlington, MA: Jones and Bartlett, 2018); Mary R. O'Brien, Karen Kinloch, Karen E. Groves and Barbara A. Jack, "Meeting Patients' Spiritual Needs during End-Of-Life Care," *Journal of Clinical Nursing* 28, no. 1–2 (January 2019: 182–189.

122. Tracy J. Carr, "Facing Existential Realities: Exploring Barriers and Challenges to Spiritual Nursing Care," *Qualitative Health Research* 20, no. 10 (2010): 1379–1392; B. Denholm, "Staff Nurses and Prayer," *AORN Journal* 88, no. 3 (2008): 451–455; Koenig, "The Spiritual Care Team"; O'Brien, *Spirituality in Nursing*; O'Brien et al., "Meeting Patients' Spiritual Needs."

123. Michael O. Emerson et al., "Houston Region Grows More Racially/Ethnically Diverse, with Small Declines in Segregation," 2012, Kinder Institute for Urban Research, Rice University, https://kinder.rice.edu/sites/default/files/documents/Houston%20Region %20Grows%20More%20Ethnically%20Diverse%204-9.pdf; Randy Capps, Michael Fix, and Chiamaka Nwosu, *A Profile of Immigrants in Houston, the Nation's Most Diverse Metropolitan Area* (Washington, DC: Migration Policy Institute, March 2015), https://www.migrationpolicy.org/research/profile-immigrants-houston-nations-most -diverse-metropolitan-area.

124. Capps, Fix, and Nwosu, *A Profile of Immigrants in Houston*.

125. See current TMC facts and figures, "About TMC," Texas Medical Center, accessed December 2016, https://www.tmc.edu/about-tmc/; "TMC Facts & Figures," Texas Medical Center, 2016, https://www.tmc.edu/wp-content/uploads/2016/08/TMC _FactsFiguresOnePager_0307162.pdf.

126. While some hospitals in the TMC obviously have personnel departments to aid foreign-born employees with their statuses and any related employment or tax paper-work (M. D. Anderson hospital, for example), others such as Michael E. DeBakey Vet-erans Hospital, a federal institution, does not have such a department and does not keep records of nativity, given that all employees must be U.S. citizens. However, analysis of nine TMC academic institutions suggest that in 2012 there were roughly 4,936 foreign-born students enrolled in the TMC with an additional 133 exchange students and 1,692 exchange visitors as professors, researchers, and short-term schol-ars and specialists from twelve different countries; see "TMC International Students, Exchange Visitors, and Employees," Texas Medical Center, March 2012, https://digital commons.library.tmc.edu/cgi/viewcontent.cgi?referer=https://www.google.com /&httpsredir=1&article=1001&context=tmcreports.

127. Emerson et al., "Houston Region Grows"; Kristen McCabe, *Foreign-born Health Care Workers*; Mary Schiflett, "The Second Downtown," *Houston Review of History and Culture* 2, no. 1 (2004): 2–7; Squires and Beltrán-Sánchez, *Strengthening Health Systems*; Siyam and dal Poz, eds., *Migration of Health Workers*; "TMC Facts and Figures."

128. John Harrington, "There Are 18.2 Million Veterans in the US. Which State Is Home to the Most of Them?," *USA Today*, July 4, 2019, https://www.usatoday.com/story /money/2019/07/04/states-with-the-most-veterans-new-york-alaska/39645251/; Alanna Moriarty, "50 Largest Veterans Hospitals by Numbers of Staffed Beds," *Definitive Healthcare* (blog), September 30, 2020, https://blog.definitivehc.com /largest-veterans-hospitals.

129. See "VA Houston Health Care," U.S. Department of Veterans Affairs, accessed Novem-ber 2020, https://www.houston.va.gov/about/index.asp.

130. "VA Houston Health Care," U.S. Department of Veterans Affairs.

131. St. John Barned-Smith and Samantha Ketterer, "Veterans: Report Validates Wait-Time Allegations at Houston VA," *Houston Chronicle*, June 28, 2016, https://www.houstonchronicle.com/news/houston-texas/houston/article/Veterans-Report-validates-wait-time-allegations-8319802.php

132. German Lopez, "The VA scandal of 2014, explained," *Vox*, May 13, 2015, https://www.vox.com/2014/9/26/18080592/va-scandal-explained.

133. See methodological appendix.

134. Methodological appendix.

135. Methodological appendix.

136. Methodological appendix.

137. Methodological appendix.

138. Methodological appendix.

2. Colonialism, Christian Culture, and Nursing Care

1. Although INA was a fairly new association at the time this study began, the core group of nurses who make up its most active membership has been together for over fifteen years.

2. Mireille Kingma, "Nurse Migration and the Global Health Care Economy," *Policy, Politics & Nursing Practice* 9, no. 4 (November 2008): 328–333; Mireille Kingma, "Nurses on the Move: A Global Overview," *Health Services Research* 42, no. 3 (June 2007): 1281–1298.

3. Rochelle E. Ball, "Divergent Development, Racialized Rights: Globalized Labour Markets and the Trade of Nurses—The Case of the Philippines," *Women's Studies International Forum* 27, no. 2 (2004): 119–133; Catherine Ceniza Choy, *Empire of Care: Nursing and Migration in Filipino American History* (Durham, NC: Duke University Press, 2003); Marie Percot, "Indian Nurses in the Gulf: Two Generations of Female Migration" (paper, Sixth Mediterranean Social and Political Research Meeting, March 2005), https://halshs.archives-ouvertes.fr/halshs-00004458/document; Nicola Yeates, *Global Care Economies and Migrant Workers: Explorations in Global Care Chains* (New York: Palgrave Macmillan, 2009).

4. Linda H. Aiken, Robyn B. Cheung, and Danielle M. Olds, "Education Policy Initiatives to Address the Nurse Shortage in the United States," *Health Affairs* 28, no. 4 (2009): w646–w656; Barbara Brush and Julie Sochalski, "International Nurse Migration: Lessons from the Philippines," *Policy, Politics & Nursing Practice* 8, no. 1 (2007): 37–46; Kingma, "Nurse Migration"; Kingma, "Nurses on the Move"; Megan Prescott and Mark Nichter, "Transnational Nurse Migration: Future Directions for Medical Anthropologist Research," *Social Science and Medicine* 107 (2014): 113–123.

5. V. N. Pasumpon, "Chennai: Nurse Strike Movement Ends in Victory," *New Socialist Alternative*, March 29, 2012, http://www.socialism.in/?p=2538.

6. Pasumpon, "Chennai." Also see Fely Marilyn E. Lorenzo et al., "Nurse Migration from a Source Country Perspective: Philippine Country Case Study," *Health Services Research* 42, no. 3 (June 2007): 1406–1418; Douglas S. Massey et al., "Theories of International Migration: A Review and Appraisal," *Population and Development Review* 19, no. 3 (September 1993): 431–466.

7. See "How Much Do RNs Make in Texas?," *Registered Nurse* online, accessed March 2020, http://www.topregisterednurse.com/salary/texas/.

8. Prescott and Nichter, "Transnational Nurse Migration."

9. Barbara Dicicco-Bloom, "The Racial and Gendered Experiences of Immigrant Nurses from Kerala, India," *Journal of Transcultural Nursing* 15, no. 1 (2004): 26–33; Massey et al., "Theories of International Migration"; Percot, "Indian Nurses in the Gulf"; Sujani Reddy, "Women on the Move: A History of Indian Nurse Migration to the United States," (PhD diss., New York University, 2008); Donald L. Redfoot and Ari N. Houser, "We Shall Travel On: Quality Care, Economic Development, and the International Migration of Long-Term Care Workers," AARP Policy Institute, 2005, https://assets.aarp.org/rgcenter/il/2005_14_intl_ltc.pdf; Yeates, *Global Care Economies*.

10. Yeates, *Global Care Economies*; Redfoot and Houser, "We Shall Travel On."

11. Marie Percot, "Indian Nurses in the Gulf: Two Generations of Female Migration," *South Asia Research* 26, no. 1 (2006): 42–62; Prescott and Nichter, "Transnational Nurse Migration."

12. Redfoot and Houser, "We Shall Travel On."

13. Rhacel Salazar Parrenas, *Servants of Globalization: Migration and Domestic Work* (Stanford, CA: Stanford University Press, 2001); Prescott and Nichter, "Transnational Nurse Migration"; James Tyner, *Made in the Philippines: Gendered Discourses and the Making of Migrants* (London: Routledge, 2004).

14. Kristen McCabe, *Foreign-born Health Care Workers in the United States* (Washington, DC: Migration Policy Institute, June 2012), http://www.migrationpolicy.org/article/foreign-born-health-care-workers-united-states; Joanne Spetz, Michael Gates, and Cheryl B. Jones, "Internationally Educated Nurses in the United States: Their Origins and Roles," *Nursing Outlook* 62, no. 1 (2014): 8–15; Allison Squires and Hiram Beltrán-Sánchez, *Strengthening Health Systems in North and Central America: What Role for Migration?* (Washington, DC: Migration Policy Institute, February 2013), https://www.migrationpolicy.org/research/strengthening-health-systems-north-and-central-america-what-role-migration?pdf=RMSG-HealthCare.pdf; Amani Siyam and Mario Roberto dal Poz, eds., *Migration of Health Workers: WHO Code of Practice and the Global Economic Crisis* (Washington, DC: Migration Policy Institute, May 2014), https://www.migrationpolicy.org/research/migration-health-workers-who-code-practice-and-global-economic-crisis.

15. McCabe, *Foreign-born Health Care Workers in the United States*.

16. See previous note. Additional data clarification provided in personal communication with Liz Heimann, Communications Coordinator, Migration Policy Institute.

17. Claire Cain Miller and Ruth Fremson, "Forget about the Stigma: Male Nurses Explain Why Nursing Is a Job of the Future for Men," *New York Times*, January 4, 2018, https://www.nytimes.com/interactive/2018/01/04/upshot/male-nurses.html; Emily Rappleye, "Gender Ratio of Nurses across 50 States," *Becher's Hospital Review*, May 29, 2015, https://www.beckershospitalreview.com/human-capital-and-risk/gender-ratio-of-nurses-across-50-states.html; American Society of Registered Nurses Staff, "Men in Nursing," *Journal of Nursing*, June 1, 2008, https://www.asrn.org/journal-nursing/374-men-in-nursing.html.

18. See further Barbara Ehrenreich and Arlie R. Hochschild, eds., *Global Woman: Nannies, Maids and Sex Workers in the New Economy* (New York: Metropolitan Books, 2002); Arlie Russell Hochschild, "The Nanny Chain" *The American Prospect* 11 (January 2000): 1–4; Margret Walton-Roberts, "Contextualizing the Global Nursing Care Chain: International Migration and the Status of Nursing in Kerala, India," *Global Networks* 12, no. 2 (April 2012): 175–194; also see criticisms in Rhacel Salazar Parrenas, "Closing Remarks" (paper, Transnational Mobilities for Care Conference, National University of Singapore, Singapore, September 10–11, 2009).

19. Nicola Yeates, "Global Care Chains: Critical Reflections and Lines of Enquiry," *International Feminist Journal of Politics* 6, no. 3 (2004): 369–391; Yeates, *Global Care Economies*; Nicola Yeates, "Global Care Chains: A State-of-the-Art Review and Future Directions in Care Transnationalism Research," *Global Networks* 12, no. 2 (2012): 135–154.

20. Prescott and Nichter, "Transnational Nurse Migration."

21. Prescott and Nichter, "Transnational Nurse Migration."

22. See further Immanuel Wallerstein, "The Rise and Future Demise of the World Capitalist System: Concepts for Comparative Analysis," *Comparative Studies in Society and History* 16, no. 4 (September 1974): 387–415. Also see Massey et al., "Theories of International Migration."

23. See Barbara Brush, "The Potent Lever of Toil: Nursing Development and Exportation in the Postcolonial Philippines," *American Journal of Public Health* 100, no. 9 (September 2010): 1572–1581; Choy, *Empire of Care*; Yin Li Espiritu, "Gender, Migration, and Work: Filipina Health Care Professionals to the United States," *Revue Européenne des Migrations Internationales* 21, no. 1 (2005): 55–75; Sheba George, *When Women Come First: Gender and Class in Transnational Migration* (Berkeley: University of California Press, 2005); Yasmin Y. Ortiga, "Professional Problems: The Burden of Producing the 'Global' Filipino Nurse," *Social Science and Medicine* 115, (August 2014): 64–71; Yeates, "Global Care Chains"; Yeates, *Global Care Economies*.

24. Notable exceptions include George, *When Women Come First*; Madelaine Healey, *Indian Sisters: A History of Nursing and the State, 1907–2007* (London: Routledge, 2013); Sujani Reddy, *Nursing and Empire: Gendered Labor and Migration from India to the United States* (Chapel Hill: University of North Carolina Press, 2015).

25. Madelaine Healey suggests that the neglect of religion in the study of nursing and the globalization of the profession after colonial rule in countries such as India and the Philippines is likely based on the perception that nurses were devoutly Christian, intensely bound to religious missions, conservative, and unlikely to challenge the orthodoxy of imperial rule; see Healey, *Indian Sisters*, 13. This likely makes nurses like Emmy, Joy, and Kareena, whose narratives open this chapter, less popular subjects for study.

26. Barbara Brush, "The Rockefeller Agenda for American/Philippines Nursing Relations," *Western Journal of Nursing Research* 17, no. 5 (1995): 540–555; Barbara Brush, *Sending for Nurses: Foreign Nurse Immigration to American Hospitals, 1945–1980* (PhD diss., University of Pennsylvania, 1994); Choy, *Empire of Care*; George, *When Women Come First*; Reddy, *Nursing and Empire*. Scholars interested in a detailed history of nursing in India and Philippines should read these works. Likewise, scholars interested in the history of colonial nursing should explore the rich field of colonial health that further contextualizes the role of medical missionaries working under or in collaboration with colonial agents. See for example, Warwick Anderson, *Colonial Pathologies: American Tropical Medicine, Race, and Hygiene in the Philippines* (Durham, NC: Duke University Press, 1987); David Arnold, *Colonizing the Body: State Medicine and Epidemic Disease in Nineteenth Century India* (Berkeley: University of California Press, 1993); Healey, *Indian Sisters*; Shula Marks, "What is Colonial about Colonial Medicine? And What Has Happened to Imperialism and Health?," *Social History of Medicine* 10, no. 2 (1997): 205–219; Radhika Ramasubban, "Imperial Health in British India, 1857–1900," in *Disease, Medicine and Empire: Perspectives on Western Medicine and Experience of European Expansion*, eds. Roy McLeod and Milton Lewis (London: Routledge, 1988), 38–60.

27. Choy, *Empire of Care*; Healey, *Indian Sisters*.
28. John Connell, *Migration and the Globalization of Health Care: The Health Worker Exodus?* (Northampton, MA: Edward Elgar, 2010); Sreelekha Nair and Madelaine Healey, "A Profession on the Margins: Status Issues in Indian Nursing," (occasional paper, Centre for Women in Developing Societies, delivered at the Centre for Women's Development Studies, New Delhi, India 2006).
29. Brush, "Potent Lever of Toil"; Brush, *Sending for Nurses*; Choy, *Empire of Care*; Espiritu, "Gender, Migration, and Work"; George, *When Women Come First*; Reddy, *Nursing and Empire*; Reddy, "Women on the Move."
30. Brush, "The Rockefeller Agenda for American/Philippines Nursing Relations"; Choy, *Empire of Care*; Reddy, *Nursing and Empire*.
31. I include in these dates the rule of the British East India Company from 1757 to 1858, which ended after the Indian Rebellion of 1857 and the eventual transfer of power to the official rule of the British Crown under Queen Victoria in 1858. Despite the fact that the so-called British Raj only lasted from 1858 to 1947, the year of Indian independence, the brief history outlined in this section is concerned with general British influence on Indian society whether it was under Crown rule or not.
32. Binumol Abraham, "Women Nurses and the Notion of Their Empowerment," (discussion paper 88, Kerala Research Programme on Local Level Development, Centre for Development Studies Thiruvananthapuram, 2004); Meera Abraham, *Caste and Gender: Missionaries and Nursing History in South India* (Bangalore, India: B. I. Publications, 1996); Choy, *Empire of Care*; George, *When Women Come First*; Anastacia Giron-Tupas, *History of Nursing in the Philippines* (Manila, PR: University Book Supply, 1952); Reddy, *Nursing and Empire*; Robert D. Woodberry, "The Missionary Roots of Liberal Democracy," *American Political Science Review* 106, no. 2 (May 2012): 244–274. On the reluctance to recognize the U.S. as an empire in public discourse see Julian Go, *Patterns of Empire: The British and American Empires, 1688 to the Present* (New York: Cambridge University Press, 2011).
33. Abraham, "Women Nurses"; Abraham, *Caste and Gender*; George, *When Women Come First*. Also see Weber on the strongly traditionalistic concept of vocation in Hinduism; Max Weber, *The Sociology of Religion* (Boston: Beacon Press, [1922] 1993).
34. Madelaine Healey, "Regarded, Paid and Housed as Menials: Nursing in Colonial India, 1900–1948," *South Asian History and Culture* 2, no. 1 (January 2011): 55–75; Sreelekha Nair and Madelaine Healey, "Transcending Boundaries: Indian Nurses in Internal and International Migration" working paper (occasional paper, Centre for Women in Developing Societies, New Delhi, India, 2007); T. K. Oommen, *Doctors and Nurses: A Study in Occupational Role Structures* (Delhi, India: MacMillan, 1978).
35. George, *When Women Come First*; Percot, "Indian Nurses in the Gulf."
36. See Healey, *Indian Sisters*, 323–325; Prema A. Kurein, *Kaleidoscopic Ethnicity: International Migration and the Reconstruction of Community Identities in India* (New Brunswick, NJ: Rutgers University Press, 2002); Abraham, "Women Nurses"; Abraham, *Caste and Gender*; George, *When Women Come First*.
37. Teodoro A. Agoncillo and Oscar M. Alphonso, *History of the Filipino People* (Quezon City, Philippines: Malaya Books, 1967), 42; Emma H. Blair and James A. Robertson, eds., *The Philippine Islands, 1493–1898* (Cleveland, OH: A.H. Clark, 1903); Stephen M. Cherry, *Faith, Family, and Filipino American Community Life* (New Brunswick, NJ: Rutgers University Press, 2014); John Nance, *The Gentle Tasadays: A Stone Age People in the Philippine Rain Forest* (New York: Harcourt, Brace, Javanovich, 1972).

38. Hazel McFerson, *Mixed Blessing: The Impact of the American Colonial Experience on Politics and Society in the Philippines* (Westport, CN: Praeger 2001); Alejandro R. Roces, "Exodus of Nurses Creates Local Shortage," *PhilStar Global*, August 8, 2002, https://www.philstar.com/opinion/2002/08/08/171262/exodus-nurses-creates-local-shortage.

39. See previous note.

40. Choy, *Empire of Care*; Giron-Tupas, *History of Nursing*; Lukas Kaelin, "A Questions of Justice: Assessing Nurse Migration from a Philosophical Perspective," *Developing World Bioethics* 11, no. 1 (2010): 30–39.

41. Cherry, *Faith, Family*; Peter Gowing, *Islands under the Cross: The Story of the Church in the Philippines* (Manila, Philippines: National Council of Churches in the Philippines, 1967); John Leddy Phelan, *The Hispanization of the Philippines: Spanish Aims and Filipino Responses, 1565–1700* (Madison: University of Wisconsin Press, [1959] 1967); Vicente Rafael, *Contracting Colonialism* (Ithaca, NY: Cornell University Press, 1998).

42. Choy, *Empire of Care*; Giron-Tupas, *History of Nursing*.

43. Jose R. Bantug, *A Short History of Nursing in the Philippines during the Spanish Regime, 1565–1898* (Manila, Philippines: Cologio Medico-Farmacentutico de Filipinas, 1953); Choy, *Empire of Care*; Roces, "Exodus of Nurses."

44. Giron-Tupas, *History of Nursing*; Roces, "Exodus of Nurses."

45. Joanna Basuray, "Nurse Miss Sahib: Colonial Culture-Bound Education in India and Transcultural Nursing," *Journal of Transcultural Nursing* 9, no. 1 (July to December 1997): 14–19; Choy, *Empire of Care*; Healey, *Indian Sisters*; Reddy, *Nursing and Empire*; Keith Watson, *Education in the Third World* (London: Croom Helm, 1982).

46. Abraham, "Women Nurses"; Abraham, *Caste and Gender*; T. Howard Somerwell, *Knife and Life in India: The Story of a Surgical Missionary at Neyyoor, Travancore* (London: Living Stone Press, 1940).

47. George, *When Women Come First*; Reema Gill, "Nursing Shortage in India with Special Reference to International Migration of Nurses," *Social Medicine* 6, no. 1 (2011): 52–59; Patricia Hill, *The World Their Housework: The American Woman's Foreign Mission Movement and Cultural Formation, 1890–1950* (Ann Arbor; University of Michigan Press, 1985); Reddy, *Nursing and Empire*; Munira Wells, "The Experience of Indian Nurses in America," (PhD diss., Seton Hall University, 2013). Also see Barbra Mann Wall and Sioban Nelson, "Our Heels Are Praying Very Hard All Day," *Holistic Nursing Practice* 17, no. 9 (2003): 320–328.

48. Healey, *Indian Sisters*.

49. Parvati Raghuram, "Global Care, Local Configuration—Challenges to Conceptualizations of Care," *Global Networks* 12, no. 2 (2012): 154–177; Caroline Osella and Filippo Osella, "Nuancing the Migrant Experience: Perspectives from Kerala, South India," in *Transnational South Asians: The Making of a Neo-Diaspora*, eds. Susan Koshy and R. Radhakrishnan (Oxford: Oxford University Press, 2008), 146–178; Walton-Roberts, "Global Nursing Care Chain."

50. Jeffery Cox, *Imperial Fault Lines: Christianity and Colonial Power in India, 1818–1949* (Stanford, CA: Stanford University Press, 2002); Reddy, "Women on the Move."

51. There are little over twenty million Catholics in India, roughly 2 percent of the total population, and the Catholic church is the largest Christian denomination in the country; see data at the Catholic Hierarchy, "Statistics by Country," November 17, 2005, http://www.catholic-hierarchy.org/country/sc3.html; data at Pew Research Center, "Global Christianity—A Report on the Size and Distribution of the World's

Christian Population," December 19, 2011, https://www.pewforum.org/2011/12/19
/global-christianity-exec/; and data at BBC, "Fact File—Roman Catholics around the
World," April 1, 2005, http://news.bbc.co.uk/2/hi/4243727.stm. There are one hundred and seventy-four Catholic archdioceses in India, of which one hundred and
thirty-two are in the Latin Catholic church (Latin rite), thirty-one are in the Syro-
Malabar Catholic church, and eleven are in the Syro-Malankara Catholic church—
each practicing their own rites but united as part of the universal Roman Catholic
Church under the pope. The Syro-Malabar church, which traces its origins in India
back to the evangelistic activity of the apostle Thomas in the first century, is the largest of the Nasrani or St. Thomas Christians denominations with over four million
adherents. See Jaisy Joseph, *The Struggle for Identity among Syro-Malabar Catholics*
(Fairfax, VA: Eastern Christian Publications, 2009); Leslie Brown, *The Indian Christians of St. Thomas: An Account of the Ancient Syrian Church of Malabar* (Cambridge: Cambridge University Press, 1956); also see overview from the Syro-Malabar
Church, "The Syro Malabar Church: An Overview," accessed March 2020, http://
www.syromalabarchurch.in/syro-malabar-church.php. It follows the East Syriac
liturgy rite. The Malankara Catholic church was established in 1930, under the leadership of Archbishop Mar Ivanios, when it split from the Malankara church and
entered into communion with the larger Roman Catholic Church; see Thomas M.
Landy, "Syro-Malankara Catholic Church Finds Identity in Liturgy," *Catholics and
Culture* online, accessed March 2020, https://www.catholicsandcultures.org/eastern
-catholic-churches/syro-malankara-catholic-church. The Malankara church itself
emerged from a split within the Saint Thomas Christian community—both of which
trace their origins back to evangelism of Thomas the Apostle. The Malankara Catholic
church also follows the East Syriac liturgy rite. It is important to note that India has
the second-largest Catholic population in Asia, second only to the Philippines. Also
see Reddy, *Nursing and Empire*, and Reddy, "Women on the Move."

52. George, *When Women Come First*; Healey, *Indian Sisters*. Note that Reddy disputes
the simplicity of this argument; see Reddy, *Nursing and Empire*.

53. Reddy, *Nursing and Empire*.

54. It is important to note that the Catholic church provided more education and created more organizational civil society in countries such as India and the Philippines
(not mentioned directly by Woodberry) where it competed directly with aggressive
competition from conversionary Protestant missionaries; see in general Woodberry,
"The Missionary Roots." Also see Elizabeth Simon, "Christianity and Nursing in
India: A Remarkable Impact," *Journal of Christian Nursing* 26, no. 2 (April 2009):
88–94; Gustav Warneck and George Robson, *Outline of History of Protestant Missions
from the Reformation to Present Time: A Contribution to Modern Church History*
(New York: Franklin Classics, [1901] 2018).

55. Christians from Kerala were also drawn to Vellore, not just because they were Christian and in large supply for Protestant missionary needs but because of the active
recruitment of Vera K. Pittman, a medical missionary originally assigned to service in
China; see Christian Medical College of Vellore, "Ten of the Many Remarkable Women
Who Made Us Who We Are Today," *Other News*, 2018, https://www.cmch-vellore
.edu/WeeklyNews/OTHERNEWS/2018/Women%20pioneers.pdf. Vellore offered tremendous opportunities for young Indian women, but it also seems that Keralites fit
what Pittman was looking for in future nurses; see Reddy, *Nursing and Empire*, and
Reddy, "Women on the Move." It is important to note that Pittman also helped to

write *A New Textbook for Nursing in India* with the assistance of Lois Marsilije and the support of the Christian Medical Association of India and its Board of Nursing Education Nurses League; see Healey, *Indian Sisters*.

56. Part of this success was the result of the patronage of public health by the princely rulers of Tarvancore and their promotion of policies that drew more women into healthcare than in other areas of India under British rule. Today, Kerala still has one of the highest, if not the highest, literacy rates, and much of this phenomena can be attributed to this historical foundation. See Abraham, "Women Nurses"; Abraham, *Caste and Gender*; Dicicco-Bloom, "Racial and Gendered Experiences"; Richard W. Franke and Barbara H. Chasin, *Kerala: Development through Radical Reform* (New Delhi, India: Promilla, 1994); Healey, *Indian Sisters*; Robin Jeffrey, *Politics, Women and Well-Being: How Kerala Became a Model* (Basingstoke, UK: McMillan, 1992); Praveena Kodoth and Tina K. Jacob, "International Mobility of Nurses from Kerala (India) to the EU: Prospects and Challenges with Special Reference to the Netherlands and Denmark" from the collected paper of the EURA_NET Project: Transnational Migration in Transition: Transformative Characteristics of Temporary Mobility of People (working paper 405, Indian Institute of Management, April 2013); Catrin Evans, Rafath Razia, and Elaine Cook, "Building Nurse Education Capacity in India: Insights from a Faculty Development Programme in Andhra Pradesh," *BMC Nursing* 12, no. 8 (2015): 1–8; Nair and Healey, "Transcending Boundaries."

57. Abraham, *Caste and Gender*; George, *When Women Come First*; Reddy, *Nursing and Empire*; Reddy, "Women on the Move"; Simon, "Christianity and Nursing."

58. See previous note. Also see Abraham, "Women Nurses"; Rosemary Fitzgerald, "Rescue and Redemption: The Rise of Female Medical Missions in Colonial India during the Late Nineteenth and Early Twentieth Centuries," in *Nursing History and the Politics of Welfare*, eds. Anne Marie Rafferty, Jane Robinson, and Ruth Elkan (London: Routledge, 1997), 64–79; Alice Williams, *A Brief History of Nursing in India And Pakistan* (New Delhi, India: Trained Nurses Association of India, 1958).

59. See previous note.

60. Cherry, *Faith, Family*.

61. The Benedictine Sisters were sent in response to the church's desire to bring Filipinas back into the fold; see Gowing, *Islands under the Cross*.

62. Laubach cited in Steffi San Buenaventura, "Filipino Religion at Home and Abroad: Historical Roots and Immigrant Transformations," in *Religions in Asian America: Building Faith Communities*, eds. Pyong G. Min and Jung H. Kim (Walnut Creek, CA: AltaMira Press, 2002), 143–184.

63. See further St. Paul University Philippines history online, "History: SPUP through the Years," St. Paul University Philippines, accessed March 2020, https://spup.edu.ph/history/.

64. Giron-Tupas, *History of Nursing*. Also see Gowing, *Islands under the Cross*.

65. See interactive data at "Philippines," Global Religious Futures Project, Pew-Templeton, http://www.globalreligiousfutures.org/countries/philippines#/?affiliations_religion_id=37&affiliations_year=2010&region_name=All%20Countries&restrictions_year=2016. Note that the source of the interactive data is "The Future of World Religions: Population Growth Projections, 2010-2050," *Pew Research Center*, April 2, 2015, https://www.pewforum.org/2015/04/02/religious-projections-2010-2050/.

66. Minority Nurse Staff, "Philippine Nurses in the U.S.—Yesterday and Today," *Minority Nurse*, March 20, 2013, https://minoritynurse.com/tag/filipino-philippine-nurses/.

67. Choy, *Empire of Care*; Healey, *Indian Sisters*; Nair and Healey, "Transcending Boundaries."

68. See further Teresa Amott and Julie Matthaei, *Race, Gender, and Work: A Multicultural Economic History of Women in the United States* (Boston: South End Press, 1991).

69. Choy, *Empire of Care*.

70. From 1863 to 1903, John D. Rockefeller made donations to 1,494 institutions and individuals. He supported two hundred and twenty churches and missionary organizations within his own Baptist denomination and over eighty institutions and one hundred and sixty social welfare and moral reform organizations of other Christian denominations (Kennith W. Rose and Darwin Stapleton, "Philanthropy and Institution-Building in the Twentieth Century," (unpublished conference paper), http://rockarch .org/publications/conferences/philcity.php. Also see, Kenneth W. Rose, Benjamin R. Shute, Jr and Darwin H. Stapleton, "Philanthropy and Institution-Building in the Twentieth Century," *Minerva* 35, no. 3 (Autumn 1997): 203–205. From a statistical survey of Rockefeller Foundation charity index cards during this time, we can gather that well over a third of all money Rockefeller contributed to groups and institutions was for church-based organizations and groups, largely doing medical work. Among the charitable gifts to some six hundred and seventy-eight individuals, one hundred and twenty-four (18 percent) were to ministers and missionaries and roughly one-fifth of all individual contributions were church related, also largely to medical missionaries. See Stapleton, "Philanthropy and Institution-Building in the Twentieth Century; also see Richard E. Brown, *Rockefeller Medicine Men: Medicine and Capitalism in America* (Berkeley: University of California Press, 1979); Reddy, *Nursing and Empire*; Reddy, "Women on the Move."

71. Stefanie Bator, "Women Are the Way Forward: The Rockefeller Foundation in the Philippines, 1923–1932," 2011, http://rockarch.issuelab.org/resources/28079/28079 .pdf; Nair and Healey, "Transcending Boundaries."

72. Choy, *Empire of Care*; Giron-Tupas, *History of Nursing*.

73. Brush, "Rockefeller Agenda"; Choy, *Empire of Care*.

74. Healey, *Indian Sisters*; Reddy, *Nursing and Empire*.

75. Reddy, "Women on the Move."

76. Reddy, "Women on the Move."

77. Historically, Philippine law has limited nurse-recruitment agencies to recruiting 25 percent of nurses for export, but this has not always been followed despite the fact that the Philippine Overseas Employment Administration works diligently to stop illegal recruitment practices; see Susan Martin et al., *The Role of Migrant Care Workers in Aging Societies: Report on Research Findings in the United States*, December 2009: http://www.ltsscenter.org/resource-library/Role_of_Migrant_Care_Workers_in_Aging _Societies.pdf; Patricia Pittman et al., "Perceptions of Employment-Based Discrimination among Newly Arrived Foreign-Educated Nurses," *American Journal of Nursing* 114, no. 1 (January 2014): 26–35.

78. Jeffrey C. Alexander, *The Meanings of Social Life: A Cultural Sociology* (New York: Oxford University Press, 2003); Philip Smith and Alexander Riley, *Cultural Theory: An Introduction* (Hoboken, NJ: Wiley-Blackwell, 2008).

79. Alexander, *Meanings of Social Life*.

80. Martin Barker, "Kant as a Problem for Weber," *British Journal of Sociology* 31, no. 2 (June 1980): 224–245; Immanuel Kant, *The Metaphysical Elements of Ethics*, trans. Thomas Kingsmill Abbott (Scotts Valley, CA: CreateSpace Independent Publishing, [1780] 2015); David Norman Smith, "Faith, Reason, and Charisma: Rudolf Sohm,

Max Weber, and the Theology of Grace," *Sociological Inquiry* 68, no. 1 (1998): 32–60. Also see Christian Smith, *Resisting Regan: The U.S. Central America Peace Movement* (Chicago: University of Chicago Press, 1996).

81. Cherry, *Faith, Family*; Paul DiMaggio, "Culture and Cognition," *Annual Review of Sociology* 23 (1997): 263–287; Elaine Howard Ecklund, *Korean American Evangelicals: New Models for Civic Life* (New York: Oxford University Press, 2006); Ann Swidler, *Talk of Love: How Americans Use Their Culture* (Chicago: University of Chicago Press, 1997); Ronald L. Jepperson and Ann Swidler, "What Properties of Culture Should We Measure?" *Poetics* 22, no. 4 (1994): 359–371; William H. Sewell Jr., "A Theory of Structure: Duality, Agency, and Transformation," *American Journal of Sociology* 98, no. 1 (1992): 1–29; Christian Smith, *Moral Believing Animals: Human Personhood and Culture* (New York: Oxford University Press, 2003).

82. Alexander, *Meanings of Social Life*; Cherry, *Faith, Family*; Kathleen Mary Carley, "The Value of Cognitive Foundations for Dynamic Social Theory," *Journal of Mathematical Sociology* 14, no. 2–3 (1989): 171–208; Kathleen Mary Carley, "A Theory of Group Stability," *American Sociology Review* 56, no. 3 (1991): 331–354; Barry Schwartz, *Vertical Classification: A Study in Structuralism and the Sociology of Knowledge* (Chicago: University of Chicago Press, 1981); Harrison C. White, *Identity and Control: A Structural Theory of Social Action* (Princeton, NJ: Princeton University Press, 1992); Robert Wuthnow, *Meaning and Moral Order* (Berkeley: University of California Press, 1987); Michael P. Young, *Bearing Witness against Sin: The Evangelical Birth of the American Social Movement* (Chicago: University of Chicago Press, 2006).

83. For more on religion, cultural frameworks and work or workplace spirituality, see Robert A. Giacalone and Carole L. Jurkiewicz, *Handbook of Workplace Spirituality and Organizational Performance* (Armonk, NY: MG Sharpe, 2003); Kathy L. Dean and Charles J. Fornaciari, "Empirical Research in Management, Spirituality and Religion during Its Founding Years," *Journal of Management, Spirituality and Religion* 4, no. 1 (2007): 3–34; Monty L. Lynn, Michael J. Naughton, and Steve VanderVeen, "Connecting Religion and Work: Patterns and Influences of Work-Faith Integration," *Human Relations* 64, no. 5 (2010): 675–701; Joan Marques, Satinder Dhiman, and Richard King, *The Workplace and Spirituality: New Perspectives on Research and Practice* (Woodstock, VT: Skylight Paths, 2009); Ian Mitroff and Elizabeth Denton, *A Spiritual Audit of Corporate America: A Hard Look at Spirituality, Religion, and Values in the Workplace* (San Francisco: Jossey-Bass, 1999).

84. Erving Goffman originally defined frames as "interpretive schemata" that form the basic frameworks of understanding available to members of society for making sense out of events and social interaction; see *Frame Analysis* (New York: Harper & Row, [1947] 1997), 155. Also see Carley, "Value of Cognitive Foundations"; Carley, "Theory of Group Stability"; DiMaggio, "Culture and Cognition"; Young, *Bearing Witness against Sin*.

85. Wendy Griswold, "The Sociology of Culture," in *The Sage Handbook of Sociology*, eds. Craig Calhoun, Chris Rojek, and Bryan S. Turner (New York: Sage, 2005); Charles Taylor, *Sources of the Self: The Making of the Modern Identity* (Cambridge, MA: Harvard University Press, 1992).

86. Pierre Bourdieu, "Structures, Habitus, Practices," in *The Logic of Practice*, trans. Richard Nice (Stanford, CA: Stanford University Press, [1980] 1990), 52–65; Ann Swidler, "Culture in Action: Symbols and Strategies," *American Sociological Review* 52, no. 2 (April 1986): 273–286; Taylor, *Sources of the Self*; Charles Tilly, "How to Detect, Describe, and Explain Repertoires of Contention" (working paper no. 150, Center for

Studies of Social Change, New School for Social Research Annual Review, New York City, NY, 1992); Robert Wuthnow, *Poor Richard's Principle: Recovering the American Dream through Moral Dimensions of Works, Business, and Money* (Princeton, NJ: Princeton University Press, 1996); Wuthnow, *Meaning and Moral Order.*

87. Alexander, *Meanings of Social Life.*

88. Pierre Bourdieu, "The Genesis of the Concepts of Habitus and Field," *Sociocriticism* 2, no. 2 (1985): 11–24; Bradford Verter, "Spiritual Capital: Theorizing Religion with Bourdieu against Bourdieu," *Sociological Theory* 21, no. 2 (2003): 150–174.

89. Samantha Ammons and Penny Edgell, "Religious Influences on Work-Family Trade-offs," *Journal of Family Issues* 28, no. 6 (2007): 794–826; Alfred Darnell and Darren E. Sherkat, "The Impact of Protestant Fundamentalism on Educational Attainment," *American Sociological Review* 62, no. 2 (1997): 306–315; Evelyn Leher, "The Effects of Religion on the Labor Supply of Married Women," *Social Science Research* 24, no. 3 (1995): 281–301; Cuiting Li and Jennifer Kerpelman, "Parental Influence on Young Women's Certainty about Their Career Aspirations," *Sex Roles* 56, no.1 (2007): 105–115; Darren E. Sherkat, "Embedding Religious Choices: Integrating Preferences and Social Constraints into Rational Choice Theories of Religious Behavior," in *Rational Choice Theory and Religion: Summary and Assessment*, ed. Lawrence A. Young (New York: Routledge, 1997), 65–86; Darren E. Sherkat, "Counterculture or Continuity? Examining Competing Influences on Baby Boomers' Religious Orientations and Participation," *Social Forces* 76, no. 3 (1998): 1087–1114; Emily Sigalow, Michelle Shain, and Meredith Bergey, "Religion and Decisions about Marriage, Residence, Occupation, and Children," *Journal for the Scientific Study of Religion* 51, no. 2 (2012): 304–323; James V. Spikard, "Rethinking Religious Social Action: What is "Rational" about Rational Choice Theory?" *Sociology of Religion* 59, no. 2 (Summer 1998): 99–115; Rodney Stark and William S. Bainbridge, *The Future of Religion: Secularization, Revival, and Cult Formation* (Berkeley: University of California Press, 1985); Rodney Stark and Laurence Iannaccone, "A Supply-Side Reinterpretation of the 'Secularization' of Europe," *Journal for the Scientific Study of Religion* 33, no. 3 (1994): 230–252; R. Stephen Warner, "Work in Progress towards a New Paradigm for the Sociological Study of Religion in the United States," *American Journal of Sociology* 98, no. 5 (1993): 1044–1093; Lawrence A. Young, *Rational Choice Theory and Religion* (New York: Routledge, 1997).

90. Colin Jerolmack and Douglas Porpora, "Religion, Rationality, and Experience: A Response to the New Rational Choice Theory of Religion," *Sociological Theory* 22, no. 1 (2004): 140–160; Smith, *Resisting Regan.*

91. Jerry Park et al., "Workplace-Bridging Religious Capital: Connecting Congregations to Work Outcomes," *Sociology of Religion* 75, no. 2 (2014): 309–331; Verter, "Spiritual Capital."

92. Bourdieu, in opposition to rational choice approaches to how individuals operate in the social world, describes this as an implicit practical logic—a sense or feel, stemming from habitus, that gives a practical sense and bodily disposition to the daily orientation and navigation of an individual (agent) through social fields. See Pierre Bourdieu, *Outline of a Theory of Practice* (Cambridge: Cambridge University Press, 1977); Verter, "Spiritual Capital."

93. Taylor, *Sources of the Self.*

94. John Tropman, *The Catholic Ethic in American Society* (San Francisco: Jossey-Bass, 1995); John Tropman, *The Catholic Ethic and the Spirit of Community* (Washington, DC: Georgetown University Press, 2002).

95. Bourdieu would use the term "field" here to describe similar understandings; see Bourdieu, "Genesis of the Concepts."

96. United States Conference of Catholic Bishops, *Health and Health Care: A Pastoral Letter of the American Catholic Bishops* (Washington, DC: USCCB, November 1982), https://www.usccb.org/issues-and-action/human-life-and-dignity/health-care /upload/health-and-health-care-pastoral-letter-pdf-09-01-43.pdf.

97. United States Conference of Catholic Bishops, *Health and Health Care.*

98. See "Mission Overview," Catholic Health Association of the United States, accessed August 2020, https://www.chausa.org/mission/overview; "Facts—Statistics," Catholic Health Association of the United States, accessed August 2020, https://www .chausa.org/about/about/facts-statistics. Also see Barbra Mann Wall, "The Role of Catholic Nurses in Women's Health Care Policy Disputes: A Historical Study," *Nursing Outlook* 61, no. 5 (2013): 367–374.

99. In the historical case of Catholic nursing schools in the United States, see Barbra Mann Wall, "Definite Lines of Influence: Catholic Sisters and Nurse Training Schools, 1890–1920," *Nursing Research* 5, no. 5 (2001): 314–321.

100. Barbra Mann Wall, "American Catholic Nursing: An Historical Analysis," *Medizinhistorisches Journal* 47, no. 2–3 (2012): 160–175.

101. See Christopher Kauffman, *Ministry and Meaning: A Religious History of Catholic Healthcare in the United States* (New York: Herder & Herder, 1995); also see chapter 8 in Barbra Mann Wall, *American Catholic Hospitals: A Century of Changing Markets and Missions* (New Brunswick, NJ: Rutgers University Press, 2011); Thomas John Paprocki, "Caring for the Sick: The Catholic Contribution and Its Relevance," *Notre Dame Journal of Law Ethics* 25, no.2 (2012): 447–461; and Mark S. Latkovic, "The Catholic Church in America, the Discipline of Bioethics, and the Culture of Life: Looking to the Encyclical Evangelium Vitae for Guidance," *Linacre Quarterly* 78, no. 4 (November 2011): 415–436. Also see Jay P. Dolan, *In Search of American Catholicism: A History of Religion and Culture in Tension* (New York: Oxford University Press, 2003). More generally, see Jay P. Dolan, *In Search of American Catholicism: A History of Religion and Culture in Tension* (New York: Oxford University Press, 2003).

102. Mann Wall, "Role of Catholic Nurses."

103. Mann Wall, "Role of Catholic Nurses"; also see Mann Wall, *American Catholic Hospitals.*

104. Myrock C. Shinall, Jr., "From the Editor: The Separation of Church and Medicine," *American Medical Association Journal of Ethics* 11, no. 10 (2009): 747–749.

105. Cherry, *Faith, Family.*

106. See David I. Auerbach, Peter I. Buerhaus, and Douglas O. Staiger, "Will the RN Workforce Weather the Retirement of the Baby Boomers?" *Medical Care* 53, no. 10 (2015): 850–856; Jessica Cortes and Patricia Pan, *Foreign-Nurse Importation to the United States and the Supply of Native Registered Nurses* (Collingdale, PA: Diane Publishing Company, 2014); C. Brett Lockhard and Michael Wolf, "Occupational Employment Projections to 2020," *Monthly Labor Review*, (January 2012): 84–108; Siyam and dal Poz, eds., *Migration of Health Workers*; U.S. Department of Health and Human Services, Health Resources and Services Administration, *The Registered Nurse Population: Findings from the 2008 National Sample Survey of Registered Nurses* (Washington, DC: U.S. Department of Health and Human Services, 2010), https://www.who.int/hrh/migration/14075_MigrationofHealth_Workers.pdf; U.S. Department of Labor Bureau of Labor and Statistics, "Occupations with the Largest

Predicted Number of Job Openings due to Growth and Replacement Needs, 2012 and Projected 2022," *Economic News Release*, last modified December 19, 2013, http://www.bls.gov/news.release/ecopro.t08.htm.

3. New American Battlefields

1. By comparison, the average registered nurse turnover from 2010 to 2014 was a little over 7 percent; see, John D. Daigh, Jr., *OIG Determination of Veterans Health Administration's Occupational Staffing Shortages FY 2019*, report #19-000346-241 (Washington D.C.: Department of Veterans Affairs, Office of Inspector General, Office of Healthcare Inspections, September 30, 2019), https://www.va.gov/oig/pubs/VAOIG -19-00346-241.pdf; Robert Goldenkoff and Debra A. Draper, "Veterans Health Administration: Actions Needed to Better Recruit and Retain Clinical and Administrative Staff," *United States Government Accountability Office Testimony before the Subcommittee on Health, Committee on Veterans' Affairs, House of Representatives GAO-17-475T* (2017), https://www.gao.gov/assets/690/683564.pdf; The Department of Veterans Affairs (VA), Veterans Health Administration (VHA), "Oversight Improvements Needed for Nurse Recruitment and Retention Initiatives," *United States Government Accountability Office Testimony before the Subcommittee on Health, Committee on Veterans' Affairs, House of Representatives GAO-15-794* (2015), https://www .gao.gov/assets/gao-15-794.pdf. Also see Meghan Hoyer and Gregg Zoroya, "VA Has 41,500 Unfilled Medical Jobs, Forcing Vets into Costly Private Care," *USA Today*, July 23, 2015, https://www.usatoday.com/story/news/nation/2015/07/23/va-has-41500 -unfilled-medical-jobs-forcing-vets-into-costly-private-care/30504525/.

2. See previous note.

3. Daigh, Jr., *OIG Determination*; Goldenkoff and Draper, "Veterans Health Administration."

4. "Nursing at Recent Hospital Conventions," *American Journal of Nursing* 36, no. 11 (1936): 1156–1162; Stella Goostray, "Supply, Demand, and Standards," *American Journal of Nursing* 41, no. 7 (1941): 745–746; "The Nursing Situation in New York State," *Trained Nurse and Hospital Review* 96 (1935): 253; Jean Whelan, *Nursing the Nation: Building the Nurse Labor Force* (New Brunswick, NJ: Rutgers University Press, 2021).

5. Deborah Judd, Kathleen Sitzman, and G. Megan Davis, *A History of American Nursing: Trends and Eras* (Boston: Jones & Bartlett Learning, 2009); Mary Roberts, *American Nursing: History and Interpretation* (New York: Macmillan Co., 1954); Arlene Keeling, John Kirchgessner, and Michele Hehman, *A History of Professional Nursing in the United States, 1610 to 2016: Toward a Culture of Health* (New York: Springer Publishing, 2018).

6. Joan E. Lynaugh, "Nursing the Great Society: The Impact of the Nurse Training Act of 1964," *Nursing History Review* 16, no. 1 (2008): 13–28; Jean C. Whelan, "Where Did All the Nurses Go?," University of Pennsylvania School of Nursing, accessed August 2016, http://www.nursing.upenn.edu/nhhc/workforce-issues/where-did-all -the-nurses-go/.

7. Roberts, *American Nursing*; Whelan, "Where Did All the Nurses Go?."

8. In 1945, General Omar Bradley took over as the head of the VA and steered its transformation into a modern organization. One year later, Public Law 293 established the Department of Medicine and Surgery within VA, along with numerous other programs like the VA Voluntary Service to meet the increasing needs of veterans returning from WWII. The law enabled the VA to recruit and retain top medical personnel

by modifying the civil service system. When General Bradley left his position at the VA in 1948, there were one hundred and twenty-five VA hospitals, nearly triple what had existed prior. See "VA History Office," Department of Veterans Affairs (VA), last updated October 14, 2021, https://www.va.gov/about_va/vahistory.asp.

9. Lynaugh, "Nursing the Great Society."

10. Lynaugh, "Nursing the Great Society."

11. Joan E. Lynaugh and Barbara L. Bush, *American Nursing from Hospitals to Health Systems* (Malden, MA: Blackwell Publishers, 1996).

12. United States Department of Labor, *The Economic Status of Registered Professional Nurses 1946-1947* (Washington, D.C.: Bureau of Labor Statistics, 1947).

13. John C. Kirchgessner, "Mid-century Transitions and Shortages, 1945-1960," in *A History of Professional Nursing in the United States, 1610 to 2016: Toward a Culture of Health*, eds. Arlene Keeling, John Kirchgessner, and Michele Hehman (New York: Springer Publishing, 2018): 285-308.

14. Lynaugh, "Nursing the Great Society"; Lynaugh and Bush, *American Nursing from Hospitals*.

15. Sister Rosemary Donley and Sister Mary Jean Flaherty, "Revisiting the American Nurses Association's First Position on Education for Nurses," *Online Journal of Issues in Nursing* 7, no. 2 (2002), http://www.nursingworld.org/ojin/topic18/tpc18_1.htm.

16. Ian R.H. Rockett and Sandra L. Putnam, "Physician-Nurse Migration to the United States: Regional and Health Status Origins in Relation to Legislation and Policy," *International Migration* 27, no. 3 (September 1989): 389-409.

17. Lynaugh, "Nursing the Great Society."

18. This further codified the classification standards for federal positions originally outlined in the Classification Act of 1949; see Daigh, Jr., *OIG Determination*.

19. See Linda H. Aiken, Robyn B. Cheung, and Danielle M. Olds, "Education Policy Initiatives to Address the Nurse Shortage in the United States," *Health Affairs* 28, no. 4 (2009): w646-w656; Peter I. Buerhaus, Douglas O. Staiger and David I. Auerbach, "Is the Current Shortage of Hospital Nurses Ending?," *Health Affairs* 22, no. 6 (2003): 191-198; Kevin Grumbach et al., "Measuring Shortages of Hospital Nurses: How Do You Know a Hospital with a Nursing Shortage when You See One?," *Medical Care Research and Review* 58, no. 4 (2001): 387-403; Lisa M. Haddad and Tammy J. Toney-Butler, *Nursing Shortage* (Treasure Island, FL: StatPearls Publishing, 2020); Mary Halter et al., "The Determinants and Consequences of Adult Nursing Staff Turnover: A Systematic Review of Systematic Reviews," *BMC Health Research Services* 17, no. 824 (2017): 1-20; B. Lindsay Lowell and Stefka Georgieva Gerova, "Immigrants and the Healthcare Workforce: Profiles and Shortages," *Work and Occupations* 31, no. 4 (2004): 474-498; Leah E. Masselink and Cheryl B. Jones, "Immigration Policy and Internationally Educated Nurses in the United States: A Brief History," *Nursing Outlook* 62, no. 1 (January-February 2014): 39-45; Patricia Prescott, "The Enigmatic Nursing Workforce," *Journal of Nursing Administration* 30, no. 2 (2000): 59-54; Robert Rosseter, "Fact Sheet: Nursing Shortage AACN Online," American Association of the Colleges of Nursing, 2019, https://www.aacnnursing.org/Portals/42/News/Factsheets/Nursing-Shortage-Factsheet.pdf.

20. See Michelle C. Hehman, "Caring in Crisis, 1980-2000," in *A History of Professional Nursing in the United States, 1610 to 2016: Toward a Culture of Health*, eds. Arlene Keeling, John Kirchgessner, and Michele Hehman (New York: Springer Publishing, 2018), 331-354; Christine T. Kovner et al., "What Does Nurse Turnover

Rate Mean and What Is the Rate?," *Policy, Politics and Nursing Practice* 15, no. 3–4 (2014): 64–71; Masselink and Jones, "Immigration Policy."

21. Goldenkoff and Draper, "Veterans Health Administration."

22. Goldenkoff and Draper, "Veterans Health Administration." Also see Department of Veterans Affairs' (VA) Veterans Health Administration's (VHA), "Oversight Improvements Needed."

23. Daigh, Jr., *OIG Determination.*

24. Ilene MacDonald, "VA Scandal: RNs Leave Program as Demand for Care Grows," *Fierce Healthcare*, November 2, 2015, https://www.fiercehealthcare.com/healthcare /va-scandal-rns-leave-program-as-demand-for-care-grows.

25. The Department of Veterans Affairs' (VA) Veterans Health Administration's (VHA), "Oversight Improvements Needed."

26. Daigh, Jr., *OIG Determination.*

27. Nicole Ogrysko, "More than 1,600 Employees at VA Medical Facilities Have Coronavirus," *Federal News Network*, April 15, 2020, https://federalnewsnetwork.com /veterans-affairs/2020/04/over-1600-employees-at-va-medical-facilities-have -coronavirus/.

28. See debate/evidence in Rodney A. Hayward, "Lessons from the Rise—and Fall?—of VA Healthcare," *Journal General Internal Medicine* 32, no. 1 (2016): 11–13; Philip Longman, *Best Care Anywhere: Why VA Health Care Would Work Better for Everyone* (San Francisco: Berrett-Koehler Publishers, 2012); Claire O'Hanlon et al., "Comparing VA and Non-VA Quality of Care: A Systematic Review," *Journal of General Internal Medicine* 32, no. 1 (2017): 105–121.

29. Jessica L. Adler, *Burdens of War: Creating the United States Veterans Health System* (Baltimore, MA: Johns Hopkins University Press, 2017); Rosemary Stevens, *A Time of Scandal: Charles R. Forbes, Warren G. Harding, and the Making of the Veterans Bureau* (Baltimore, MA: Johns Hopkins University Press, 2016). Also see Michael Pearson, "The VA's Troubled History," *CNN*, May 23, 2014, https://www.cnn.com /2014/05/23/politics/va-scandals-timeline/index.html.

30. See previous note.

31. See for example, "Lufkin Veterans Speak Out about VA Scandal," *KTRE ABC 9*, July 28, 2014, https://www.ktre.com/story/25545811/lufkin-veterans-speak-out-about -va-scandal/; St. John Barned-Smith and Samantha Ketterer, "Veterans: Report Validates Wait-Time Allegations at Houston VA," *Houston Chronicle*, June 28, 2016, https://www.houstonchronicle.com/news/houston-texas/houston/article/Veterans -Report-validates-wait-time-allegations-8319802.php.

32. Note that Texas has the second-largest veteran population in the United States. In Texas, the average veteran is less White than the national average (60 percent in Texas versus 77 percent nationally) but otherwise matches this national profile. See Texas Workforce Investment Council, "Veterans in Texas: A Demographic Study," *Office of the Texas Governor 2019 Update*, accessed January 2020, https://gov.texas.gov/uploads /files/organization/twic/Veterans-in-Texas-2019.pdf. Also see United Health Foundation and the Military Officer's Association of America (MOAA), "Health of Those Who Have Served Report, 2016," *America's Health Ranking*, November 2016, http:// assets.americashealthrankings.org/app/uploads/htwhs_report_r3.pdf.

33. United Health Foundation and MOAA, "Health of Those Who Have Served"; also see previous assessments, Ellen A. Kramarow and Patricia N. Pastor, "The Health of Male Veterans and Nonveterans Aged 25–64: United States, 2007–2010," *NCHS Data Brief* 101 (August 2012): 1–8, https://www.ncbi.nlm.nih.gov/pubmed/23101789.

34. See previous note.

35. United Health Foundation and MOAA, "Health of Those Who Have Served"; Krama-row and Pastor, "The Health of Male Veterans and Nonveterans Aged 25–64."

36. See, for example, Dave Philipps, "In Unit Stalked by Suicide, Veterans Try to Save One Another," *New York Times*, September 19, 2015, https://www.nytimes.com /2015/09/20/us/marine-battalion-veterans-scarred-by-suicides-turn-to-one-another -for-help.html?_r=0.

37. See, for example, Lisa K. Richardson, B. Christopher Frueh, and Ronald Acierno, "Prevalence Estimates of Combat-Related PTSD: A Critical Review," *Australia and New Zealand Journal of Psychiatry* 44, no. 1 (2010): 4–19.

38. Terri Tanielian and Lisa H. Jaycox, *Invisible Wounds of War: Psychological and Cogni-tive Injuries, Their Consequences, and Services to Assist Recovery* (Santa Monica, CA: RAND, 2008), with summary updates online, http://www.veteransandptsd.com /PTSD-statistics.html; also see Hannah Fischer, "A Guide to U.S. Military Casualty Statistics: Operation Freedom's Sentinel, Operation Inherent Resolve, Operation New Dawn, Operation Iraqi Freedom, and Operation Enduring Freedom," *Congressional Research Service*, August 7, 2008, https://fas.org/sgp/crs/natsec/RS22452.pdf.

39. See previous note.

40. Elizabeth Ralevski, Lening A. Olivera-Figueroa, and Ismene Petrakis, "PTSD and Comorbid AUD: A Review of Pharmacological and Alternative Treatment Options," *Substance Abuse and Rehabilitation* 5 (March 2014): 25–36.

41. See Susan V. Eisen et al., "Mental and Physical Health Status and Alcohol and Drug Use Following Return from Deployment to Iraq or Afghanistan," *American Journal of Public Health* 102, supplement 1 (2012): S66–S73.

42. James Dao, "As Suicides Rise in U.S., Veterans Are Less of Total," *New York Times*, February 1, 2013, http://www.nytimes.com/2013/02/02/us/veterans-make-up-shrink ing-percentage-of-suicides.html?_r=0.

43. United States Department of Veterans Affairs, "VA Suicide Prevention Program Facts about Veteran Suicide," *VA Online*, July 2016, https://www.va.gov/opa/publications /factsheets/Suicide_Prevention_FactSheet_New_VA_Stats_070616_1400.pdf.

44. United States Department of Veterans Affairs, "VA Suicide Prevention Program Facts."

45. United States Department of Veterans Affairs, "VA Suicide Prevention Program Facts."

46. Joan Mazzolini, "Foreign Medical Graduates Are Major Crutch for VA System," August 6, 2004, https://www.valuemd.com/relaxing-lounge/21484-foreign-medical-graduates -major-crutch-va-system.html. First posted here, http://www.newhouse.com/archive /story1c013001.html. Note that I was never able to find the original article and its source publication.

47. Mazzolini, "Foreign Medical Graduates."

48. Mazzolini, "Foreign Medical Graduates. Mazzolini uses the Deasy malpractice case as a supposed example to highlight her argument but the connection to foreign-born concerns is unclear. See, the lawsuit cited in the article, John F. Deasy, Jr., Plaintiff-Appellee, v. United States of America, Denver Veterans Administration Medical Cen-ter (the "Denver VAMC") Baltimore Veterans Administration Medical Center (the Baltimore VAMC) and Perry Point Veterans Administration Medical Center (Perry Point VAMC), case no. 95-1276 October 28, 1996 (United States Court of Appeals, Tenth Circuit), https://caselaw.findlaw.com/us-10th-circuit/1361836.html.

49. Soldier1 (screen name). Comment date May 14, 2013. Comment on Soldier. "Tired of all the foreign doctors." *Topix*, May 31, 2013, http://www.topix.com/forum/city /beckley-wv/TT95LLLHDTH7UVQIR/p2. Note that forum is no longer online.

50. SoldierUS (screen name). Comment date May 15, 2013. Comment on Soldier. "Tired of all the foreign doctors." *Topix*, May 31, 2013, http://www.topix.com/forum/city /beckley-wv/TT95LLLHDTH7UVQIR/p2. Note that forum is no longer online.

51. DonaldDuck (screen name). Comment date May 15, 2013. Comment on Soldier. "Tired of all the foreign doctors." *Topix*, May 31, 2013, http://www.topix.com/forum/city /beckley-wv/TT95LLLHDTH7UVQIR/p2. Note that forum is no longer online.

52. Dunadd (screen name). Comment date May 15, 2013. Comment on Soldier. "Tired of all the foreign doctors." *Topix*, May 31, 2013, http://www.topix.com/forum/city /beckley-wv/TT95LLLHDTH7UVQIR/p2. Note that forum is no longer online.

53. VetNurse (screen name). Comment date May 15, 2013. Comment on Soldier. "Tired of all the foreign doctors." *Topix*, May 31, 2013, http://www.topix.com/forum/city /beckley-wv/TT95LLLHDTH7UVQIR/p2. Note that forum is no longer online.

54. Josh (screen name). Comment date May 15, 2013. Comment on Soldier. "Tired of all the foreign doctors." *Topix*, May 31, 2013, http://www.topix.com/forum/city/beckley -wv/TT95LLLHDTH7UVQIR/p2. Note that forum is no longer online.

55. Hameems mother's lover (screen name). Comment date May 15, 2013. Comment on Soldier. "Tired of all the foreign doctors." *Topix*, May 31, 2013, http://www.topix .com/forum/city/beckley-wv/TT95LLLHDTH7UVQIR/p2. Note that forum is no longer online.

56. See Office of Diversity & Inclusion, Human Resources & Administration, U.S. Department of Veterans Affairs, "Diversity & Inclusion Strategic Plan FY 2017–2020," *VA Online*, 2020, accessed December 2020, https://www.diversity.va.gov/products/files /StrategicPlan.pdf.

57. This data includes all work domains, including doctors and nurses—permanent and temporary employees in full-time, part-time, and intermittent pay statuses. Specific data on the racial/ethnic diversity of VA nurses are not publicly available. See Office of Diversity & Inclusion, Human Resources & Administration, U.S. Department of Veterans Affairs, "Diversity & Inclusion Annual Report FY 2015," *VA Online*, 2015, accessed December 2020 https://www.diversity.va.gov/products/files/DIAR.pdf.

58. The civil labor force (CLF) consists of all people sixteen years of age or over, excluding those in the armed forces, who are employed or seeking employment. The CLF contains all occupations and is an accurate comparative basis for federal government–wide comparison, which is the largest employer in the U.S. with all occupations represented. Although the VA tracks hiring of Individuals with Targeted Disabilities, there is no CLF or RCLF (Relevant Civil Labor Force) for this group. See Office of Diversity & Inclusion, Human Resources & Administration, U.S. Department of Veterans Affairs, "Diversity & Inclusion Annual Report FY 2015."

59. Relevant Civil Labor Force (RCLF) reflects all people sixteen years of age or older, excluding those in the armed forces, who are employed in or actively seeking employment in a specific occupation—the occupations representative of the VA workforce. The RCLF compares the applicants seeking specific VA occupations such as doctors, nurses, human resources workers, veterans benefits claims examiners, etc. See Office of Diversity & Inclusion, Human Resources & Administration, U.S. Department of Veterans Affairs, "Diversity & Inclusion Annual Report FY 2015."

60. Office of Diversity & Inclusion, Human Resources & Administration, U.S. Department of Veterans Affairs, "Diversity & Inclusion Annual Report FY 2015.

61. See "VA Houston Health Care," U.S. Department of Veterans Affairs, accessed November 2020, https://www.houston.va.gov/about/index.asp.

62. Note that the VA Provider Portal has changed since the years of the study. Comparable information/ demographic data is available at *U.S. News Health Portal*, https:// health.usnews.com/best-hospitals/area/tx/michael-e-debakey-va-medical-center -6742035#doctors, accessed October 2021.

63. Note that Kemal Budak, my former MA student and research assistant, logged every entry on the portal and looked up each university for all 848 cases. Although I thanked Kemal in the acknowledgments, I want to draw further attention to his efforts here.

64. See, for example, "Texas Board of Nursing: Nurse Portal," Texas Board of Nursing, accessed February 2020, https://www.bon.texas.gov/forms/rninq.asp. All you have to do is type in a nurse's first and last name or license number, which may be posted on paperwork or name badges, and any potential information about where they obtained their license or went to college is often posted, open access.

65. Note that the educational/training locations of the interview sample were nearly identical to the survey sample, with less than a two-percent difference in each domain—US Only, Home Country Only, or Both. See methodological appendix on sample selection and other demographic comparisons.

66. See "Weams Institution Search," United States Department of Veterans Affairs, last updated May 1, 2020, https://inquiry.vba.va.gov/weamspub/buildSearchCountry Criteria.do.

67. In 2009, for example, President Obama issued an executive order, Veterans Employment Initiative 13518, which directed the federal government and its agencies— including the VA system—to increase employment initiatives for veterans.

68. See, for example, Be Be, "Discrimination against Hiring Veterans," *All Nurses* (blog), June 18, 2014, https://allnurses.com/discrimination-hiring-veterans-t531634/.

69. Jie Zong and Jeanne Batalova, "Immigrant Veterans in the United States," *Migration Policy Institute*, May 5, 2016, https://www.migrationpolicy.org/article/immigrant -veterans-united-states.

70. Zong and Batalova, "Immigrant Veterans."

71. See Mona Chalabi, "What Percentage of Americans Have Served in the Military?," *Five Thirty Eight*, March 19, 2015, https://fivethirtyeight.com/features/what-percen tage-of-americans-have-served-in-the-military/; Zong and Batalova, "Immigrant Veterans."

72. See U.S. Bureau of Labor Statistics calculations, "Occupational Employment and Wages, May 2019: 29–1141 Registered Nurses," Bureau of Labor Statistics, accessed January 2020, https://www.bls.gov/oes/current/oes291141.htm, compared to review of VA nurse locality pay schedules available at "Title 38 Pay Schedules," U.S. Department of Veterans Affairs, accessed January 2020, https://www.va.gov/OHRM /Pay/; for further calculations, also see U.S. Department of Veterans Affairs Registered Nurse Salaries," Glassdoor, accessed January 2020, https://www.glassdoor .com/Salary/US-Department-of-Veterans-Affairs-Registered-Nurse-Salaries-E41429 _D_KO34,50.htm.

73. See VA Nurse locality pay schedules for Texas specifically, "Title 38 Pay Schedules."

74. Texas ranks seventeenth in the nation for nurse salary. See calculations at U.S. Bureau of Labor Statistics, "Occupational Employment and Wages, May 2019."

75. U.S. Department of Veterans Affairs, "Nurse Honored During National Nurses Week," press release, May 7 2013, accessed December 2014, http://stylemagazine .com/news/2013/may/07/houston-va-nurses-honored-during-national-nurses-w/. Also see Stephen M. Cherry and Kody Alred, "Models of Disaster Response: Lessons

Learned from Filipino Immigrant Mobilizations for Hurricane Katrina Victims," *Criminal Justice Studies* 25 (2012): 391–408.

76. Adams, "Salute to Nurses: Top 10 Area Nurses Receive Recognition for Dedicated Care of Those in Need," *Houston Chronicle*, May 8, 2014, http://www.chron.com /jobs/article/Salute-to-Nurses-Top-10-area-nurses-receive-5463680.php.

77. Alice Adams, "Salute to Nurses."

78. I was not able to directly observe nurses, foreign-born or American-born, at the hospital directly nor did I interview a wide-enough sample of American-born nurses to evaluate the degree to which this is a perception or if real differences exist in their nursing approaches. See methodological appendix.

79. Foreign-born Filipino American nurses in one study have been shown to be more committed to serving their organizations/hospitals than nurses from any other Asian countries, including India. Although no explanation is given for this finding, it is likely that it is a result of the United States's long, complicated historical relationship to the Philippines and the degree to which American culture and language have penetrated the social fabric of the islands. See Shwu-Ru Liou, Hsiu-Min Tsai, and Ching-Yu Cheng, "Acculturation, Collectivist Orientation and Organizational Commitment among Asian Nurses Working in the US Healthcare System," *Journal of Nursing Management* 21, no. 4 (2013): 614–623.

80. I was not able to interview a large-enough sample of foreign-born nurses to make true analytical comparisons between those who left the VA and those who stayed/ retired. Many of those who left the hospital were also unwilling to commit to an interview or were suspicious of who I was/how I was given their contact information by their peers. Hence, the focus of the study is on those who stay or have retired. See the methodological appendix for more details.

81. Robert Bellah, "Civil Religion in America," *Daedalus* 96, no. 1 (1967): 1–21; N. J. Demerath III and Rhys Williams, "Civil Religion in an Uncivil Society," *Annals of the American Academy of Political and Social Science* 480, no. 1 (1985): 154–166; Phillip E. Hammond et al., "Religion and American Culture," *Journal of Interpretation* 4, no. 1 (1994): 1–23. Also see transcript of Pew Research Center panel discussion, "God Bless America: Reflections on Civil Religion After September 11," Pew Research Center, February 6, 2002, https://www.pewforum.org/2002/02/06/god -bless-america-reflections-on-civil-religion-after-september-11/.

82. See Philip Jenkins, *The Next Christendom: The Coming of Global Christianity* (New York: Oxford University Press, 2002), 118.

4. Understanding and Coping with the Trauma of War

1. In Texas the veteran population is less White (60 percent are White) but otherwise matches this national profile. See Texas Workforce Investment Council, *Veterans in Texas: A Demographic Study* (Austin: Office of the Texas Governor, 2019), https:// gov.texas.gov/uploads/files/organization/twic/Veterans-in-Texas-2019.pdf. Also see United Health Foundation and the Military Officer's Association of America (MOAA), *Health of Those Who Have Served Report 2016* (Minnetonka, MN: America's Health Ranking, 2016), http://assets.americashealthrankings.org/app/uploads/htwhs_report _r3.pdf.

2. Eryn Brown, "CDC: Emergency Room Visits Surged in 2009," *Los Angeles Times*, October 18, 2011, http://articles.latimes.com/2011/oct/18/news/la-heb-emergency -room-visits-up-20111018; Kimani Paul-Emile, "Patients' Racial Preferences and the Medical Culture of Accommodation," *UCLA Law Review* 60, no. 462 (2012): 462–504;

Kimani Paul-Emile et al., "Dealing with Racist Patients," *New England Journal of Medicine* 374 (February 2016): 708–711.

3. Robin Farmer, "The Impact of Racist Patients," *Minority Nurse*, October 15, 2014, https:// minoritynurse.com/impact-racist-patients/; Emilia Benton, "Should EPs Accommodate Patient Requests for a Specific Doctor? Many Do," *Emergency Medicine News*, April 2011, accessed January 2017, http://journals.lww.com/emnews/Fulltext/2011 /04000/Breaking_News__Should_EPs_Accommodate_Patient.3.aspx; Vida Foubister, "Requests by Patients Can Put Doctors in Ethical Bind," *American Medical Association News*, January 22, 2001, http://www.ama-assn.org/amednews/2001/01/22/prsb0122 .htm; Jacqueline Howard, "Racism in Medicine: An 'Open Secret,'" *CNN*, October 26, 2016, https://www.cnn.com/2016/10/26/health/doctors-discrimination-racism/index .html; Kenneth Kipnis, "Quality Care and the Wounds of Diversity," *APA News* 97, no. 112 (1998): 112–113; Aasim I. Padela et al., "Patient Choice of Provider Type in the Emergency Department: Perceptions and Factors Relating to Accommodation of Requests for Care Providers," *Emergency Medical Journal* 27, no. 6 (2010): 465–469; Paul-Emile et al., "Dealing with Racist Patients." See full legal discussion in Paul-Emile, "Patients' Racial Preferences."

4. Bob Tedeschi, "6 in 10 Doctors Report Abusive Remarks from Patients, and Many Get Little Help Coping with the Wounds," *STAT*, October 18, 2017, https://www.statnews .com/2017/10/18/patient-prejudice-wounds-doctors/; WebMD News Staff, "Patient Prejudice Survey Results," *WebMD*, October 18, 2017, https://www.webmd.com/a-to -z-guides/news/20171018/patient-prejudice-survey-results?ecd=stat. The survey sample in this study was 1,186 healthcare providers, comprising 822 physicians, 100 registered nurses, 160 nurse practitioners, and 104 physician assistants.

5. See previous note.

6. It is important to note that the majority of previous research has focused on minority patients and majority White physicians. Minority patients routinely rate their doctor visits with White doctors lower than visits with doctors of their same background. See Lisa A. Cooper et al., "Patient-Centered Communication, Ratings of Care, and Concordance of Patient and Physician Race," *Annals of Internal Medicine* 139, no. 11(2003): 907–915; Marsha Lillie-Blanton and Caya B. Lewis, "Policy Challenges and Opportunities in Closing the Racial/Ethnic Divide in HealthCare," *Kaiser Family Foundation Issue Brief* 3 (March 2005): 1–11; Nicole Lurie and Tamara Dubowitz, "Health Disparities and Access to Health," *Journal of the American Medical Association* 297, no. 10 (2007): 1118–1121; Malat and Hamilton, "Preference for Same-Race Health Care Providers"; Padela et al., "Patient Choice of Provider Type," 465. Also see the extensive legal review in Paul-Emile, "Patients' Racial Preferences."

7. Catherine Ceniza Choy, *Empire of Care: Nursing and Migration in Filipino American History* (Durham, NC: Duke University Press, 2003); Catherine Ceniza Choy, "The Export of Womanpower: A Transnational History of Filipino Nurse Migration to the United States" (PhD diss., University of California, Los Angeles, 1998); Barbara Dicicco-Bloom, "The Racial and Gender Experiences of Immigrant Nurses from Kerala, India," *Journal of Transcultural Nursing* 15, no. 1 (January 2004): 26–33; Paul-Emile, "Patients' Racial Preferences"; Paul-Emile et al., "Dealing with Racist Patients"; Yu Liang Xu, "Racism and Discrimination in Nursing: Reflection on Multicultural Nursing Conference," *Home Health Care Management & Practice* 20, no. 3 (2008): 284–286; Yu Liang Xu, Antonio Gutiérre, and Su Hyun Kim, "Adaptation and Transformation through (Un)Learning: Lived Experiences of Immigrant Chinese Nurses in US Healthcare Environment," *Advances in Nursing Science* 31, no. 2 (April–June 2008): E33–E47.

8. Damon Adams, "Patients Say Best Doctors Are Ones Who Look Like Them," *American Medical News*, January 12, 2004, https://amednews.com/article/20040112/profession /301129960/7/; David H. Thom, "Physician Behaviors That Predict Patient Trust," *Journal of Family Practice* 50, no. 4 (2001): 323–328; Paul-Emile, "Patients' Racial Preferences."

9. Lisa A. Cooper et al., "Patient-Centered Communication, Ratings of Care, and Concordance of Patient and Physician Race," *Annals of Internal Medicine* 139, no. 11 (December 2003): 907–915.

10. Howard, "Racism in Medicine"; Farah Khan, "How I Deal with Racist Patients," *Daily Beast*, April 14, 2017, https://www.thedailybeast.com/how-i-deal-with-racist-patients; Padela et al., "Patient Choice of Provider Type"; Paul-Emile, "Patients' Racial Preferences"; Paul-Emile et al., "Dealing with Racist Patients"; Mireille Kingma, "Nurses on the Move: Diversity and the Work Environment," *Contemporary Nurse* 28, no. 1–2 (2008): 198–206; Stacy Newton, Jennifer Pillay, and Gina Higginbottom, "The Migration and Transition of Internationally Educated Nurses: A Global Perspective," *Journal of Nursing Management* 20, no. 4 (2012): 534–550; Xu, Gutiérre, and Kim, "Adaptation and Transformation."

11. Valerie Vestal and Donald Kautz, "International Perspectives: Responding to Similarities and Differences between Filipino and American Nurses," *Journal of Nursing Administration* 39, no. 1 (January 2009): 8–10; also see Naty Lopez, "The Acculturation of Selected Filipino Nurses to Nursing Practice in the United States" (PhD diss., University of Pennsylvania, 1990).

12. Pauline W. Chen, "When the Doctor Doesn't Look Like You," *New York Times*, April 12, 2010, https://www.nytimes.com/2010/08/12/health/12chen.html.

13. Chen, "When the Doctor."

14. Linda Flynn, "Does International Nurse Recruitment Influence Practice Values in U.S. Hospitals?," *Journal of Nursing Scholarship* 34, no. 1 (2002): 67–73; Hayley Germack, "U.S. Hospital Employment of Foreign-Educated Nurses and Patient Experience: A Cross-Sectional Study," *Journal of Nursing Regulation* 8, no. 3 (October 2017): 26–35; Donna Felber Neff, Utilization of Non-US Educated Nurses in US hospitals: Implications for Hospital Mortality," *International Journal for Quality in Health Care* 25, no. 4 (September 2013): 366–372.

15. Paul-Emile, "Patients' Racial Preferences"; Paul-Emile et al., "Dealing with Racist Patients."

16. Also see Sachin H. Jain, "The Racist Patient," *Annals of Internal Medicine* 158, no. 8 (2013): 632. Dr. Jain is an attending doctor at the Boston VA medical center. For further examples see Scott McDonald, "Doctor Says Minority Professionals Often Face Discrimination from Patients," *Newsweek*, March 7, 2019, https://www.newsweek .com/minority-doctors-continue-facing-racism-patients-other-doctors-1356027.

17. Title VII of the Civil Rights Act of 1964, Pub. L. 88-352, Title VII (1964), U.S. Equal Employment Opportunity Commission (EEOC), https://www.eeoc.gov/laws/statutes /titlevii.cfm, and "Patient Bill of Rights," National Institutes of Health, last updated May 24, 2021, https://clinicalcenter.nih.gov/participate/patientinfo/legal/bill_of_rights .html; see also Paul-Emile, "Patients' Racial Preferences"; Paul-Emile et al., "Dealing with Racist Patients."

18. See previous note.

19. See Thom, "Physician Behaviors."

20. Paul-Emile, "Patients' Racial Preferences"; Paul-Emile et al., "Dealing with Racist Patients"; Jennifer Malat and Mary Ann Hamilton, "Preference for Same-Race Health

Care Providers and Perceptions of Interpersonal Discrimination in Health Care," *Journal of Health & Social Behavior* 47, no. 2 (2006): 173–187; Thom, "Physician Behaviors."

21. Beyond point-of-care satisfaction or happiness, racial bias across healthcare also appears to have a severe impact on overall minority patient care, treatment, and mortality; see for example Paul-Emile et al., "Dealing with Racist Patients"; Michael O. Schroeder, "Racial Bias in Medicine Leads to Worse Care for Minorities," *U.S. News and World Report*, February 11, 2016, https://health.usnews.com/health-news/patient-advice/articles/2016-02-11/racial-bias-in-medicine-leads-to-worse-care-for-minorities; Monique Tello, "Racism and Discrimination in Health Care: Providers and Patients," *Harvard Health Publishing, Harvard Medical School*, January 16, 2017, https://www.health.harvard.edu/blog/racism-discrimination-health-care-providers-patients-2017011611015.

22. Gordon Allport, *The Nature of Prejudice* (Cambridge, MA: Addison-Wesley, 1954); Lincoln Quillian, "New Approaches to Understanding Racial Prejudice and Discrimination," *Annual Sociological Review* 32 (2006): 299–328; Joe R. Feagin and Douglas L. Eckberg, "Discrimination: Motivations, Action, Effects and Context," *Annual Sociological Review* 6 (1980): 1–20; Marylee Taylor and Thomas F. Pettigrew, "Prejudice," in *Encyclopedia of Sociology*, 2nd ed., eds. Edgar F. Borgatta and Rhonda J. Montgomery (New York: Macmillan Reference, 2000), 2242–2248.

23. Quillian, "New Approaches."

24. Quillian, "New Approaches."

25. Feagin and Eckberg, "Discrimination."

26. Feagin and Eckberg, "Discrimination."

27. Feagin and Eckberg, "Discrimination."

28. Elizabeth Adams and Annette Kennedy, *Positive Practice Environments: Key Considerations for the Development of a Framework to Support the Integration of International Nurses* (Geneva, Switzerland: International Council of Nurses, 2006); Kingma, "Nurses on the Move."

29. Kingma, "Nurses on the Move."

30. See related concepts/theory in Patricia Hill Collins, "Intersectionality's Definitional Dilemmas," *Annual Sociological Review* 41 (2015): 1–20.

31. Eighty-eight percent of foreign-born Filipino Americans and 93 percent of foreign-born Indian Americans stated in interviews that they had experienced some form of racism or discrimination with their patients at the VA in the last twelve months, when asked to answer *yes* or *no*. This is nearly identical to the survey findings.

32. No supplemental or secondary data allow me to confirm this beyond interviews. Since this study was conducted outside the VA through a snowball sample, a systematic analysis of a generalizable sample of foreign-born nurses by grade, step, and unit/location was not possible. See further comments on study limitations in the methodological appendix.

33. Unlike the survey data previously reported on the frequency of discrimination foreign-born nurses experienced with veterans (patients) in figure 4.1, the data presented here come from the interview sample (N=87). I asked foreign-born nurses whether they experienced any form of racism or discrimination with peers and superiors in the last year—*yes* or *no*.

34. Another study of foreign-born nurses found that 68 percent of those recruited by a staffing agency reported at least one form of discrimination in the last year; see Patricia Pittman et al., "Perceptions of Employment Based Discrimination Among

Newly Arrived Foreign-Educated Nurses," *American Journal of Nursing* 114, no. 1 (2014): 26–35; Kenneth Quinnell, "Foreign-Born Nurses Discriminated against in the United States," AFL-CIO, December 20, 2013, https://aflcio.org/Blog/Corporate -Greed/Study-Foreign-Born-Nurses-Discriminated-Against-in-the-United-States.

35. See previous note; also see Newton et al., "Migration and Transition."

36. Linda A. Beechinor and Joyce J. Fitzpatrick suggest that Filipino American nurses who worked together with fellow Filipinos reported significantly lower levels of stress compared to those who did not have similar social networks of like peers; see Linda A. Victorino Beechinor and Joyce J. Fitzpatrick, "Demands of Immigration among Nurses from Canada and the Philippines," *International Journal of Nursing Practice* 14, no. 2 (2008): 78–187. See further Newton et al., "Migration and Transition."

37. It is important to remember the number of lawsuits brought against prominent hospitals across the country, particularly in California, by foreign-born Filipino American nurses because they were fired for speaking their native languages on breaks. Some hospitals have even written policies that prevent Filipinos from speaking non-English languages anywhere on hospital grounds, often highlighting Tagalog in the description; see Catherine A. Traywick, "Medical Malpractice? Filipino Nurses Fight Back against Discrimination in the Workplace," *Hyphen Asia America Unabridged*, November 7, 2011, https://hyphenmagazine.com/magazine/issue-24-survival-winter -2011/medical-malpractice. Also see discussion in chapter 1.

38. See, for example, Mackenzie Bean, "Racial Discrimination Widespread at Missouri VA Hospital, Employees Allege," *Becker's Hospital Review*, March 19, 2002, https:// www.beckershospitalreview.com/patient-safety-outcomes/racial-discrimination -widespread-at-missouri-va-hospital-employees-allege.html; Chris Levister, "Black Loma Linda VA Nurses Paid to Drop Job Bias Complaints," *Black Voice News*, December 18, 2014, https://www.blackvoicenews.com/2004/12/18/black-loma-linda-va -nurses-paid-to-drop-job-bias-complaints/; Margaret Stafford, "Widespread Discrimination Alleged at Kansas City VA Hospital," *Associated Press*, March 18, 2020, https://www.usnews.com/news/us/articles/2020-03-18/widespread-discrimination -alleged-at-kansas-city-va-hospital. Note that data do not allow for a systematic and comparative analysis of nurse pay, benefits, and shifts across rank, and location/unit worked at the hospital. See further study limitations in methodological appendix.

39. See previous note.

40. See Harold Blumer, "Race Prejudice as a Sense of Group Position," *Pacific Sociological Review* 1, no. 1 (1958): 3–7. Also see Lawrence Bobo, "Prejudice as Group Position: Microfoundations of a Sociological Approach to Racism and Race Relations," *Journal of Social Issues* 55, no. 3 (1999): 445–472; Carol A. Tuttas, "Perceived Racial and Ethnic Prejudice and Discrimination Experiences of Minority Migrant Nurses: A Literature Review," *Journal of Transcultural Nursing* 26, no. 5 (2015): 514–520.

41. See previous note.

42. One study at the VA suggests that nurses' cultural competency is significantly higher after they attend training programs, but this does not mean that higher administration is doing anything about discrimination; see Dale Louis Gradel, "The Effectiveness of an Asynchronous Cultural Competency Training Program for Registered Nurses" (PhD diss., Walden University, 2014).

43. See Pew Research Center, "Attendance at Religious Services among Catholics," *Pew Religion & Public Life*, accessed January 2020, https://www.pewforum.org/religious -landscape-study/religious-tradition/catholic/attendance-at-religious-services/.

44. Also see Arlene N. Hayne, Clara Gerhardt, and Jonathan Davis, "Filipino Nurses in the United States: Recruitment, Retention, Occupational Stress and Job Satisfaction," *Journal of Transcultural Nursing* 20, no. 3 (2009): 313–322.

45. Mary Elaine Koren, "Interventional Studies to Support Spiritual Self-Care of Health Care Practitioners," *Holistic Nursing Practice* 28, no. 5 (2014): 291–300.

46. Diane Applebaum et al., "The Impact of Environmental Factors on Nursing Stress, Job Satisfaction, and Turnover Intention," *Journal of Nursing Administration* 40, no. 7–8 (July–August 2014): 323–328; Andrew B. McGrath, Norma Reid, and Jeffery Boore, "Occupational Stress in Nursing," *International Journal of Nursing Studies* 40, no. 5 (July 2003): 555–565; Andrew McVicar, "Workplace Stress in Nursing: A Literature Review," *Journal of Advanced Nursing* 44, no. 6 (2003): 633–642; Sherrill R. Snellgrove, "Occupational Stress and Job Satisfaction: A Comparative Study of Health Visitors, District Nurses and Community Psychiatric Nurses," *Journal of Nursing Management* 6, no. 2 (1998): 97–104.

47. Linda Aiken et al., "Hospital Nurse Staffing and Patient Mortality, Nurse Burnout, and Job Satisfaction," *Journal of the American Medical Association* 288, no. 16 (2002): 1987–1993; Diane Applebaum et al., "Impact of Environmental Factors"; Timothy Bartram et al., "Do Perceived High Performance Work Systems Influence the Relationship between Emotional Labour, Burnout, and Intention To Leave? A Study of Australian Nurses," *Journal of Advanced Nursing* 68, no. 7 (2012): 1567–1578; Carol S. Brewer and Christine T. Kovner, "Intersection of Migration and Turnover Theories—What Can We Learn?," *Nursing Outlook* 62, no. 1 (2014): 29–38; Christina Anne Bridgeman, "Caregiver Burnout and Job Satisfaction Among Palliative and Non-Palliative Nurses: A Mixed-Methods Study" (PhD diss., University of Phoenix, 2013); Rodger W. Griffeth et al., "The Development of a Multidimensional Measure of Job Market Cognitions: The Employment Opportunity Index (EOI)," *Journal of Applied Psychology* 90, no. 2 (2005): 335–349; Natasha Khamisa et al., "Work Related Stress, Burnout, Job Satisfaction and General Health of Nurses," *International Journal of Environmental Research and Public Health* 12, no. 91 (2013): 652–666; Peter Van Bogaert et al., "The Relationship between Nurse Practice Environment, Nurse Work Characteristics, Burnout and Job Outcome and Quality of Nursing Care: A Cross-Sectional Survey," *International Journal of Nursing Studies* 50, no. 12 (December 2013): 1667–677.

48. Bridgeman, "Caregiver Burnout."

49. Obrey Alexis, Voss Vydelingum, and Ian Robbins, "Engaging with a New Reality: Experiences of Overseas Minority Ethnic Nurses in the NHS," *Journal of Clinical Nursing* 16, no. 12 (2007): 2221–2228; Kate Gerrish and Vanessa Griffith, "Integration of Overseas Registered Nurses: Evaluation of an Adaptation Programme," *Journal of Advanced Nursing* 45, no. 6 (2004): 579–587; John A. Larsen, "Embodiment of Discrimination and Overseas Nurses Career Progression," *Journal of Clinical Nursing* 16, no. 12 (2007): 2187–2195; Newton et al., "Migration and Transition"; Xu, Gutiérre, and Kim, "Adaptation and Transformation."

50. Isabella Aboderin, "Contexts, Motives and Experiences of Nigerian Overseas Nurses: Understanding Links to Globalization," *Journal of Clinical Nursing* 16, no. 12 (2007): 2237–2245; Newton et al., "Migration and Transition."

51. Alexis et al., "Engaging with a New Reality"; Jorgia Briones Connor and Arlene Michaels Miller, "Occupational Stress and Adaptation of Immigrant Nurses from the Philippines," *Journal of Research Nursing* 19, no. 6 (2014): 504–515; Gerrish and Griffith, "Integration of Overseas Registered Nurses"; Larsen, "Embodiment of

Discrimination"; Newton et al., "Migration and Transition"; Xu et al., "Adaptation and Transformation."

52. McGrath, Reid, and Boore, "Occupational Stress in Nursing"; James C. Quick et al., *Preventative Stress Management in Organisations* (Washington DC: American Psychological Association, 1997).

53. C. Daniel Batson, Patricia A. Schoenrade, and W. Larry Ventis, *Religion and the Individual: A Social-Psychological Perspective* (New York: Oxford University Press, 1993); Maryanne Ekedahl and Yvonne Wengstrom, "Caritas, Spirituality and Religiosity in Nurses' Coping," *European Journal of Cancer Care* 19, no. 4 (2010): 530–537; Maryanne Ekedahl and Yvonne Wengstrom, "Coping Processes in a Multidisciplinary Healthcare Team—A Comparison of Nurses in Cancer Care and Hospital Chaplains," *European Journal of Cancer Care* 17, no. 1 (2007): 42–48; Roy F. Baumeister, "Religion and Psychology: Introduction to the Special Issue," *Psychological Inquiry* 13, no. 3 (2002): 165–167; Peter C. Hill and Kenneth I. Pargament, "Advances in the Conceptualization and Measurement of Religion and Spirituality," *American Psychologist* 58, no. 1 (2003): 64–74; Harold G. Koenig, *Spirituality in Patient Care: Why, How, When, and What* (Philadelphia, PA: Templeton Foundation Press, [2002] 2007); Harold Koenig, "The Spiritual Care Team: Enabling the Practice of Whole Person Medicine," *Religions* 5, no. 4 (2014): 1161–1174; Harold G. Koenig, Dana E. King, and Verna B. Carson, *Handbook of Religion and Health*, 2nd ed. (New York: Oxford University Press, 2012); Harold G. Koenig, *Medicine, Religion, and Health: Where Science and Spirituality Meet* (Philadelphia, PA: Templeton Foundation Press, 2008); Kenneth I. Pargament et al., "Religious Coping Methods as Predictors of Psychological, Physical and Spiritual Outcomes among Medically Ill Elderly Patients: A Two-Year Longitudinal Study," *Journal of Health Psychology* 9, no. 6 (2004): 713–730; Kenneth Pargament, "Living with Rheumatoid Arthritis: The Role of Daily Spirituality and Daily Religious and Spiritual Coping," *Journal of Pain* 2, no. 2 (2001): 101–110; Crystal L. Park, "Religion as a Meaning-Making Framework in Coping with Life Stress," *Journal of Social Issues* 61, no. 4 (2005): 707–729; Andrew J. Weaver, Harold G. Koenig, and Laura T. Flannelly, "Nurses and Healthcare Chaplains: Natural Allies," *Journal of Health Care Chaplaincy* 14, no. 2 (2008): 91–98.

54. Mark A. Schuster et al., "A National Survey of Stress Reactions after the September 11, 2001, Terrorist Attacks," *New England Journal of Medicine* 345, no. 20 (2001): 1507–1512.

55. Schuster et al., "National Survey of Stress Reactions."

56. Verna Benner Carson and Harold G. Koenig, *Spiritual Dimensions of Nursing Practice* (West Conshohocken, PA: Templeton Foundation Press, 2008); Judith Allen Shelly and Arlene B. Miller, *Called to Care: A Christian Worldview for Nursing* (Downers Grove, IL: IVP Academic, 2006); Barbra Mann Wall and Sioban Nelson, "Our Heels Are Praying Very Hard All Day," *Holistic Nursing Practice* 17, no. 6 (2003): 320–328.

57. Shanshan Li et al., "Religious Service Attendance and Lower Depression Among Women—A Prospective Cohort Study," *Annals of Behavioral Medicine* 50, no. 6 (July 8, 2016): 876–884; Tyler J. VanderWeele, "Religion and Health: A Synthesis," in *Spirituality and Religion within the Culture of Medicine: From Evidence to Practice*, eds. J. R. Peteet and Michael J. Balboni (New York: Oxford University Press, 2017), 357–402.

58. Stephen M. Cherry, *Faith, Family, and Filipino American Community Life* (New Brunswick, NJ: Rutgers University Press, 2014); Paul DiMaggio, "Culture and Cognition,"

Annual Review of Sociology 23 (1997): 263–287; Erving Goffman, *Frame Analysis* (New York: Harper & Row, [1947] 1997); Hill and Pargament, "Advances in the Conceptualization"; Park, "Religion as a Meaning-Making Framework"; Ralph W. Hood Jr., Peter C. Hill, and Bernard Spilka, *The Psychology of Religion: An Empirical Approach*, 5th ed. (New York: Guilford, 2018); Daniel N. McIntosh, "Religion as Schema, with Implications for the Relation Between Religion and Coping," *International Journal for the Psychology of Religion* 5, no. 1 (1995): 1–16; William H. Sewell Jr., "A Theory of Structure: Duality, Agency, and Transformation," *American Journal Sociology* 98, no. 1 (1992): 1–29; Michael P. Young, *Bearing Witness Against Sin: The Evangelical Birth of the American Social Movement* (Chicago: University of Chicago Press, 2006).

59. Tatsuya Morita et al., "Emotional Burden of Nurses in Palliative Sedation Therapy," *Palliative Medicine* 18, no. 6 (2004): 550–557; Doug Oman, "Unique and Common Facets of Religion and Spirituality: Both Are Important," *Journal of Religion, Spirituality and Aging* 21, no. 4 (2009): 275–286; Doug Oman, John Hedberg, Carl E. Thoresen, "Passage Meditation Reduces Perceived Stress in Health Professionals: A Randomized, Controlled Trial," *Journal of Consulting and Clinical Psychology* 74, no. 4 (2006): 714–719; Christina G. Shinbara and Lynn Olson, "When Nurses Grieve: Spirituality's Role in Coping," *Journal of Christian Nursing* 27, no. 1 (January–March 2010): 32–37; Karran Thorpe and Jeannette Barsky, "Healing through Self-Reflection," *Journal of Advanced Nursing* 35, no. 5 (2001): 760–768.

60. Ekedahl and Wengstrom, "Coping Processes."

5. Faith and the Practice of Care

1. This is also the case historically in American Catholic nursing schools. See Barbra Mann Wall, "Definite Lines of Influence," *Nursing Research* 50, no. 5 (2001): 314–320.

2. Barbara L. Brush and Julie Sochalski, "International Nurse Migration: Lessons From the Philippines," *Policy, Politics and Nursing Practice* 8, no. 1 (2007): 37–46; Fely Lorenzo et al., "Nurse Migration from a Source Country Perspective: Philippine Country Case Study," *Health Services Research* 42, no. 3 (2007): 1406–1418; Megan Prescott and Mark Nichter, "Transnational Nurse Migration: Future Directions for Medical Anthropological Research," *Social Science and Medicine* 107 (April 2014): 113–123; Staff, "Nursing Their Grievances," *Hindu*, July 31, 2015, https://www.thehindu.com/news/cities/Delhi/nursing-their-grievances/article7483581.ece.

3. See Rochelle Ball and Nicola Piper, "Globalisation and Regulation of Citizenship: Filipino Migrant Workers in Japan," *Political Geography* 21, no. 8 (2002): 1013–1034; Prescott and Nichter, "Transnational Nurse Migration."

4. See Leodoro Labrague et al., "Filipino Nurses' Spirituality and Provision of Spiritual Nursing Care," *Clinical Nursing Research* 25, no. 6 (2016): 607–625.

5. Passing rates for all state-certified nursing programs are posted in regional and national newspapers every year as per Section 7 (m) in the law R.A. 8981, otherwise known as the PRC Modernization Act of 2000. Also note that many schools with fewer students, such as University of Saint Louis–Tuguerrao (98.53 percent passing rate) are religious institutions; see "May 2014 Nursing Board Exam (NLE) Performance of Schools," *Philippine News*, June 27, 2014, https://philnews.ph/2014/06/27/may-2014-nursing-board-exam-nle-performance-of-schools/.

6. Fredrick Vincent Doherty, for example, helped establish the first English-speaking school on the island of Mindanao and also helped build a small Catholic chapel there as a testament to his faith and devotion. See Peter Gowing, *Islands under the Cross: The Story of the Church in the Philippines* (Manila, Philippines: National

Council of Churches in the Philippines, 1967); Marvin A. Tort, "Education Is about Quality, Not Quantity," *Business World Online*, October 5, 2017, http://bworldonline .com/education-quality-not-quantity/.

7. See website "College of Nursing," Silliman University, accessed August 2019, https://su.edu.ph/schools-colleges/college-of-nursing/.

8. See websites "College of Nursing," University of Santo Tomas, accessed August 2019, http://www.ust.edu.ph/nursing/; "Vision and Mission," Xavier University, accessed August 2019, http://www.xu.edu.ph/vision-and-mission; Xavier University Vison and Mission, Saint Paul University–Iloilo, accessed August 2019, http://spuiloilo .edu.ph/?page_id=94.

9. See Paulinian Nurses Take the Oath, *St. Paul University Iloilo*, 2014, https://spuiloilo .edu.ph/?p=2179 accessed August 2019.

10. Catherine Ceniza Choy, *Empire of Care: Nursing and Migration in Filipino American History* (Durham, NC: Duke University Press, 2003); Yasmin Y. Ortiga, "Professional Problems: The Burden of Producing the 'Global' Filipino Nurse," *Social Science and Medicine* 115 (August 2014): 64–71; also see "Nov. 2014 Nursing Board Exam Top Performing & Performance of Schools," *Philippine News*, January 23, 2015, https:// philnews.ph/2015/01/23/nov-2015-nursing-board-exam-top-performing-performance -of-schools/.

11. Indulekha Aravind, "Kerala's Nurses: Taking Care of the World," *Business Standard*, July 26, 2014, http://www.business-standard.com/article/beyond-business/kerala-s -nurses-taking-care-of-the-world-114072501466_1.html; Sheba George, *When Women Come First: Gender and Class in Transnational Migration* (Berkeley: University of California Press, 2005); Sreelekha Nair and Marie Percot, *Transcending Boundaries: Indian Nurses in Internal and International Migration* (New Delhi, India: Centre for Women's Development Studies, 2007); J. Pazhanilats, "NURSE-ing NRI Dreams, They Flock to Cochi," *Hindu*, September 29, 2003, https://www.thehindu.com/thehindu/mp /2003/09/29/stories/2003092900320100./; S. Iruday Rajan and Udaya S. Mishra, "Managing Migration in the Philippines: Lessons for India" (working paper no. 393, Centre for Development Studies, Trivandrum, India, 2007); Margaret Walton-Roberts, "Contextualizing the Global Nursing Care Chain: International Migration and the Status of Nursing in Kerala, India," *Global Networks* 12, no. 2 (2012): 175–194; Nicola Yeates, *Globalizing Care Economies and Migrant Workers: Explorations in Global Care Chains* (Basingstoke, UK: Palgrave Macmillan, 2009).

12. See, for example, "Karnataka Religion Census 2011," Census 2011, India, accessed August, 2019, http://www.census2011.co.in/data/religion/state/29-karnataka.html; also see Bhuvaneshwari G. Devangamath and Sudha A. Raddi, "A Descriptive Study to Assess the Knowledge Regarding Nursing Management of First Stage of Labour among Final Year GNM Students of Selected School of Nursing, Belgaum, Karnataka," *International Journal of Science and Research* 6, no. 14 (2013): 2199–2220; Prescott and Nichter, "Transnational Nurse Migration."

13. Barbara Dicicco-Bloom, "The Racial and Gendered Experiences of Immigrant Nurses from Kerala, India," *Journal of Transcultural Nursing* 15, no. 1 (2004): 26–33; George, *When Women Come First*; Robin Jeffrey, *Politics, Women, and Well-Being: How Kerala Became a Model* (London: Macmillan, 1992); Joyce Jose, "Demands of Immigration of Indian Nurses" (PhD diss., Frances Payne Bolton School of Nursing, Case Western Reserve University, 2006); Seelekha Nair, "Rethinking Citizenship, Community, and Rights: The Case of Nurses from Kerala in Delhi," *Indian Journal of Gender*

Studies 14, no. 1 (2007): 137–156; Elizabeth Simon, "Christianity and Nursing in India: A Remarkable Impact," *Journal of Christian Nursing* 26, no. 2 (April 2009): 88–94.

14. See "A Brief History," Holy Cross College of Nursing, 2012, accessed December 2017http://holycrosscollegeofnursing.org/history.html, and "About Us," Lourdes College of Nursing, 2017, accessed August 2019, http://lourdescollegeofnursing.in /about-us.

15. "A Brief History," Holy Cross College of Nursing, 2012, accessed December 2017, http://holycrosscollegeofnursing.org/history.html, and "About Us," Lourdes College of Nursing, 2017, accessed August 2019, http://lourdescollegeofnursing.in/about-us.

16. Binumol Abraham, "Women Nurses and the Notion of Their 'Empowerment'" (discussion paper no. 88, Kerala Research Programme on Local Level Development, Centre for Development Studies, Thiruvananthapuram, India, 2004); Madelaine Healey, *Indian Sisters: A History of Nursing and the State, 1907–2007* (New York: Routledge, 2013).

17. Since the Philippines is overwhelmingly Christian, with upwards of 94 percent of the population as Christian, of which 86 percent are Catholic, the same religious exclusion problems do not exist, especially considering how many programs are state run or the extent to which the state regulates all others. See Jack Miller, "Religion in the Philippines," Asia Society, Center for Global Education, accessed August 2019, https:// asiasociety.org/education/religion-philippines. For further research on Indian nurses see Dicicco-Bloom, "Racial and Gendered Experiences"; Nair and Percot, *Transcending Boundaries*" (New Delhi, India: Centre for Women's Development Studies, 2007); Munira Wells, "The Experiences of Indian Nurses in America," (PhD diss., Seton Hall University, 2013).

18. Don Grant, "Spiritual Interventions: How, When, and Why Nurses Use Them," *Holistic Nursing Practice* 18, no. 1 (2004): 36–41; Sharon S. Hadacek, "Dimensions of Caring: A Qualitative Analysis of Nurses' Stories," *Journal of Nursing Education* 47, no. 3 (2008): 124–129.

19. See for example Mary Elaine Koren and Christina Papamiditriou, "Spirituality of Staff Nurses, Application of Modeling and Role Modeling Theory," *Holistic Nursing Practice* 27, no. 1 (2013): 37–44.

20. Farr A. Curlin et al., "The Association of Physicians' Religious Characteristics with their Attitudes and Self-Reported Behaviors Regarding Religion and Spirituality in the Clinical Encounter," *Medical Care* 44, no. 5 (2006): 446–453; Farr A. Curlin et al., "How Are Religion and Spirituality Related to Health? A Study of Physicians' Perspectives," *Southern Medical Journal* 98, no. 8 (August 2005): 761–766; Harold Koenig, "The Spiritual Care Team: Enabling the Practice of Whole Person Medicine," *Religions* 5, no. 4 (2014): 1161–1174; Harold G. Koenig, *Medicine, Religion, and Health: Where Science and Spirituality Meet* (Philadelphia, PA: Templeton Foundation Press, 2008).

21. Note this is not an exhaustive review of the literature on religion and health. See, for example, Christopher G. Ellison and Jeffery Levin, "The Religion-Health Connection: Evidence, Theory, and Future Directions," *Health Education Behavior* 25, no. 6 (1998): 700–720; Curlin et al., "How Are Religion and Spirituality?"; Koenig, "Spiritual Care Team"; Raymond Lawrence, "The Witches' Brew of Spirituality and Medicine," *Annals of Behavioral Medicine* 24, no. 1 (2002): 74–76; Bruce Y. Lee and Andrew B. Newberg, "Religion and Health: A Review and Critical Analysis," *Zygon* 40,

no. 2 (2005): 443–468; Stephen Post, Christina Puchalski, and David Larson, "Physicians and Patient Spirituality: Professional Boundaries, Competency, and Ethics," *Annals of Internal Medicine* 132, no. 7 (2000): 578–583; Neil Scheurich, "Reconsidering Spirituality and Medicine," *Academic Medicine* 78, no. 4 (2003): 356–360.

22. Richard P. Sloan, *Blind Faith: The Unholy Alliance of Religion and Medicine* (New York: Macmillan, 2015); Richard P. Sloan, Emilia Bagiella, and Tia Powell, "Religion, Spirituality, and Medicine," *Lancet* 353 (1999): 664–667.

23. See Leonard Hummel et al., "Defining Spiritual Care: An Exploratory Study," *Journal of Health Care Chaplaincy* 15, no. 1 (2008): 40–51. For further research, see Wendy Cadge, *Paging God: Religion in the Halls of Medicine* (Chicago: University of Chicago Press, 2012).

24. See endnote 21 of this chapter. Also see Anna Buck et al., "An Examination of the Relationship between Multiple Dimensions of Religiosity, Blood Pressure, and Hypertension," *Social Science and Medicine* 68, no. 2 (2009): 314–322; Arndt Bussing et al., "Are Spirituality and Religiosity Resources for Patients with Chronic Pain Conditions?," *Pain Medicine* 10, no. 2 (2009): 327–339; Marlene Z. Cohen et al., "A Platform for Nursing Research on Spirituality and Religiosity: Definitions and Measures," *Western Journal of Nursing Research* 34, no. 6 (2012): 795–817; June M. Como, "Spiritual Practice, a Literature Review Related to Spiritual Health and Health Outcomes," *Holistic Nursing Practice* 21, no. 5 (2007): 224–236; Salvatore Giaquinto, Cristiana Spiridigliozzi, and Barbara Caracciolo, "Can Faith Protect from Emotional Distress after Stroke?," *Stroke* 38, no. 3 (2007): 993–997; Ellen L. Idler, Stanislav V. Kasl, and Judith C. Hays, "Patterns of Religious Practice and Belief in the Last Year of Life," *Journals of Gerontology: Series B* 56, no. 6 (2001): S326–S334; Paul S. Mueller, David J. Plevak, and Teresa A. Rummans, "Religious Involvement, Spirituality, and Medicine: Implications for Clinical Practice," *Mayo Clinic Proceedings* 76, no. 12 (2001): 1766–1771; Kenneth I. Pargament et al., "Religious Coping Methods as Predictors of Psychological, Physical and Spiritual Outcomes among Medically Ill Elderly Patients: A Two-Year Longitudinal Study," *Journal of Health Psychology* 9, no. 6 (2004): 713–730; William J. Strawbridge et al., "Religious Attendance Increases Survival by Improving and Maintaining Good Health Behaviors, Mental Health, and Social Relationships," *Annals of Behavioral Medicine* 23, no. 1 (2001): 68–74; Leslie Tepper et al., "The Prevalence of Religious Coping among Persons with Persistent Mental Illness," *Psychiatric Services* 52, no. 5 (2001): 660–665; Andrew P. Tix and Patricia A. Frazier, "The Use of Religious Coping during Stressful Life Events," *Journal of Consulting and Clinical Psychology* 66, no. 2 (1997): 411–422; Andrew J. Weaver, Harold G. Koenig, and Laura T. Flannelly, "Nurses and Healthcare Chaplains: Natural Allies," *Journal of Health Care Chaplaincy* 14, no. 2 (2008): 91–98; Li-Fen Wu and Lih-Ying Lin, "Exploration of Clinical Nurses' Perceptions of Spirituality and Spiritual Care," *Journal of Nursing Research* 19, no. 4 (2011): 250–256.

25. C. Cheryl Clark et al., "Spirituality: Integral to Quality Care," *Holistic Nursing Practice* 5, no. 3 (1991): 67–76; Grant, "Spiritual Interventions"; Melanie McEwen, "Spiritual Nursing Care: State of the Art," *Holistic Nursing Practice* 19, no. 4 (2005): 161–168; Aru Narayanasamy, "A Review of Spirituality as Applied to Nursing," *International Journal of Nursing Studies* 36 (1999): 117–125; Linda Ross, "The Spiritual Dimensions: Its Importance to Patients' Health, Well-being and Quality of Life and Its Implications for Nursing Practice," *International Journal of Nursing Studies* 32, no. 5 (1995): 67–76; Leslie J. Van Dover and Jane M. Bacon, "Spiritual Care in Nursing Practice: A Close-up View," *Nursing Forum* 36, no. 3 (2001): 18–30.

26. Harold Koenig, "Religion, Spirituality, and Health" *Religions* 5, 2014: 1161–1174; Koenig, *Medicine, Religion, and Health*; also see Elizabeth Johnston Taylor, *Spiritual Care: Nursing Theory, Research and Practice* (Upper Saddle River, NJ: Prentice-Hall, 2002).

27. See previous note.

28. Michael J. Balboni et al., "Religion, Spirituality, and the Hidden Curriculum: Medical Student and Faculty Reflections," *Journal of Pain Symptom Management* 50, no. 4 (October 2005): 507–515; Cadge, *Paging God*; Roberta Cavendish, "Patients' Perceptions of Spirituality and the Nurse as a Spiritual Care Provider," *Holistic Nursing Practice* 20, no. 1 (2006): 41–47; Roberta Cavendish et al., "Spiritual Perspectives of Nurses in the United States Relevant for Education and Practice," *Western Journal of Nursing Research* 26, no. 2 (2004): 219–221; Don Grant, Kathleen O'Neil, and Laura Stephens, "Spirituality in the Workplace: New Empirical Directions in the Study of the Sacred," *Sociology of Religion* 65, no. 3 (2004): 265–283; Susan Stranahan, "Spiritual Perception, Attitudes about Spiritual Care, and Spiritual Care Practices among Nurse Practitioners," *Western Journal of Nursing Research* 23, no. 1 (2001): 90–104; Elizabeth Johnston Taylor, Martha E. Farrar Highfield, and Madalon D. Amenta, "Attitudes and Beliefs regarding Spiritual Care. A Survey of Cancer Nurses," *Cancer Nursing* 17, no. 6 (1994): 479–487; Weaver, Koenig, and Flannelly, "Nurses and Healthcare Chaplains"; Angelika A. Zollfrank et al., "Teaching Health Care Providers to Provide Spiritual Care: A Pilot Study," *Journal of Palliative Medicine* 18, no. 5 (2015): 1–7.

29. See discussion in chapter 1. Also see Michael J. Balboni et al., "Why Is Spiritual Care Infrequent at the End of Life? Spiritual Care Perceptions among Patients, Nurses, and Physicians and the Role of Training," *Journal of Clinical Oncology* 31, no. 4 (February 2013): 461–467; Karen A. Boutell and Frederick W. Bozett, "Nurses' Assessment of Patients' Spirituality: Continuing Education Implications," *Journal of Continuing Education* 21, no. 4 (1987): 172–176; Julian D. Emblem, "Religion and Spirituality Defined According to Current Use in Nursing Literature," *Journal of Professional Nursing* 8, no. 1 (1992): 41–47; Grant, "Spiritual Interventions"; Aru Narayanasamy, "Nurse Awareness and Preparedness in Meeting Their Patients Spiritual Needs," *Nursing Education Today* 13, no. 3 (1992): 196–201; Aru Narayanasamy, "Recognizing Spiritual Needs," in *Spiritual Assessment in Healthcare Practice*, eds. Linda Ross and Wilfred McSherry (Keswick, UK: M&K Update Ltd., 2010), 37–55; Aru Narayanasamy, "Nurse Awareness and Preparedness in Meeting Their Patients Spiritual Needs," *Nursing Education Today* 13, no. 3 (1992): 196–201; Aru Narayanasamy, "Palliative Care and Spirituality," *Indian Journal of Palliative Care* 13, no. 2 (December 2007): 32–41.

30. Corinne Lemmer, "Teaching the Spiritual Dimensions of Nursing Care," *Journal of Nursing Education* 41, no. 11 (November 2002): 482–497.

31. Bonnie Weaver Battey, "Perspectives on Spiritual Care for Nurse Managers," *Journal of Nursing Management* 20, no. 8 (2012): 1012–1020; Harold G. Koenig, Dana E. King, and Verna B. Carson, *Handbook of Religion and Health*, 2nd ed. (New York: Oxford University Press, 2012); Harold G. Koenig et al., "Spirituality in Medical School Curricula: Findings from a National Survey," *International Journal of Psychiatry in Medicine* 40, no. 4 (2001): 391–398.

32. Lemmer, "Teaching the Spiritual Dimensions." Note that medical schools in Lemmer's study most likely to demonstrate an interest in teaching spiritual care were in states that tended to be more religious. See further Koenig et al., "Spirituality in Medical School Curricula."

33. Melanie McEwen "Analysis of Spirituality Content in Nursing Textbooks," *Journal of Nursing Education* 43, no. 1 (2004): 20–30. Also see Barbara Pesut, "Spirituality and Spiritual Care in Nursing Fundamentals Textbooks," *Journal of Nursing Education* 47, no. 4 (2008): 167–173; Fiona Timmins, Maryanne Murphy, Freda Neill, Thelma Begley, and Greg Sheaf, "An Exploration of the Inclusion of Spirituality and Spiritual Care Concepts in Core Nursing Textbooks *Nursing Education Today* 35, no. 1 (January 2015): 277-282,"; Diana L. Vance, "Nurses' Attitudes towards Spirituality and Patient Care," *Medical-Surgical Nursing* 10, no. 5 (2001): 264–268.

34. See previous note.

35. Lynn Clark Callister et al., "Threading Spirituality throughout Nursing Education," *Holistic Nursing Practice* 18, no. 3 (2004): 160–166; "Does the Joint Commission Specify What Needs to Be Included in a Spiritual Assessment?," Joint Commission on Accreditation of Healthcare Organizations, Spiritual Assessment 2017, last updated March 16, 2021, https://www.jointcommission.org/en/standards/standard-faqs/critical-access-hospital/provision-of-care-treatment-and-services-pc/000001669/; Cheryl M. Lantz, "Teaching Spiritual Care in a Public Institution: Legal Implications, Standards of Practice, and Ethical Obligations," *Journal of Nursing Education* 46, no. 1 (2007): 33–38; Lemmer, "Teaching the Spiritual Dimensions"; Sheryl Reimer-Kirkham et al., "Discourses of Spirituality and Leadership in Nursing: A Mixed Methods Analysis," *Journal of Nursing Management* 20, no. 8 (2012): 1029–1038; International Council of Nurses, *The ICN Code of Ethics for Nurses* (Geneva, Switzerland: International Council of Nurses, 2012), https://www.icn.ch/sites/default/files/inline-files/2012_ICN_Codeofethicsfornurses_%20eng.pdf; Pat Staten, "Spiritual Assessment Required in All Settings," *Hospital Peer Review* 28, no. 4 (2003): 55–56; Wu and Lin, "Exploration of Clinical Nurses' Perceptions"; Li-Fen, Yu-Chen Liao, and Dah-Cherng Yeh, "Nursing Student Perceptions of Spirituality and Spiritual Care," *Journal of Nursing Research* 20, no. 3 (September 2012): 219–227.

36. Bonnie Weaver Battey, *Spiritual–Communication–Satisfaction–Importance (SCSI) Questionnaire Survey Manual* (Bloomington, IN: Xlibris Corporation, 2011); Bonnie Weaver Battey, *Spirituality in Nursing Practice: A Computer Assisted Instruction Program and Course Manual* (St. Louis, MO: ASK Data Systems Inc., 2011); Battey, "Perspectives on Spiritual Care"; Audrey Berman et al., *Kozier & Erbs Fundamentals of Nursing: Concepts, Process, and Practice*, 8th ed. (Upper Saddle River, NJ: Prentice Hall Health, 2007); Harold G. Koenig, "Editors Comment On Abstract of Ozbasaran et al. CROSSROADS . . . Exploring Research on Religion, Spirituality and Health," *Newsletter of the Center for Spirituality, Theology & Health* 1, no. 3 (September 2011):1–3, http://www.spiritualityandhealth.duke.edu/resources/pdfs/CSTH%20Newsletter%20Sept%202011.pdf; McEwen "Analysis of Spirituality Content"; Pesut, "Spirituality and Spiritual Care"; Timmins et al., "Exploration of the Inclusion"; Diana L. Vance, "Nurses' Attitudes towards Spirituality and Patient Care," *Medical-Surgical Nursing* 10, no. 5 (2001): 264–268.

37. See Lantz, "Teaching Spiritual Care." Also see Battey, "Perspectives on Spiritual Care"; Koenig, King, and Carson, *Handbook of Religion and Health*; Koenig, "Editors Comment"; Wilfred McSherry, *Making Sense of Spirituality in Nursing and Health Care Practice: An Interactive Approach* (Philadelphia, PA: Jessica Kingsley Publishers, 2006); Timmins et al., "Exploration of the Inclusion."

38. Lantz, "Teaching Spiritual Care." Also see discussion in chapter 2 of this book.

39. Ann Belcher and Margaret Griffiths, "The Spiritual Care Perspectives and Practices of Hospice Nurses," *Journal of Hospice & Palliative Nursing* 7, no. 5 (2005): 271–279;

Verna Benner Carson and Ruth Stoll, "Defining the Indefinable and Reviewing Its Place in Nursing," in *Spiritual Dimensions of Nursing Practice*, eds. Verna Benner Carson and Harold G. Koenig (West Conshohocken, PA: Templeton Press, 2008), 3–61; Cavendish et al., "Patients' Perceptions"; Moon Fai Chan, "Factors Affecting Nursing Staff in Practicing Spiritual Care," *Journal of Clinical Nursing* 19, no. 15–16 (2010): 2128–2136; Loretta Chung, Francis Wong, and Moon Chan, "Relationship of Nurses' Spirituality to Their Understanding and Practice of Spiritual Care," *Journal of Advanced Nursing* 58, no. 2 (2007): 158–170; Leodoro Labrague et al., "Filipino Nurses' Spirituality."

40. John Tropman, *The Catholic Ethic in American Society* (San Francisco: Jossey-Bass, 1995); John Tropman, *The Catholic Ethic and the Spirit of Community* (Washington, DC: Georgetown University Press, 2002).

41. Andrew J. Weaver, "A Systematic Review of Research on Religion and Spirituality in the Journal of Traumatic Stress: 1990–1999," *Mental Health, Religion & Culture* 6, no. 3 (2003): 215–228.

42. Jane Dyson, Mark Cobb, and Dyson Forman, "The Meaning of Spirituality: A Literature Review," *Journal of Advanced Nursing* 26, no. 6 (1997): 1183–1188; Monir Ramezani et al., "Spiritual Care in Nursing: A Concept Analysis," *International Nursing Review* 61, no. 2 (2014): 211–219; Jean Stallwood and Ruth Stoll, "Spiritual Dimensions of Nursing Practice," in *Clinical Nursing*, 3rd ed., eds. Irene L. Beland and Joyce Y. Passos (New York: Macmillan, 1975), 1086–1098.

43. Ewan Kelly "Preparation for Providing Spiritual Care," *Scottish Journal of Healthcare Chaplaincy* 5, no. 2 (2002): 11–15; McSherry, *Making Sense of Spirituality*; Wilfred McSherry and Steve Jamieson, "An Online Survey of Nurses' Perceptions of Spirituality and Spiritual Care," *Journal of Clinical Nursing* 20, no. 11–12 (June 2011): 1757–1767; Christina M. Puchalski and Betty Ferrell, *Making Health Care Whole: Integrating Spirituality into Patient Care* (West Conshohocken, PA: Templeton Press, 2010); Christina M. Puchalski et al., "Interdisciplinary Spiritual Care for Seriously Ill and Dying Patients: Collaborative Model," *Cancer Journal* 12, no. 5 (2006): 398–416; Ramezani et al., "Spiritual Care in Nursing"; Rick Sawatzky and Barbara Pesut, "Attributes of Spiritual Care in Nursing Practice," *Journal of Holistic Nursing* 23, no. 1 (2005): 19–33.

44. After 2019, the VA changed its policy in response to the Supreme Court verdict in the case of *The American Legion vs. American Humanist Association*. The new policy allowed (1) the inclusion in appropriate circumstances of religious content in publicly accessible displays at VA facilities; (2) patients and their guests to request and be provided religious literature, symbols, and sacred texts during visits to VA chapels and during their treatment; and (3) acceptance of donations of religious literature, cards, and symbols at its facilities and distribution to VA patrons under appropriate circumstances or to a patron who requests them. The VA essentially relaxed its prior standards. See discussion in chapter 1. Also see Charles Dervarics, "VA Chaplains Play a Key Role in Providing Spiritual and Comprehensive Care," *Defense Media Network*, December 3, 2017, https://www.defensemedianetwork.com/stories/va-chaplains-play-key-role-providing-spiritual-comprehensive-care/.

45. Lisa Burkhart et al., "Spiritual Care in Nursing Practice in Veteran Health Care," *Global Qualitative Nursing Research* (January–December 2019): 1–9.

46. Reimer-Kirkham et al., "Discourses of Spirituality."

47. Keith G. Meador, "When Patients Say, It's in God's Hands," *Virtual Mentor* 11, no. 10 (2009): 750–754.

48. Anna Merlan, "The Depressed Lesbian Vet and the Allegedly Homophobic VA Nurse: A Match Made in Hell," *Dallas Observer*, November 18, 2011, https://www .dallasobserver.com/news/the-depressed-lesbian-vet-and-the-allegedly-homophobic -va-nurse-a-match-made-in-hell-7135436.

49. Amy Ai et al., "Prayer and Reverence in Naturalistic, Aesthetic, and Sociomoral Contexts Predicted Fewer Complications Following Coronary Artery Bypass," *Journal of Behavioral Medicine* 32, no. 6 (2009): 570–581; Luciano Bernardi et al., "Effect of Rosary Prayer and Yoga Mantras on Autonomic Cardiovascular Rhythms: Comparative Study," *British Medical Journal* 323, no. 7327 (2001): 1446–1449; Grant, "Spiritual Interventions"; Elizabeth Johnston Taylor, "Prayer's Clinical Issues and Implications," *Holistic Nursing Practice* 17, no. 4 (2003): 179–188.

50. The most commonly used scale to assess spiritual well-being was developed in 1983 by Craig W. Ellison, and then further elaborated by Ellison and Raymond F. Paloutzian. It uses twenty items and has two subscales—"Religious Well-Being" and "Existential Well-Being"; see Craig W. Ellison, "Spiritual Well-Being: Conceptualization and Measurement," *Journal of Psychology and Theology* 11, no. 4 (1983): 330–340; Craig W. Ellison and Joel Smith, "Toward an Integrative Measure of Health and Well-Being," *Journal of Psychology and Theology* 19, no. 1 (1991): 35–48; Raymond F. Paloutzian and Craig W. Ellison, "Loneliness, Spiritual Well-Being and the Quality Of Life," in *Loneliness: A Sourcebook of Current Theory, Research and Therapy*, eds. Letitia A. Peplau and Daniel Perlman (New York: Wiley, 1982), 224–237. For further research see Balboni et al., "Why Is Spiritual Care Infrequent?"; Verna Benner Carson and Harry Green, "Spiritual Well-Being: A Predictor of Hardiness in the AIDS Patient," *Journal of Professional Nursing* 8, no. 4 (1992): 209–220; Carson and Stoll, "Defining the Indefinable"; Verna Benner Carson, Karen L. Soeken, and Patricia M. Grimm, "Hope and Its Relationship to Spiritual Well-Being," *Journal of Psychology and Theology* 16, no. 2 (1988): 159–167; Richard H. Fehring, Joan F. Miller, and Chuck Shaw, "Spiritual Well-Being, Religiosity, Hope, Depression, and Other Mood States," *Oncology Nursing Forum* 24, no. 4 (1997): 663–671; Koenig, *Medicine, Religion, and Health*; B. J. Landis, "Uncertainty, Spiritual Well-Being and Psychosocial Adjustment to Chronic Illness," *Issues in Mental Health Nursing* 17, no. 3 (1996): 217–223; Koenig, "Religion, Spirituality, and Health"; Colleen S. McClain, Barry Rosenfeld, and William Breitbart, "Effect of Spiritual Well-Being on End-of-Life Despair in Terminally-Ill Cancer Patients," *Lancet* 361, no. 9369 (May 2003): 1603–1607; Jaqueline R. Mickley and Karen Soeken, "Religiousness and Hope in Hispanic and Anglo-American Women with Breast Cancer," *Oncology Nursing Forum* 20, no. 8 (1993): 1171–1176; Jaqueline R. Mickley, Karen Soeken, and Anne Belcher, "Spiritual Well-Being, Religiousness and Hope among Women with Breast Cancer," *Image: Journal of Nursing Scholarship* 24, no. 4 (Winter 1992): 267–272; Karen Soeken and Verna Benner Carson, "Responding to the Spiritual Needs of the Chronically Ill," *Nursing Clinics of North America* 22, no. 3 (1987): 603–611; Stallwood and Stoll, "Spiritual Dimensions of Nursing Practice"; Zollfrank et al., "Teaching Health Care Providers."

51. For other expressions of this sentiment or ones like it, see Michael S. Goldstein, "The VA and Limits on Veterans' Religious Freedom," *American Thinker*, December 4, 2015, https://www.americanthinker.com/articles/2015/12/the_va_and_limits _on_veterans_religious_liberty.html.

52. Karen S. Dunn, Cecilia Otten, and Elizabeth Stephens, "Nursing Experience and the Care of Dying Patients," *Oncology Nursing Forum* 32, no. 1 (2005): 97–104; Susan Irvin, "The Experiences of the Registered Nurse Caring for the Person Dying of

Cancer in a Nursing Home," *Collegian* 7, no. 4 (2000): 30–34; Shelia A. Payne, S. J. Dean, and C. Kalus, "A Comparative Study of Death Anxiety in Hospice and Emergency Nurses," *Journal of Advanced Nursing* 28, no. 4 (1998): 700–706; Eva M. Roman, Eva Sorribes, and Olga Ezquerro, "Nurses' Attitudes To Terminally Ill Patients," *Journal of Advanced Nursing* 34, no. 3 (2001): 338–345.

53. Robin Lally, "Oncology Nurses Share Their Experiences with Bereavement and Self-Care," *Oncology Nursing Society News* 20, no. 10 (2005): 4–11; Tatsuya Morita et al., "Family Experience with Palliative Sedation Therapy for Terminally Ill Cancer Patients," *Journal of Pain and Symptom Management* 28, no. 6 (December 2004): 557–565; Danai Papadatou, "A Proposed Model of Health Professionals' Grieving Process," *Omega* 41, no. 1 (2002): 59–77; Christina G. Shinbara and Lynn Olson, "When Nurses Grieve: Spirituality's Role in Coping," *Journal of Christian Nursing* 27, no. 1 (January–March 2010): 32–37.

54. Grant, "Spiritual Interventions"; McEwen, "Spiritual Nursing Care"; Narayanasamy, "Review of Spirituality"; Ross, "Spiritual Dimensions"; Van Dover and Bacon, "Spiritual Care in Nursing Practice."

55. See review of studies in Taylor, "Prayer's Clinical Issues."

56. Taylor, "Prayer's Clinical Issues." Also see Kenneth Pargament, *The Psychology of Religion and Coping* (New York: Guilford, 1997).

57. Grant, "Spiritual Interventions."

58. See review of studies in Taylor, "Prayer's Clinical Issues."

59. Taylor, "Prayer's Clinical Issues."

60. Boutell and Bozett, "Nurses' Assessment"; Grant, "Spiritual Interventions"; McEwen, "Spiritual Nursing Care"; Narayanasamy, "Review of Spirituality"; Narayanasamy, "Nurse Awareness"; Ross, "Spiritual Dimensions"; Van Dover and Bacon, "Spiritual Care in Nursing Practice."

61. See previous note. Also see Koenig, "Spiritual Care Team."

62. Koenig, "Religion, Spirituality, and Health"; Balboni et al., "Support of Cancer Patients' Spiritual Needs and Associations with Medical Care Costs at the End of Life," *Cancer* I117, no. 23 (December 2011): 5383–5391.

63. See discussion in Taylor, "Prayer's Clinical Issues."

6. Extending Heath and Care to Community

1. See "History of Star of Hope Mission," Star of Hope Mission, accessed May 2019, https://www.sohmission.org/about-us/history/.

2. See National Coalition for Homeless Veterans, Annual Homeless Assessment Reports (AHAR) by Year: https://www.hudexchange.info/homelessness-assistance/ahar/#reports.

3. Mary Jo Bane, "The Catholic Puzzle: Parishes and Civic Life," in *Taking Faith Seriously*, eds. Mary Jo Bane, Brent Coffin, and Richard Higgins (Cambridge, MA: Harvard University Press, 2005), 63–93; Nancy Burns, Kay Lehman Schlozman, and Sidney Verba, *The Private Roots of Public Action* (Cambridge, MA: Harvard University Press, 2001); Marc Musick and John Wilson, *Volunteers: A Social Profile* (Bloomington: Indiana University Press, 2008); Robert Putnam, *Bowling Alone: The Collapse and Revival of American Community* (New York: Simon and Schuster, 2000); Bradford Smith et al., *Philanthropy in Communities of Color* (Bloomington: Indiana University Press, 2009); Yuying Tong, "Foreign-born Concentration and Acculturation to Volunteering among Immigrant Youth," *Social Forces* 89, no. 1 (2010): 117–144; S. Karthick Ramakrishnan and Irene Bloemraad, *Civic Hopes and*

Political Realities: Immigrants, Community Organizations, and Political Engagement (Thousand Oaks, CA: Sage, 2011).

4. Josue Lopez and R. Dale Safrit, "Hispanic American Volunteering," *Journal of Extension* 39, no. 6 (2001): 206–219; Musick and Wilson, *Volunteers*; Colin Rochester et al., *Volunteering and Society in the Twenty-First Century* (New York: Palgrave Macmillan, 2010).

5. Musick and Wilson, *Volunteers*.

6. See David Card and John E. DiNardo, "Do Immigrant Flows Lead to Native Outflows?," *American Economic Review* 90, no. 2 (2009): 360–367; Samuel P. Huntington, "Jose Can You See? . . . How Hispanic Immigrants Threaten America's Identity, Values, and Way of Life," *Foreign Policy*, March/April 2004, 30–45; Samuel P. Huntington, *Who Are We? The Challenges to America's National Identity* (New York: Simon and Schuster, 2004); Jeffrey S. Passel, *Estimates of the Size and Characteristics of the Undocumented Population, Research Report of the Pew Hispanic Center* (Washington, DC: Pew Hispanic Center, 2005), http://www.pewhispanic.org/2005/03/21/estimates-of-the-size-and -characteristics-of-the-undocumented-population/; Robert Rector, Christin Kim, and Shanea Watkins, *The Fiscal Cost of Low-Skill Households to the U.S. Taxpayer*, Special Report No. 12 (Washington, DC: Heritage Foundation, 2007).

7. Robert Serow and Julia Dreyden, "Community Service among College and University Students: Individual and Institutional Relationships," *Adolescence* 25, no. 99 (1990): 553–566; Tong, "Foreign-born Concentration"; John Wilson and Marc Musick, "Who Cares? Toward an Integrated Theory of Volunteer Work," *American Sociological Review* 62, no. 5 (1997): 694–713; Min Zhou, "Segmented Assimilation: Issues, Controversies, and Recent Research on the New Second Generation," *International Migration Review* 31, no. 4 (1997): 975–1008.

8. Miller McPherson and Thomas Rotolo, "Diversity and Change in Voluntary Groups," *American Sociological Review* 61, no. 2 (1996): 179–202; Richard D. Sundeen, Cristina Garcia, and Lili Wang, "Volunteer Behavior among Asian American Groups in the United States," *Journal of Asian American Studies* 10, no. 3 (2007): 3243–3281; John J. Wilson, "Volunteering," *Annual Review of Sociology* 26, no. 1 (2000): 215–240.

9. Henry Brady, Sidney Verba, and Kay L. Schlozman, "Beyond SES: A Resource Model of Political Participation," *American Political Science Review* 89, no. 2 (1995): 269–295; Saul Rosenthal, Candice Feiring, and Michael Lewis, "Political Volunteering from Late Adolescence to Young Adulthood: Patterns and Predictions," *Journal of Social Sciences* 54, no. 4 (1998): 471–493.

10. Elton F. Jackson et al., "Volunteering and Charitable Giving: Do Religious and Associational Ties Promote Helping Behavior?," *Nonprofit Voluntary Sector Quarterly* 24, no. 1 (1995): 59–78; Gerald Marwell and Pamela Oliver, *The Critical Mass in Collective Action* (Cambridge: Cambridge University Press, 1993); McPherson and Rotolo, "Diversity and Change"; David H. Smith, "Determinants of Voluntary Association Participation and Volunteering," *Non-profit Voluntary Sector Quarterly* 23, no. 3 (1994): 243–263; Wilson, "Volunteering"; Nancy Wolff, Burton Weisbrod, and Edward Bird, "The Supply of Volunteer Labor: The Case Of Hospitals," *Nonprofit Management and Leadership* 4, no. 1 (Winter 1993): 23–45.

11. Tong, "Foreign-born Concentration."

12. Tong, "Foreign-born Concentration."

13. Milton Gordon, *Assimilation in American Life* (New York: Oxford University Press, 1964).

14. Penny E. Becker and Pawan H. Dhingra, "Religious Involvement and Volunteering: Implications for Civil Society," *Sociology of Religion* 62, no. 3 (2001): 315–335; Valerie Lewis, Carol Ann MacGregor, and Robert D. Putnam, "Religion, Networks, and Neighborliness: The Impact of Religious Social Networks on Civic Engagement," *Social Science Research* 42, no. 2 (2013): 331–346; Pamela Paxton, Nicholas E. Reith, and Jennifer L. Glanvill, "Volunteering and the Dimensions of Religiosity: A Cross-National Analysis," *Review of Religious Research* 56 (2014): 597–625; Putnam, *Bowling Alone*; Robert Putnam and David Campbell, *American Grace: How Religion Divides and Unites Us* (New York: Simon and Schuster, 2010); Jerry Z. Park and Christian Smith, "To Whom Much Has Been Given . . . Religious Capital and Community Voluntarism among Churchgoing Protestants," *Journal for the Scientific Study of Religion* 39, no. 3 (2000): 272–286.

15. Putnam, *Bowling Alone*.

16. Musick and Wilson, *Volunteers*; Virginia A. Hodgkinson, "The Connection between Philanthropic Behavior Directed to Religious Institutions and Small Religious Nonprofit Organizations" (presentation, Conference on Small Religious Nonprofits: From Vulnerability to Viability, DePaul University, Chicago, IL, October 1995); Wilson and Musick, "Who Cares?."

17. See previous note; also see David E. Campbell and Stephen J. Yonish, "Religion and Volunteering in America," in *Religion and Social Capital*, ed. Corwin E. Schmidt (Waco, TX: Baylor University Press, 2003), 87–106.

18. Campbell and Yonish, "Religion and Volunteering"; Musick and Wilson, *Volunteers*; Putnam, *Bowling Alone*; Wilson and Musick, "Who Cares?"; Robert Wuthnow and Conrad Hackett, "The Social Integration of Practitioners of Non-western Religions in the United States," *Journal for the Scientific Study of Religion* 42, no. 4 (2003): 651–657.

19. See previous note; also see Christopher G. Ellison, "Are Religious People Nice People: Evidence from the National Survey of Black Americans," *Social Forces* 71, no. 2 (1992): 411–430; Robert Wuthnow, "Religion and the Voluntary Spirit in the United States," in *Faith and Philanthropy in America*, eds. Robert Wuthnow, Virginia Hodgkinson, and Associates (San Francisco: Jossey-Bass, 1991), 3–21; Robert Wuthnow, *Acts of Compassion* (Princeton, NJ: Princeton University Press, 1991).

20. Bane, "Catholic Puzzle."

21. Several scholars have proposed that a distinctive Catholic ethic exists that fosters a more communitarian spirit than Protestantism. For these scholars, the Catholic ethic emphasizes communal relationships through what Ferdinand Tonnies defined as more personal or *Gemeinschaft* orientations. See Ferdinand Tonnies, *Community and Society/Gemeinschaft und Gesellschaft* (New Brunswick, NJ: Transaction Publishers, [1887] 1998); Bane, "Catholic Puzzle"; Andrew Greely, *The Catholic Imagination* (Berkeley: University of California Press, 2000); Daniel Rigney, Jerome Matz, and Armando Abney, "Is There a Catholic Sharing Ethic? A Research Note," *Sociology of Religion* 65, no. 2 (2004): 155–165; John Tropman, *The Catholic Ethic in American Society* (San Francisco: Jossey-Bass, 1995); John Tropman, *The Catholic Ethic and the Spirit of Community* (Washington, DC: Georgetown University Press, 2002).

22. Bane, "Catholic Puzzle"; William V. D'Antonio et al., *American Catholics: Gender, Generation, and Commitment* (Walnut Creek, CA: AltaMira Press, 2001); William V. D'Antonio et al., *American Catholics Today: New Realities of Their Faith and Their Church* (Lanham, MD: Rowman & Littlefield, 2007); James D. Davidson and Mark McCormick, "Catholics and Civic Engagement: Empirical Findings at the Individual

Level," in *Civil Society, Civic Engagement and Catholicism in the U.S.*, eds. Antonius Liedhegener and Werner Kremp (Germany: WVT Wissenschaftlicher Verlag Trier, 2007), 119–134; Dean R. Hoge et al., *Young Adult Catholics: Religion in the Culture of Choice* (Notre Dame, IN: University of Notre Dame Press, 2001); Rigney et al., "Catholic Sharing Ethic." Note there is some disagreement over the extent to which Catholic youth are receiving and acting on messages of community service; see further Christian Smith and Melinda L. Denton, *Soul Searching: The Religious and Spiritual Lives of American Teenagers* (New York: Oxford University Press, 2005).

23. David Carlin, *The Decline and Fall of the Catholic Church in America* (Manchester, NH: The Sophia Institute, 2003); Meghan Davis and Antonius Liedhegener, "Catholic Civic Engagement at the Local Level: The Parish and Beyond," in *Civil Society, Civic Engagement and Catholicism in the U.S.*, eds. Antonius Liedhegener and Werner Kremp (Germany: WVT Wissenschaftlicher Verlag Trier, 2007): 135–160; Joseph A. Varacalli, *The Catholic Experience in America* (Westport, CT: Greenwood Press, 2005).

24. Brady et al., "Beyond SES"; Pui-Yan Lam, "As the Flocks Gather: How Religion Affects Voluntary Association Participation," *Journal for the Scientific Study of Religion* 41, no. 3 (2002): 405–422; Pui-Yan Lam, "Religion and Civic Culture: A Cross-National Study of Voluntary Association Membership," *Journal for the Scientific Study of Religion* 45, no. 2 (2006): 177–293; Musick and Wilson, *Volunteers*; Mark Regnerus, Christian Smith, and David Sikkink, "Who Gives to the Poor? The Role of Religious Tradition and Political Location on the Personal Generosity of Americans Toward the Poor," *Journal for the Scientific Study of Religion* 37, no. 3 (1998): 481–493. Also see discussions on Asian American civic life in Stephen M. Cherry, "Engaging the Spirit of the East: Asian American Christians and Civic Life," *Sociological Spectrum* 29, no. 2 (2009): 249–272; Elan H. Ecklund and Jerry Z. Park, "Asian American Community Participation and Religion," *Journal of Asian American Studies* 8, no. 1 (2007): 1–21.

25. This argument builds on a larger theoretical argument I have made in previous research looking specifically at the civic life of first-generation Filipino American Catholics; see Cherry, *Faith, Family.*

26. Tropman, *The Catholic Ethic* (2002).

27. Ninety-eight percent of those I interviewed (N=87) stated that they had volunteered in the community at least once in the last year—answering *yes* or *no*—not including mandatory projects/programs as part of their job at the hospital.

28. "Percentage of Americans Who Give, Volunteer Is Falling, Study Finds," *Philanthropy News Digest*, November 22, 2018, https://philanthropynewsdigest.org/news/percentage-of-americans-who-give-volunteer-is-falling-study-finds.

29. Ninety-four percent of those I interviewed (N=87) stated that they had given money to charitable causes at least once in the last year—answering *yes* or *no.*

30. See, for example, "Fewer Americans Are Giving Money to Charity but Total Donations Are at Record Levels Anyway," *Conversation*, July 3, 2018, http://theconversation.com/fewer-americans-are-giving-money-to-charity-but-total-donations-are-at-record-levels-anyway-98291.

31. See for example, David Nakamura, "Filipinos Who Fought to Aid U.S. in World War II Still Await Green Cards for Grown Children," *Washington Post*, January 3, 2015, https://www.washingtonpost.com/politics/filipinos-who-fought-to-aid-us-in-world-war-ii-still-await-green-cards-for-grown-children/2015/01/03/a370e704-913d-11e4-ba53-a477d66580ed_story.html.

32. The Lady's Ministry is a church group organized to address community needs, headed and organized by the women of the church.
33. Cherry, *Faith, Family*.
34. Cherry, *Faith, Family*.
35. Cherry, *Faith, Family*.
36. See further details on the scandal discussed in chapter 1 and the methodological appendix.
37. See Eric Westervelt, "For VA Whistleblowers, a Culture of Fear and Retaliation, *National Public Radio*, June 21, 2018, https://www.npr.org/2018/06/21/601127245/for-va-whistleblowers-a-culture-of-fear-and-retaliation.
38. This should not be all that surprising given the history of religious activism, especially in Christian communities; see Christian Smith, *Disruptive Religion* (New York: Routledge, 1996).
39. Ninety-eight percent of those I interviewed (N=87) stated that they voted in the last presidential election (2012)—answering *yes* or *no*. The overwhelming majority of those that I interviewed or spoke with in follow-up discussions after November 2016 stated that they voted in the subsequent election as well.
40. Thom File, "Voting in America: A Look at the 2016 Presidential Election," *U.S. Census*, May 10, 2017, https://www.census.gov/newsroom/blogs/random-samplings/2017/05/voting_in_america.html.
41. See Karthick Ramakrishnan, "The Asian American Vote in 2016: Record Gains, but Also Gaps," *Asian American and Pacific Islanders Data Bits*, May 19, 2017, http://aapidata.com/blog/voting-gains-gaps/.
42. It is important to note that these findings are complicated by both the overwhelmingly high religiosity of the survey sample and the frequency of their civic engagement. Given the overwhelmingly high church attendance of both populations of nurses, at rates that far exceed those of average American Catholics, the impact of their religiosity was diminished statistically. There was simply very little variance. Likewise, when roughly 90 percent of your sample states that they volunteered and gave to charitable causes at least once in the last year, the same issues arise. However, the findings presented in figure 6.3 are for the most part statistically significant.
43. Ecklund and Park, "Asian American Community Participation"; Elaine H. Ecklund and Jerry Z. Park, "Religious Diversity and Community Volunteerism among Asian Americans," *Journal for the Scientific Study of Religion* 46, no. 2 (2007): 233–244.
44. See Sydney K. Verba, Kay Lahmen Schlozman, and Henry Brady, *Voice and Equality* (Cambridge, MA: Harvard University Press, 1995).
45. Ecklund and Park, "Asian American Community Participation"; Ecklund and Park, "Religious Diversity."
46. Putnam, *Bowling Alone*. Also see, Karin Aguilar-San Juan, ed., *The State of Asian America: Activism and Resistance in the 1990s* (Boston, MA: South End Press, 1994); Joaquin L. Gonzalez III and Andrea Maison, "We Do Not Bowl Alone: Social and Cultural Capital from Filipinos and Their Church," in *Asian American Religions: The Making and Remaking of Borders and Boundaries*, eds. Tony Carnes and Fenggang Yang (New York: New York University Press, 2004): 21–38.
47. See previous note.
48. See for example Pamela Gehrke, "Civic Engagement and Nursing Education," *Advances in Nursing Science* 31, no. 1 (January–March 2008): 52–66; Musick and Wilson, *Volunteers*; Carrie Rewakowski, Maria MacPherson, and Helen Clancy,

"Advocacy: Civic Engagement among Nurses" (presentation, 45th Biennial Convention of Sigma Theta Tau International, Washington, DC, November 17, 2019); Robert Wood Johnson Foundation, *From Action To Vision: Measures to Mobilize a Culture of Health* (Princeton, NJ: Robert Wood Johnson Foundation, 2015), https:// www.rwjf.org/content/dam/files/rwjf-web-files/Research/2015/From_Vision_to _Action_RWJF2015.pdf; Staff, "How Nurses Can Promote Civic Engagement," *Nurse Journal*, September 30, 2021, https://nursejournal.org/community/how-nurses-can -promote-civic-engagement/.

7. Who Will Care for America?

1. See, for example, Steve Cohen, "The Real VA Scandal: No Will to Help Veterans," *Hill*, February 20, 2018, https://thehill.com/opinion/healthcare/374542-the-real-va-scandal -no-will-to-help-veterans; Debra A. Draper, "Veterans Health Care, Opportunities Remain to Improve Appointment Scheduling within VA and through Community Care," *Washington, DC: United States Government Accountability Office, Testimony Before the Committee on Veterans' Affairs, House of Representatives*, GAO-19-687T (July 24, 2019), https://www.gao.gov/assets/710/700574.pdf; Joe Davidson, "Four Years after Scandal, VA Gets Praise for Health Care But Falls Short on Access," *Washington Post*, November 13, 2018, https://www.washingtonpost.com/politics/2018/11/13/four-years -after-scandal-va-gets-praise-health-care-falls-short-access/#comments-wrapper; Larry M. Reinkemeyer, *Unwarranted Medical Reexaminations for Disability Benefits*, report #17-04966-201 (Washington, DC: Department of Veterans Affairs, Office of the Inspector General, Office of Audits and Evaluations, July 17, 2018), https://www .va.gov/oig/pubs/VAOIG-17-04966-201.pdf; Donovan Slack, "Thousands of Medical Tests Delayed, Improperly Canceled at VA Facilities, Audit Finds," *USA Today*, December 11, 2019, https://www.usatoday.com/story/news/nation/2019/12/11/thousands -veteran-medical-tests-delayed-improperly-canceled-va/4387520002/.

2. Joe Davidson, "VA Struggles to Fill Hospital Jobs and 49,000 Openings across the Country," *Washington Post*, November 5, 2019, https://www.washingtonpost.com /politics/va-struggles-to-fill-hospital-jobs-it-has-49000-openings-across-the-country /2019/11/05/91fbd4fe-ff4f-11e9-9777-5cd51c6fec6f_story.html+&cd=1&hl=en&ct =clnk&gl=us.

3. See GAO data presented in Stephen Spotswood, "VA Facing Critical Healthcare Staffing Shortages in Near Future," *U.S. Medicine*, October 22, 2019, https://www .usmedicine.com/agencies/department-of-veterans-affairs/va-facing-critical -healthcare-staffing-shortages-in-near-future/.

4. See "Community Care," U.S. Department of Veterans Affairs, last updated February 2, 2021, https://www.va.gov/COMMUNITYCARE/programs/veterans/VCP/index.asp.

5. Ben Kesling, "VA Issues New Rules Expanding Access to Private Care; Move Is Seen Costing Billions and Igniting Debate over Effect on Veteran's Public Services," *Wall Street Journal*, January 31, 2019, https://www.wsj.com/articles/va-will-issue-new -rules-expanding-access-to-private-care-11548866605.

6. Suzanne Gordon and Jasper Craven, "The Trump Administration is Sabotaging Veterans' Access to Health Care," *Washington Monthly*, September 13, 2019, https:// washingtonmonthly.com/2019/09/13/the-trump-administration-is-sabotaging -veterans-access-to-health-care/; Also see Editorial Staff, "Veterans Are Freer to Choose; Look Who's Objecting to Faster Access to Private Health Care," *Wall Street Journal*, February 6, 2019, https://www.wsj.com/articles/veterans-are-freer-to-choose -11549411413?mod=searchresults&page=1&pos=2.

7. See "Projections of Occupational Employment, 2016–2026," Bureau of Labor Statistics, October 2017, https://www.bls.gov/careeroutlook/2017/article/occupational-projections-charts.htm; Peter I. Buerhaus et al., "Four Challenges Facing the Nursing Workforce in the United States," *Journal of Nursing Regulation* 8, no. 2 (July 2017): 40–46. It is also important to note that as of 2018, over 50 percent of the nursing workforce is age fifty or older; see Richard A. Smiley et al., "The 2017 National Nursing Workforce Survey," *Journal of Nursing Regulation* 9, no. 3 (October 2018): s1–s88.

8. David I. Auerbach, Peter I. Buerhaus, and Douglas O. Staiger, "Will the RN Workforce Weather the Retirement of the Baby Boomers?," *Medical Care* 53, vol. 10 (2015): 850–856.

9. See breakdown by state at "The Places with the Largest Nursing Shortages," *Registered Nursing*, September 24, 2021, https://www.registerednursing.org/largest-nursing-shortages/.

10. See, for example, Peter Buerhaus, "What Is the Harm in Imposing Mandatory Hospital Nurse Staffing Regulations?," *Nursing Economics* 15, no. 2 (1997): 66–72; Heather L. Tubbs-Cooley et al., "An Observational Study of Nurse Staffing Ratios and Hospital Readmission among Children Admitted for Common Conditions," *BMJ Quality & Safety* 22 (2013): 735–742; Jack Needleman et al., "Nurse Staffing and Inpatient Hospital Mortality," *New England Journal of Medicine* 364, no. 11 (2011): 1037–1045.

11. Top officials have suggested that if the VA runs out of doctors, it should turn to nurses to treat veterans; see Lisa Rein, "Top VA Doc: If There Aren't Enough Doctors, Have Nurses Treat Our Vets," *Washington Post*, June 2, 2016, https://www.washingtonpost.com/news/powerpost/wp/2016/06/02/top-va-doc-if-there-arent-enough-doctors-have-nurses-treat-our-vets/.

12. President Trump eliminated all funding to Title VIII Nursing Workforce Development Programs with the exception of the NURSE Corps; see American Association of College of Nursing, "AACN Opposes President's Budget Cuts to Nursing Workforce, Education, and Research," press release, February 10, 2020, AACN Opposes President's Budget Cuts to Nursing Workforce, Education, and Research, https://www.aacnnursing.org/News-Information/Press-Releases/View/ArticleId/24568/Oppose-FY21-President-Budget; statement from the American Healthcare Association, accessed August 2020, https://www.ahcancal.org/advocacy/solutions/Pages/ImmigrationReform.aspx; Portia Wofford, "Nursing Shortage: Foreign Nurses Provide Aid to U.S. Hospitals," *Nurse.org*, August 1, 2019, https://nurse.org/articles/foreign-nurses-help-us-nursing-shortage/.

13. See Ed Yong, "Why Health-Care Workers Are Quitting in Droves," *Atlantic*, November 18, 2021, https://www.theatlantic.com/health/archive/2021/11/the-mass-exodus-of-americas-health-care-workers/620713/

14. Yong, "Why Health-Care Workers Are Quitting in Droves."

15. The emergency stimulus acts passed by Congress in response to COVID-19 do not address these larger immigration/staffing concerns. See further, Nicole Narea, "A Rare Bipartisan Agreement on Immigration Reform Has Tanked in the Senate," *Vox*, September 19, 2019, https://www.vox.com/policy-and-politics/2019/9/19/20873985/bipartisan-immigration-green-card-bill-senate.

16. See Fairness for High-Skilled Immigrants Act of 2020, H.R. 1044, 116th Congress (2019–2020), https://www.congress.gov/bill/116th-congress/house-bill/1044/text.

17. Narea, "Rare Bipartisan Agreement."

18. Narea, "Rare Bipartisan Agreement."

19. See, for example, Dartunorro Clark, "Trump Says Hire American. These Businesses Say They Can't—and Foreign Labor Limits Are Killing Them," *NBC*, August 6, 2018,

https://www.nbcnews.com/politics/white-house/trump-says-hire-american-these-businesses-say-they-can-t-n896766; Camilo Montoyo-Galvez, "Republicans Will Buck Trump on Immigration if 'They Feel the Heat,' Schumer Says," *CBS*, March 13, 2019, https://www.cbsnews.com/news/republicans-will-buck-trump-on-immigration-if-they-feel-the-heat-schumer-says/.

20. Research continues to suggest that immigrant nurses do not have negative long-term impacts on American wages and native employment. See for example Hyeran Chung and Mary Arends-Kuenning, "Do Foreign-Educated Nurses Displace Native-Educated Nurses?," *IZA Journal of Labor Policy* 10, no. 14 (2020): 1–28; Edward J. Schumacher, "Foreign-Born Nurses in the US Labor Market," *Health Economics* 20, no. 3 (2011): 362–378.

21. See Jeanne Batalova, Michael Fix, and Jose Ramon Fernandez-Pena, *The Integration of Immigrant Health Professionals: Looking Beyond the COVID-19 Crisis* (Washington, DC: Migration Policy Institute, April 2021), https://www.migrationpolicy.org/sites/default/files/publications/mpi-immigrant-health-workers-beyond-pandemic_final.pdf.

22. See Jens Manuel Krogstad, "Reflecting a Demographic Shift, 109 U.S. Counties Have Become Majority Nonwhite since 2000," *Pew Research Center*, August 21, 2019, https://www.pewresearch.org/fact-tank/2019/08/21/u-s-counties-majority-nonwhite/.

23. White births in the United States are now outnumbered by white deaths in twenty-six states; see Ezra Klein, "White Threat in a Browning America, How Demographic Change Is Fracturing Our Politics," *Vox*, July 30, 2018, https://www.vox.com/policy-and-politics/2018/7/30/17505406/trump-obama-race-politics-immigration.

24. The country's growing racial and ethnic diversity is increasingly driven by the birth rates of foreign-born individuals and overall population death patterns. Americans, especially its recent immigrants, have more children on average than people in most other so-called advanced nations. The growing percentage of individuals identifying with two or more racial/ethnic groups also has a tremendous impact on these demographic patterns. See Leslie Aun, "What the 2020 U.S. Census Will Tell Us About a Changing America," *Population Reference Bureau*, June 12, 2019, https://www.prb.org/what-the-2020-u-s-census-will-tell-us-about-a-changing-america/; Klein, "White Threat"; Mark Mather, *America's Changing Population, What to Expect in the 2020 Census: Population Bulletin* 74, no. 1 (Washington, DC: Population Reference Bureau, June 2019), https://www.prb.org/wp-content/uploads/2019/06/PRB-PopBulletin-2020-Census.pdf; Kim Parker, Rich Morin, and Juliana Horowitz, "Looking to the Future, Public Sees an America in Decline on Many Fronts," *Pew Research Center*, March 21, 2019, https://www.pewresearch.org/social-trends/2019/03/21/public-sees-an-america-in-decline-on-many-fronts/.

25. See Klein, "White Threat"; Erika Lee, *America for Americans: A History of Xenophobia in the United States* (New York: Basic Books, 2019).

26. United States Census Bureau, *Overview of Race and Hispanic Origin: 2010* (Washington DC: Bureau of the Census, 2010).

27. Gustavo Lopez, Neil G. Ruiz, and Eileen Patten, "Key Facts about Asian Americans, a Diverse and Growing Population," *Pew Research Center*, September 8, 2017, https://www.pewresearch.org/fact-tank/2017/09/08/key-facts-about-asian-americans/; "The Rise of Asian Americans," Pew Research Center, last updated April 4, 2013, https://www.pewsocialtrends.org/2012/06/19/the-rise-of-asian-americans/.

28. See previous note.

29. See Gustavo Lopez et al., "Key Facts about Asian Americans." As of 2015, 24 percent of Asian Americans (4.9 million) were of Chinese origin, followed by Indian-origin Asians, who accounted for 20 percent of the national Asian population (4.0 million), and Filipinos, who accounted for 19 percent of the national Asian population (3.9 million).

30. Edward J. Schumacher, for example, finds no impact on wages; see Schumacher, "Foreign-Born Nurses." Also see mixed/inconclusive results in Robert Kaestner and Neeraj Kaushal, "Effect of Immigrant Nurses on Labor Market Outcomes of US Nurses," *Journal of Urban Economics* 71, no. 2 (March 2012): 219–229.

31. See discussion in chapter 1.

32. Maureen Newman and Jane Williams, "Educating Nurses in Rhode Island: A Lot of Diversity in a Little Place," *Journal of Cultural Diversity* 10, no. 3 (2003): 91–95.

33. Amanda Barroso, "The Changing Profile of the U.S. Military: Smaller in Size, More Diverse, More Women in Leadership," *Pew Research Center,* September 10, 2019, https://www.pewresearch.org/fact-tank/2019/09/10/the-changing-profile-of-the-u-s-military/.

34. Barroso, "Changing Profile."

35. For legal discussions on the importance of providing diverse care for diverse patients see arguments made in the school admission case of Abigail Noel Fisher v. the University of Texas at Austin et al; Brief for Amici Curiae Association of American Medical Colleges et al. in Support of Respondents, Abigail Noel Fisher v. the University of Texas at Austin et al., 570 U.S. 297 (5th Cir 2013), https://www.aamc.org/system/files/c/1/447744-aamcfilesamicusbriefinfishervutaustin.pdf.

36. Mark Doescher, "Racial and Ethnic Disparities in Perceptions of Physician Style and Trust," *Archives of Family Medicine* 9, no. 10 (2009): 1156–1163; L. Ebony Boulware et al., "Race and Trust in the Health Care System," *Public Health Reports* 118, no. 4 (2003): 358–365.

37. See, for example, Megha Amrith, *Caring for Strangers: Filipino Medical Workers in Asia* (Copenhagen, Denmark: NIS Press, 2016); Patricia Cortés and Jessica Pan, "The Relative Quality of Foreign-Educated Nurses in the United States," *Journal of Human Resources* 50, no. 4 (2015): 1009–1050; Ergie Pepito Inocian et al., "Cultural Competency among Expatriate Nurses in Saudi Arabia," *International Journal of Nursing* 4, no. 1 (2015): 58–65.

38. See U.S. census data presented in Karen Zeigler and Steven A. Camarota, "Almost Half Speak a Foreign Language in America's Largest Cities," *Center for Immigration Studies,* September 19, 2018, https://cis.org/Report/Almost-Half-Speak-Foreign-Language-Americas-Largest-Cities.

39. Ziegler and Camarota, "Almost Half."

40. Ziegler and Camarota, "Almost Half."

41. Ziegler and Camarota, "Almost Half."

42. Michael O. Emerson, "Houston Region Grows More Racially/Ethnically Diverse, with Small Declines in Segregation," Kinder Institute for Urban Research, 2012, https://kinder.rice.edu/sites/g/files/bxs1676/f/documents/Houston%20Region%20Grows%20More%20Ethnically%20Diverse%204-9.pdf; Randy Capps, Michael Fix, and Chiamaka Nwosu, *A Profile of Immigrants in Houston, the Nation's Most Diverse Metropolitan Area* (Washington, DC: Migration Policy Institute, March 2015), https://www.migrationpolicy.org/research/profile-immigrants-houston-nations-most-diverse-metropolitan-area.

43. Newman and Williams, "Educating Nurses."

44. Parker, Morin, and Horowitz, "Looking to the Future"; United States Census Bureau, "An Aging Nation: Projected Number of Children and Older Adults," United States Census Bureau, March 13, 2018, https://www.census.gov/library/visualizations/2018/comm/historic-first.html.

45. See, for example, Maricar C. P. Hampton, "Filipino Health Workers Struggle in Filling Eldercare Gap," *New America Media/Philippine News*, September 16, 2010, http://haunurses.blogspot.com/2010/07/filipino-health-workers-struggle-in.html.

46. Caitlin Yoshiko Kandil, "For Filipino American Nurses on COVID-19 Front Lines, Faith Is Stronger than Fear," *Angelus News*, July 16, 2020, https://angelusnews.com/local/la-catholics/for-filipino-american-nurses-treating-local-covid-19-patients-faith-is-stronger-than-fear/.

47. It is estimated that during this time the number of foreign-born immigrants rose to 3.5million in 1890 to well over nine million by 1910, with the overwhelming majority being Catholic. See James D. Davidson, *Catholicism in Motion: The Church in American Society* (Ligouri, MO: Ligouri and Triumph, 2005); Roger Finke and Rodney Stark, *The Churching of America, 1776–1990* (New Brunswick, NJ: Rutgers University Press, 1992); Andrew M. Greely, *American Catholic: A Social Portrait* (New York: Basic Books, 1977).

48. Two of the largest American immigrant communities are Mexicans (25 percent of all immigrants) and Filipinos (4.5 percent of all immigrants). Both Mexico and the Philippines are predominately Catholic countries and represent the two largest sources of Catholic immigration to the United States today. See Guillermina Jasso et al., "Exploring Religious Preferences of Recent Immigrant to the United States: Evidence from the New Immigrant Survey Pilot," in *Religion and Immigration: Christian, Jewish, and Muslim Experiences in the United States*, eds. Yvonne Yazbeck Haddad, Jane I. Smith, and John L. Esposito (Lanham, MD: AltaMira Press, 2003), 217–253; "Largest U.S. Immigrant Groups over Time, 1960–Present," Migration Policy Institute, 2018, accessed August 2020, https://www.migrationpolicy.org/programs/data-hub/charts/largest-immigrant-groups-over-time.

49. See previous note.

50. Jay P. Dolan, *In Search of American Catholicism: A History of Religion and Culture in Tension* (New York: Oxford University Press, 2003).

51. Russell Jeung, Manjusha P. Kulkarni, and Cynthia Choi, "Op-Ed: Trump's Racist Comments Are Fueling Hate Crimes against Asian Americans. Time for State Leaders to Step In," *LA Times*, April 3, 2020, https://www.latimes.com/opinion/story/2020-04-01/coronavirus-anti-asian-discrimination-threats. Also see Russell Jeung et al., *Stop AAPI Hate National Report*, 3/19/20–2/28/21 (San Francisco: Stop AAPI Hate, 2021), https://secureservercdn.net/104.238.69.231/a1w.90d.myftpupload.com/wp-content/uploads/2021/03/210312-Stop-AAPI-Hate-National-Report-.pdf.

52. Jeung et al., "*Stop AAPI Hate National Report*." Also see Craig Timberg and Allyson Chiu, "As the Coronavirus Spreads, So Does Online Racism Targeting Asians, New Research Shows," *Washington Post*, April 8, 2020, https://www.washingtonpost.com/technology/2020/04/08/coronavirus-spreads-so-does-online-racism-targeting-asians-new-research-shows/.

53. Roughly 39 percent of American adults say it is more common for people to express racist or racially insensitive views about people who are Asian after the coronavirus outbreak than it was before. See Neil G. Ruiz, Juliana Menasce Howowitz, and

Christine Tamir, "Many Black and Asian Americans Say They Have Experienced Discrimination amid the COVID-19 Outbreak," *Pew Research Center*, July 1, 2020, https://www.pewresearch.org/social-trends/2020/07/01/many-black-and-asian-americans-say-they-have-experienced-discrimination-amid-the-covid-19-outbreak/. Also see Kimmy Yam, "Anti-Asian Hate Crimes Increased by Nearly 150% in 2020, Mostly in N.Y. and L.A., New Report Says," *NBC News*, March 9, 2021, https://www.nbcnews.com/news/asian-america/anti-asian-hate-crimes-increased-nearly-150-2020-mostly-n-n1260264; "Fact Sheet," Center for the Study of Hate & Extremisms CSUSB, accessed March 2021, https://www.csusb.edu/sites/default/files/FACT%20SHEET-%20Anti-Asian%20Hate%202020%203.2.21.pdf.

54. Alexandra Kelley, "Attacks on Asian Americans Skyrocket to Over 100 per Day during Coronavirus Pandemic," *Hill*, March 31, 2020, https://thehill.com/changing-america/respect/equality/490373-attacks-on-asian-americans-at-about-100-per-day-due-to.

55. Bob D'Angelo, "Coronavirus: Indiana Gas Station Owner Apologizes after Clerk Kicks Out Doctor for Being Asian," *WFTV News*, April 1, 2020, https://www.wftv.com/news/trending/coronavirus-indiana-gas-station-owner-apologizes-after-clerk-kicks-out-doctor-being-asian/TNT2MVQEFZGZTI2QZWT6Q5RRZE/.

56. See Kirk Semple, "Afraid to Be a Nurse: Health Workers under Attack," *New York Times*, April 27, 2020, https://www.nytimes.com/2020/04/27/world/americas/coronavirus-health-workers-attacked.html; Ricky Manalo, "When the Racist Response to Covid-19 Hits Home," *American Jesuit Review*, March 30, 2020, https://www.americamagazine.org/faith/2020/03/30/when-racist-response-covid-19-hits-home.

57. Lee, *America for Americans*, 7.

58. Tucker Doherty, "Biden Urged to Change Immigration Policy to Send More Health Workers to Covid Hot Spots," *Politico*, December 3, 2020, https://www.politico.com/news/2020/12/03/biden-immigration-policy-health-workers-442411; Laura Romero, "Hospitals Say Staffing Shortages Creating 'Dire Need' for Foreign Nurses: Demand Is High but Immigration Limitations Are Slowing the Process," *ABC News*, December 15, 2020, https://abcnews.go.com/US/hospitals-staffing-shortages-creating-dire-foreign-nurses/story?id=74736237.

59. Ryan Abello, "Philippines Brain Drain: Health Professionals Leaving for Greener Pastures Filipinos Seeking Employment Overseas," *VIA News*, August 24, 2018, https://via.news/asia/philippines-brain-drain-health-professionals-leaving/; Michael Hawkes et al., "Nursing Brain Drain from India," *Human Resources for Health* 7, no. 5 (2009), https://human-resources-health.biomedcentral.com/track/pdf/10.1186/1478-4491-7-5.pdf; C. R. Hooper, "Adding Insult to Injury: The Healthcare Brain Drain," *Journal of Medical Ethics* 34, no. 9 (2008): 684–687.

Methodological Appendix

1. Michael O. Emerson et al., "Houston Region Grows More Racially/Ethnically Diverse, with Small Declines in Segregation," 2012, https://kinder.rice.edu/sites/default/files/documents/Houston%20Region%20Grows%20More%20Ethnically%20Diverse%204-9.pdf; Randy Capps, Michael Fix, and Chiamaka Nwosu, *A Profile of Immigrants in Houston, the Nation's Most Diverse Metropolitan Area* (Washington, DC: Migration Policy Institute, March 2015), https://www.migrationpolicy.org/research/profile-immigrants-houston-nations-most-diverse-metropolitan-area.

2. See "About TMC," Texas Medical Center, 2016, accessed August 2017, https://www.tmc.edu/about-tmc/; also "TMC Facts and Figures," Texas Medical Center, accessed

December 2016, https://www.tmc.edu/wp-content/uploads/2016/08/TMC_Facts
FiguresOnePager_0307162.pdf.

3. Some hospitals in the TMC, such as M.D. Anderson hospital have personnel departments to aid foreign-born employees with their statuses and any related employment
or tax paperwork. The Michael E. DeBakey VA Medical Center, a federal institution,
does not have such a department and does not keep records of nativity, given that all
employees must be U.S. citizens. However, analysis of nine TMC academic institutions suggest that in 2012 there were roughly 4,936 foreign-born students enrolled in
the TMC, with an additional 133 exchange students and 1,692 exchange visitors as
professors, researchers, and short-term scholars and specialists from twelve different
countries; see information on TMC international students, exchange visitors, and
employees from at "TMC at a Glance," Texas Medical Center, accessed January 2014,
https://www.tmc.edu/about-tmc/.

4. Emerson et al., "Houston Region Grows"; Kristen McCabe, *Foreign-born Health Care
Workers in the United States* (Washington, DC: Migration Policy Institute, 2012):
http://www.migrationpolicy.org/article/foreign-born-health-care-workers-united
-states; Mary Schiflett, "The Second Downtown," *Houston Review of History and
Culture* 2, no. 1 (2004): 2–7; Allison Squires and Hiram Beltrán-Sánchez, *Strengthening Health Systems in North and Central America: What Role for Migration?* (Washington, DC: Migration Policy Institute, February 2013), https://www.migrationpolicy
.org/research/strengthening-health-systems-north-and-central-america-what-role
-migration?pdf=RMSG-HealthCare.pdf; Amani Siyam and Mario Roberto dal Poz, eds.,
Migration of Health Workers: WHO Code of Practice and the Global Economic Crisis
(Washington, DC: Migration Policy Institute, May 2014), https://www.migrationpolicy
.org/research/migration-health-workers-who-code-practice-and-global-economic
-crisis; "TMC Facts and Figures," Texas Medical Center.

5. John Harrington, "There Are 18.2 Million Veterans in the US. Which State Is Home
to the Most of Them?," *USA Today*, July 4, 2019, https://www.usatoday.com/story
/money/2019/07/04/states-with-the-most-veterans-new-york-alaska/39645251/;
Alanna Moriarty, "50 Largest Veterans Hospitals by Numbers of Staffed Beds,"
Definitive Healthcare (blog), September 30, 2020, https://blog.definitivehc.com
/largest-veterans-hospitals.

6. See Homer S. Black and Glenn R. Cunningham, *A Brief History of the Houston Veterans Hospital and Its Research Program, 1949–2003* (Washington, DC: U.S. Department of Veterans Affairs, 2005), https://www.homersblack.com/VA%20History%20
Pamphlet.html.

7. Black and Cunningham, *Brief History.*

8. Black and Cunningham, *Brief History.*

9. Black and Cunningham, *Brief History.*

10. Black and Cunningham, *Brief History.*

11. See WOC details, https://www.va.gov/houston-health-care/research-and-development
-rd/research-resources/, accessed December 2014.

12. Wendy Cadge, *Paging God: Religion in the Halls of Medicine* (Chicago: University of
Chicago Press, 2012). Also see, Wendy Cadge and Mary Ellen Konieczny, "Hidden in
Plain Sight: The Significance of Religion and Spirituality in Secular Organizations,"
Sociology of Religion 75, no. 4 (2014): 551–563.

13. See chapter 2 in Charles Bosk, *All God's Mistake: Genetic Counseling in a Pediatric
Hospital* (Chicago: University of Chicago Press, 1992).

14. See "Biomedical Research and Assurance Information Network," *BRAIN*, accessed August 2017, https://brain.bcm.edu/Login.aspx?ReturnUrl=%2fbrainlogin.asp.

15. See discussion in Catherine Ceniza Choy, *Empire of Care: Nursing and Migration in Filipino American History* (Durham, NC: Duke University Press, 2003).

16. Sandra Acker "In/Out/Side: Positioning the Research in Feminist Qualitative Research," *Resources for Feminist Research* 28, no. 1–2 (2000): 189. Also see Sonya Corbin Dwyer and Jennifer L. Buckle, "The Space Between: Being an Insider-Outsider in Qualitative Research," *International Journal of Qualitative Methods* 8, no. 1 (2009): 45–63.

17. See, for example, McCabe, *Foreign-born Health Care Workers*; Joanne Spetz et al., "Internationally Educated Nurses in the United States: Their Origins and Roles," *Nursing Outlook* 62, no. 1 (2014): 8–15; Squires and Beltrán-Sánchez, *Strengthening Health Systems*.

18. See previous note.

19. McCabe, *Foreign-born Health Care Workers*.

20. McCabe, *Foreign-born Health Care Workers*.

21. McCabe, *Foreign-born Health Care Workers*.

22. McCabe, *Foreign-born Health Care Workers*.

23. See Pew Research Center, "Asian Americans: A Mosaic of Faith," *Pew Research Center: Social and Demographic Trends*, July 19, 2012, https://www.pewforum.org/2012/07/19/asian-americans-a-mosaic-of-faiths-overview/; Michael Lipka, "5 Facts about Catholicism in the Philippines," *Fact Tank: News in the Numbers*, January 9, 2015, https://www.pewresearch.org/fact-tank/2015/01/09/5-facts-about-catholicism-in-the-philippines/.

24. Pew Research Center, "Asian Americans." Also see data and history cited in chapter 2 of this book.

25. On the value/importance of life histories in conducting sociological research with religious people and engaging their spiritual lives, see Karen McCarthy Brown, *Mama Lola: A Vodou Priestess in Brooklyn* (Berkeley: University of California Press, 2001). Also see review of other studies using this approach in James V. Spickard, "Micro Qualitative Approaches to the Sociology of Religion: Phenomenologies, Interviews, Narratives, and Ethnographies" in *The Sage Handbook of the Sociology of Religion*, eds. James A. Beckford and Jay Demerath (Thousand Oaks, CA: Sage, 2007), 121–143.

26. For more on the hermeneutic approach(es) to conducting interviews, see Jurgen Habermas, *Knowledge and Human Interests*, trans. J. J. Shapiro (Boston: Beacon Press, 1971), and a general review in Andres Wernet, "Hermeneutics and Objectives Hermeneutics," in *The Sage Handbook of Qualitative Data Analysis*, ed. Uwe Flick (Thousand Oaks, CA: Sage, 2014), 234–246. This methodological approach is widely used in the sociology of religion. For methodological approaches similar to my current study, see the work of Robert Wuthnow on American religious life such as *Meaning and Moral Order* (Berkeley: University of California Press, 1987) and *Sharing the Journey: Support Groups and America's New Quest for Community* (New York: Free Press, 1994) or Christian Smith and Melinda L. Denton, *Soul Searching: The Religious and Spiritual Lives of American Teenagers* (New York: Oxford University Press, 2005). Also see review of other studies using this approach in Spickard, "Micro Qualitative Approaches."

27. Clifford Geertz, *The Interpretation of Cultures: Select Essays* (New York: Basic Books, 1973); Habermas, *Knowledge and Human Interests*; Natasha S. Mauthner and

Andrea Doucet, "Reflexive Accounts and Accounts of Reflexivity in Qualitative Data Analysis," *Sociology* 37, no. 3 (2003): 413–431. See review of similar approaches in Rosaline S. Barbour, "Analysis of Focus Groups," in *The Sage Handbook of Qualitative Data Analysis*, ed. Uwe Flick (Thousand Oaks, CA: Sage, 2014), 313–326; Susan E. Kelly, "Qualitative Interviewing Techniques and Styles," *The Sage Handbook of Qualitative Methods in Health Research*, eds. Ivy Bourgeault, Robert Dingwall, and Ray de Vries (Thousand Oaks, CA: Sage, 2010), 307–326; Katheryn Roulston, "Analysing Interviews," in *The Sage Handbook of Qualitative Data Analysis*, ed. Uwe Flick (Thousand Oaks, CA: Sage, 2014), 297–312. Also see review of other sociology of religion studies using this approach in Spickard, "Micro Qualitative Approaches."

28. See review of this approach in Margrit Schreier, "Qualitative Content Analysis," in *The Sage Handbook of Qualitative Data Analysis*, ed. Uwe Flick (Thousand Oaks, CA: Sage, 2014), 170–183. Also see specific approaches to the sociology of religion in work such as Lynn Davidman, *Tradition in a Rootless World: Women Turn to Orthodox Judaism* (Berkeley: University of California Press, 1993)."

29. See a review to this approach in Dorothy Pawluch and Elena Neiterman, "What is Grounded Theory and Where Does It Come From," in *The Sage Handbook of Qualitative Methods in Health Research*, eds. Ivy Bourgeault, Robert Dingwall, and Ray de Vries (Thousand Oaks, CA: Sage, 2010), 174–192, and Robert Thornberg and Kathy Charmaz, "Grounded Theory and Theoretical Coding," in *The Sage Handbook of Qualitative Data Analysis*, ed. Uwe Flick (Thousand Oaks, CA: Sage, 2014), 153–169.

30. On general parameters and debates about response rates, see Richard Curtin, Stanley Presser, and Eleanor Singer, "The Effects of Response Rate Changes on the Index of Consumer Sentiment," *Public Opinion Quarterly* 64, no. 4 (2000): 413–428.

31. See, for example, McCabe, *Foreign-born Health Care Workers*; Spetz et al., "Internationally Educated Nurses"; Squires and Beltrán-Sánchez, *Strengthening Health Systems*.

32. In Texas the veteran population is less White (60 percent are White) but otherwise matches this national profile. For a further comparison of Texas veterans to national demographics, see Texas Workforce Investment Council, "Veterans in Texas: A Demographic Study," *Office of the Texas Governor*, June 2019, https://gov.texas.gov/uploads /files/organization/twic/Veterans-in-Texas-2019.pdf. Also see Jesse Bennett, "Veteran Households in U.S. Are Economically Better Off than Those of Non-Veterans," *Pew Research Center*, December 9, 2019, https://www.pewresearch.org/fact-tank/2019 /12/09/veteran-households-in-u-s-are-economically-better-off-than-those-of-non -veterans/#:~:text=In%202017%2C%20the%20median%20annual,difference%20 of%20more%20than%20%2412%2C000.

33. See previous note.

34. See study by Emily Ignacio, *Building Diaspora: Filipino Cultural Community Formation on the Internet* (New Brunswick, NJ: Rutgers University Press, 2005) for details on the importance of studying immigrant communities online.

Index

About the Author

STEPHEN M. CHERRY is an associate professor of sociology at the University of Houston–Clear Lake. He is the author of *Faith, Family, and Filipino American Community Life* (Rutgers University Press, 2014) and the coeditor of *Global Religious Movements Across Borders: Sacred Service*.

Available titles in the Critical Issues in Health and Medicine series:

Rachel Grob, *Testing Baby: The Transformation of Newborn Screening, Parenting, and Policymaking*

Mark A. Hall and Sara Rosenbaum, eds., *The Health Care "Safety Net" in a Post-Reform World*

Laura L. Heinemann, *Transplanting Care: Shifting Commitments in Health and Care in the United States*

Rebecca J. Hester, *Embodied Politics: Indigenous Migrant Activism, Cultural Competency, and Health Promotion in California*

Laura D. Hirshbein, *American Melancholy: Constructions of Depression in the Twentieth Century*

Laura D. Hirshbein, *Smoking Privileges: Psychiatry, the Mentally Ill, and the Tobacco Industry in America*

Timothy Hoff, *Practice under Pressure: Primary Care Physicians and Their Medicine in the Twenty-first Century*

Beatrix Hoffman, Nancy Tomes, Rachel N. Grob, and Mark Schlesinger, eds., *Patients as Policy Actors*

Ruth Horowitz, *Deciding the Public Interest: Medical Licensing and Discipline*

Powel Kazanjian, *Frederick Novy and the Development of Bacteriology in American Medicine*

Claas Kirchhelle, *Pyrrhic Progress: The History of Antibiotics in Anglo-American Food Production*

Rebecca M. Kluchin, *Fit to Be Tied: Sterilization and Reproductive Rights in America, 1950–1980*

Jennifer Lisa Koslow, *Cultivating Health: Los Angeles Women and Public Health Reform*

Jennifer Lisa Koslow, *Exhibiting Health: Public Health Displays in the Progressive Era*

Susan C. Lawrence, *Privacy and the Past: Research, Law, Archives, Ethics*

Bonnie Lefkowitz, *Community Health Centers: A Movement and the People Who Made It Happen*

Ellen Leopold, *Under the Radar: Cancer and the Cold War*

Barbara L. Ley, *From Pink to Green: Disease Prevention and the Environmental Breast Cancer Movement*

Sonja Mackenzie, *Structural Intimacies: Sexual Stories in the Black AIDS Epidemic*

Stephen E. Mawdsley, *Selling Science: Polio and the Promise of Gamma Globulin*

Frank M. McClellan, *Healthcare and Human Dignity: Law Matters*

Michelle McClellan, *Lady Lushes: Gender, Alcohol, and Medicine in Modern America*

David Mechanic, *The Truth about Health Care: Why Reform Is Not Working in America*

Richard A. Meckel, *Classrooms and Clinics: Urban Schools and the Protection and Promotion of Child Health, 1870–1930*

Terry Mizrahi, *From Residency to Retirement: Physicians' Careers over a Professional Lifetime*

Manon Parry, *Broadcasting Birth Control: Mass Media and Family Planning*

Alyssa Picard, *Making the American Mouth: Dentists and Public Health in the Twentieth Century*

Heather Munro Prescott, *The Morning After: A History of Emergency Contraception in the United States*

Sarah B. Rodriguez, *The Love Surgeon: A Story of Trust, Harm, and the Limits of Medical Regulation*

David J. Rothman and David Blumenthal, eds., *Medical Professionalism in the New Information Age*

Andrew R. Ruis, *Eating to Learn, Learning to Eat: School Lunches and Nutrition Policy in the United States*